Selected Applications of Computed Tomography

Selected Applications of Computed Tomography

Edited by **Marcus Lewis**

hayle
medical

New York

Published by Hayle Medical,
30 West, 37th Street, Suite 612,
New York, NY 10018, USA
www.haylemedical.com

Selected Applications of Computed Tomography
Edited by Marcus Lewis

International Standard Book Number: 978-1-63241-348-2 (Hardback)

Contents

Preface

All the selected applications of computed tomography are described in this insightful book. Computed tomography is a crucial imaging method in clinical practice. It was introduced in 1970s and since then, it has advanced and improved to a great extent. For instance, the introduction of helical systems has allowed the development of the "volumetric CT" concept. Even the anthropomorphic, forensic, paleontological and archeological applications of CT have emerged. Such applications make it a versatile diagnostic technology for non-destructive material testing and 3D imaging, beyond its medical use.

After months of intensive research and writing, this book is the end result of all who devoted their time and efforts in the initiation and progress of this book. It will surely be a source of reference in enhancing the required knowledge of the new developments in the area. During the course of developing this book, certain measures such as accuracy, authenticity and research focused analytical studies were given preference in order to produce a comprehensive book in the area of study.

This book would not have been possible without the efforts of the authors and the publisher. I extend my sincere thanks to them. Secondly, I express my gratitude to my family and well-wishers. And most importantly, I thank my students for constantly expressing their willingness and curiosity in enhancing their knowledge in the field, which encourages me to take up further research projects for the advancement of the area.

Editor

Part 1

Non-Radiological Application

1

Application of CT for the Study of Pathology of the Jaws

Tatsurou Tanaka et al.*
*Department of Oral Diagnostic Science, Kyushu Dental College, Kitakyushu
Japan*

1. Introduction

Computed tomography (CT) scanning is very useful in identifying and evaluating the location, size, and suspected pathological diagnosis of lesions such as cysts, tumors, and infections. At the same time, it aids in the elucidation of bone and surrounding soft tissue invasion of lesions with high resolution.[1, 2] In the maxilla and mandible, teeth are included and the CT capacity there can distinguished a foreign body of only 30 μm. Precise size and location are needed in the evaluation of lesions in the maxilla and mandible based on a high resolution in addition to the suspected pathological diagnosis based on CT findings.

Therefore, multi-detector CT (MDCT) scanning is commonly applied for various kinds of lesions in the maxilla and mandible because of its precision and diagnostic accuracy. Multi-detector CT scanning provides rapid acquisition of numerous thin axial images and more accurate reconstruction images. Multi-detector CT scanning provides accurate information about the height, width, and three-dimensional (3D) evaluation of the maxilla and mandible, as well as detailed information about the location of normal anatomical structures, such as the mandibular canal, mental foramen, mandibular foramen, incisive foramen, and maxillary sinus. In addition, the relationship between lesions and anatomical landmarks, including cortical margins and roots of teeth, can be established. These images are also excellent because MDCT eliminates streak artifacts from dental restorations that degrade direct coronal CT scans. With MDCT, axial images are used to reformat the cross-sectional images, projecting the artifact along the crowns of the teeth rather than over the bone that is the region of interest.[3] At the same time, CT readings of lesions in the maxilla and mandible measured by MDCT can reflect the nature and inclusion within lesions, from which

Yasuhiro Morimoto[1,6], Shinji Kito[1], Ayataka Ishikawa[2], Shinya Kokuryo[3], Noriaki Yamamoto[3], Manabu Habu[3], Ikuya Miyamoto[3], Masaaki Kodama[3], Shinobu Matsumoto-Takeda[1], Masafumi Oda[1], Nao Wakasugi-Sato[1], Kozue Otsuka[1], Shunji Shiiba[4], Yuji Seta[2], Yoshihiro Yamashita[3], Izumi Yoshioka[5], Kou Matsuo[2], Tetsu Takahashi[3] and Kazuhiro Tominaga[3]

[1] *Department of Oral Diagnostic Science, Kyushu Dental College, Kitakyushu, Japan,*
[2] *Department of Oral Bioscience, Kyushu Dental College, Kokurakita-ku, Kitakyushu, Japan,*
[3] *Department of Oral and Maxillofacial Surgery, Kyushu Dental College, Kitakyushu, Japan,*
[4] *Department of Control of Physical Functions, Kyushu Dental College, Kokurakita-ku, Kitakyushu, Japan,*
[5] *Department of Sensory and Motor Organs, Faculty of Medicine, Miyazaki University, Miyazaki, Japan.*
[6] *Center for Oral Biological Research, Kyushu Dental College, Kitakyushu, Japan*
* *Correspondence author*

suspected pathological diagnosis can be estimated. Multi-detector CT scanning could improve the performance of CT angiograms and dynamic contrast and maneuver imaging.[4, 5] Multi-detector CT angiography is used to delineate the blood vessels **(Fig. 1)** and to provide information about the exact location of neoplasms, lymphadenopathy, and their vascular infiltration or spread.

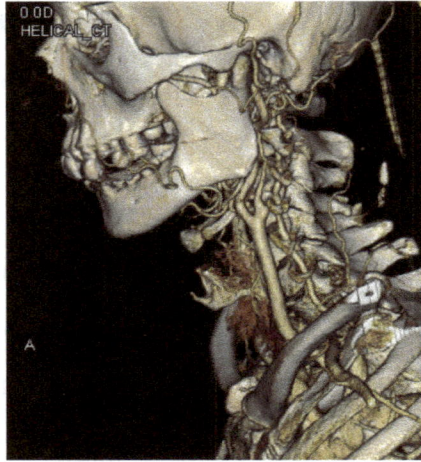

Fig. 1. CT angiography image in the oral and maxillofacial regions of a patient with oral cancer.

In the case of dental lesions such as dental caries **(Fig. 2A)**, marginal and/or periapical periodontitis **(Fig. 2B)**, or an impacted tooth **(Fig. 2C)**, cone-beam CT (CBCT), with its better resolution, may also be applied, but without CT readings. In addition, this modality has endodontic and orthodontic applications.[6, 7] For orthodontic tooth movements, CBCT offers a 3D image that can be used to visualize all three planes of space.[7] Cone-beam CT is especially useful for the evaluation of 3D alveolar bone volumes and the relationship between anatomical landmarks before dental implant surgery **(Fig. 2D)**.[8, 9] However, the disadvantage of CBCT is that soft tissues with different densities cannot be visualized on the images, which explains why there is no whole-body CBCT. This modality is best applied for identifying the calcification of hard tissues.

2. CT findings for various kinds of lesions in jaws

Characteristic CT findings of lesions commonly encountered in our clinical practice, such as cysts, tumors including fibro-osseous lesions, and infections in the maxilla and mandible, are described.

2.1 Cysts in jaws
Most cyst-like lesions occurring in the maxilla and mandible are odontogenic cysts, such as radicular cysts, and some are non-odontogenic cysts, such as nasopalatine duct cysts.[10] Also found are pseudo-cysts without cystic epithelium, such as simple bone cysts. In this report, CT images of odontogenic cysts, non-odontogenic cysts, and pseudo-cysts in jaws are shown and interpreted.

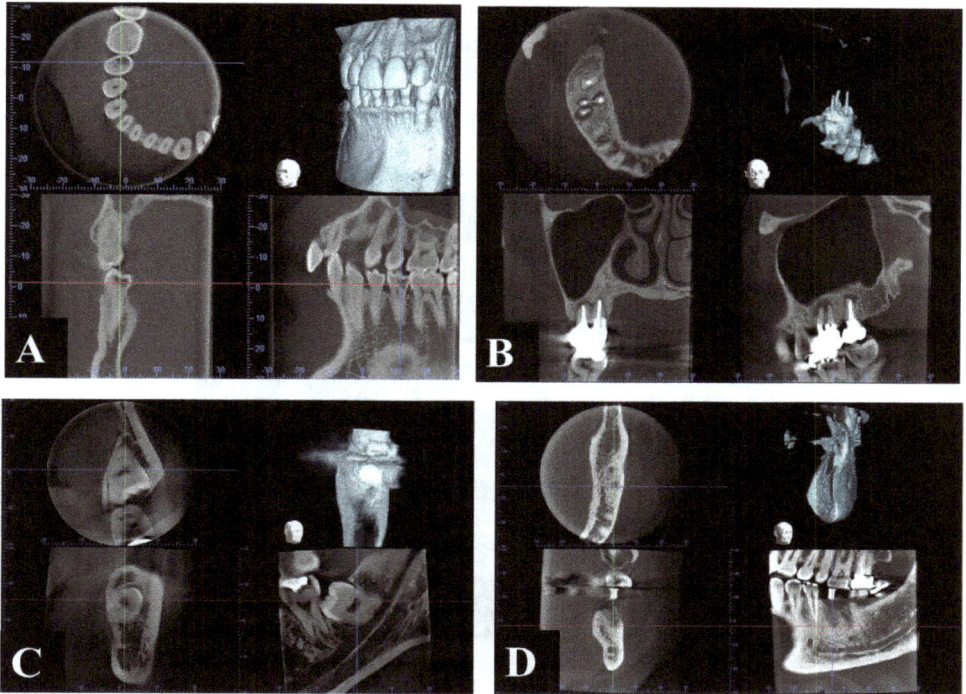

Fig. 2. CBCT images of dental caries in the right second premolar (A). CBCT images of marginal and/or periapical periodontitis in the maxillary molar region (B). CBCT images of an impacted tooth in the mandibular third molar region (C). CBCT images of the evaluation before dental implant surgery in the mandibular molar region (D).

2.2 Odontogenic cysts in jaws

Representative odontogenic cysts in the maxilla and mandible are radicular cysts and dentigerous cysts. Therefore, CT images of both types of cysts are demonstrated.

2.3 Radicular cysts, including residual cysts and periapical granulomas

Radicular cysts are the most common odontogenic cyst, which is a post-inflammatory lesion related to the apex of a non-vital tooth root.[11] The characteristic clinical locations of the cysts are adjacent to the apex of a carious or heavily restored non-vital tooth. The cyst is a cavity in the bone that contains fluid. Radiographically, the radicular cyst is a well-circumscribed radiolucency arising from the apex of the tooth and bounded by a thin rim of cortical bone **(Fig. 3A)**. On CT imaging, the cyst is shown as a water-dense mass with a well-defined margin **(Fig. 3B)**. In addition, the cyst is located around the apex of a causative tooth, including it. If the cyst occurs in the maxilla, extension into the maxillary sinus from the maxillary sinus floor may be observed **(Fig. 3C)**. At the upper border of the lesion, the bone line may be observed **(Fig. 3C)**. A periapical granuloma and radicular cyst may have identical radiographic appearances, but a radicular cyst sometimes may be differentiated from the granuloma by its size. An apical granuloma is usually smaller than 1 cm in diameter, whereas a radicular cyst may become as large as 10 cm.[12] One type of radicular cyst is a residual cyst that remains after or develops subsequence to extraction of an infected tooth. Therefore, its radiological findings including CT images are similar to those of radicular cysts without the causative teeth **(Fig. 3D, E)**.

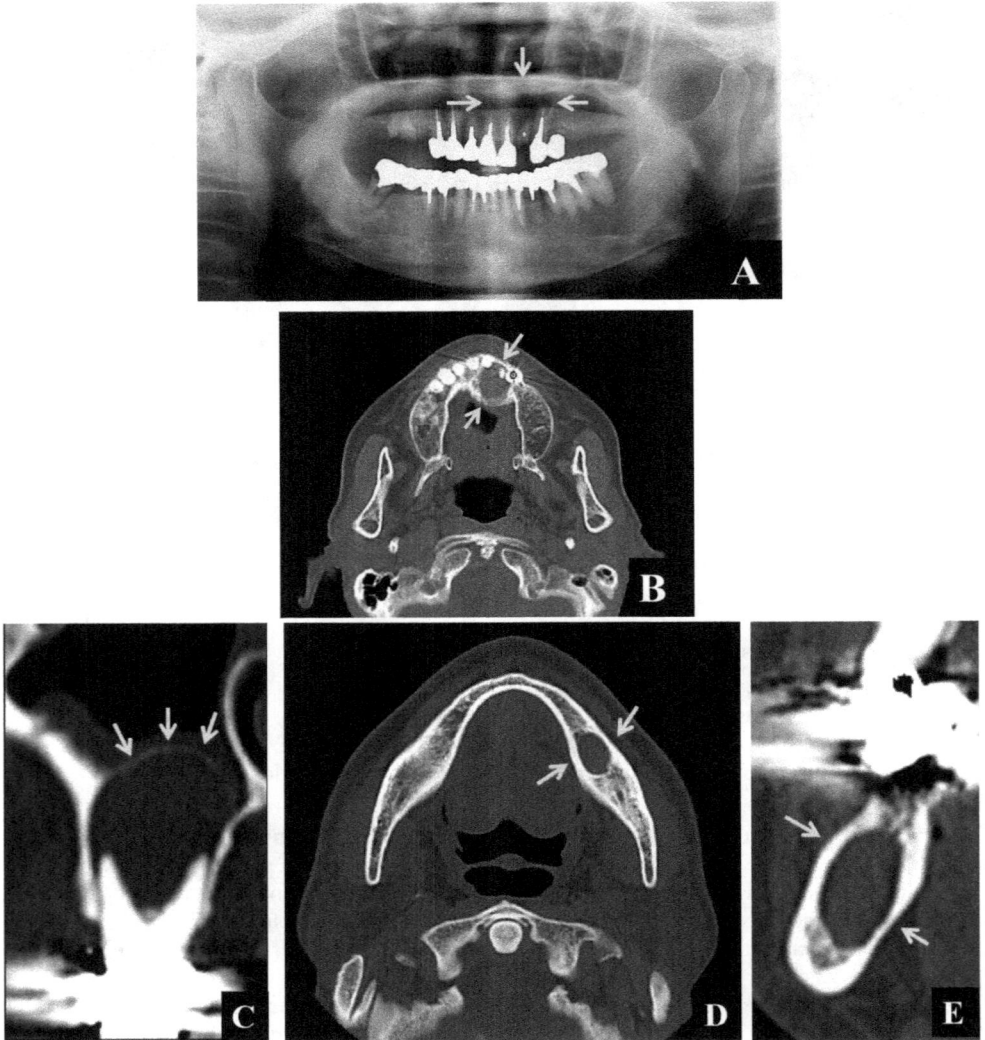

Fig. 3. Panoramic radiograph image (A), axial CT image (B) of a radicular cyst in the maxilla (arrows). Oblique coronal CT image (C) of a radicular cyst extension into the maxillary sinus from the maxillary sinus floor (arrows). Axial (D) and oblique coronal (E) CT images of the residual cyst in the left mandible (arrows).

2.4 Dentigerous cysts (follicular cysts)

The dentigerous cyst is the second most common type of odontogenic cyst; its pericoronal position around the crown of an unerupted tooth is its characteristic clinical finding. Therefore, the dentigerous cyst is the most common pathologic pericornal radiolucency in the jaws according to Ackermann et al.[13] Radiologically, the dentigerous cyst consists of an well-corticated pericoronal radiolucency exceeding about 2.5 mm on CT images, which is a criterion between cystic change and a normal dental follicular sac **(Fig. 4)**. The common teeth related to dentigerous cysts are the mandibular third molars, maxillary canines, and supernumerary teeth. Among supernumerary teeth, mesio-dens are most commonly associated with dentigerous cysts. Radiographically, the dentigerous cyst is a well-circumscribed radiolucency bounded by a thin rim of cortical bone including the crown of an unerupted tooth **(Fig. 4A)**. On CT images, this cyst is shown as a water-density mass with a well-defined margin including the crown of an unerupted tooth **(Fig. 4B)**. It is often difficult to differentiate between dentigerous cysts and odontognic benign tumors such as ameloblastomas. Dentigerous cysts cannot strongly absorb the contiguous teeth roots by knife-edge resorption **(Fig. 4C)**, but odontogenic tumors can. In addition, dentigerous cysts do not tend to expand the buccolingual cortical bone, but odontogenic tumors do.

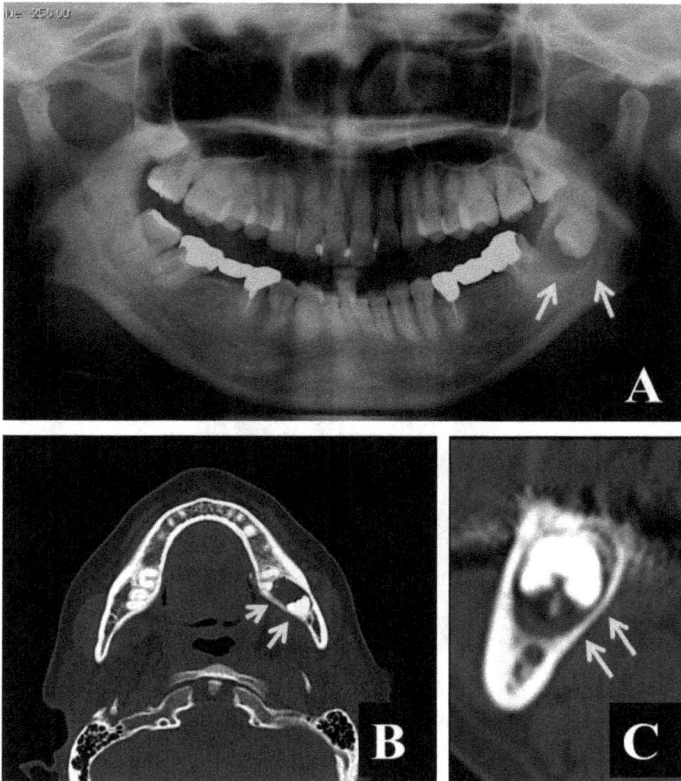

Fig. 4. Panoramic radiograph image (A), axial (B) and oblique coronal (C) CT images of a dentigerous cyst in the left mandibular third molar region (arrows).

3. Non-odontogenic cysts in jaws

3.1 Nasopalatine duct cysts (incisive canal cysts)

A nasopalatine duct cyst is a representative non-odontogenic developmental cyst (one of the fissural cysts).[10] The cyst occurs in the incisive canal near the anterior palatine papilla. Pathologically, the epithelium of the cyst may originate from remnants in the incisive canals. The nasopalatine cyst has a unique heart-shaped appearance **(Fig. 5)**. In addition, the cyst is a well-circumscribed radiolucency bounded by a thin rim of cortical bone including the incisive canals **(Fig. 5A)**. On CT images, this cyst is indicated as a water-dense mass with a well-defined margin including the incisive canals **(Fig. 5B, C)**. This cyst has intra-osseous and extra-osseous variants. It sometimes is difficult to differentiate between radicular cysts and nasopalatine duct cysts if contiguous teeth are non-vital. We base the diagnosis on whether the lesions have expanded over the median palatine suture and whether the lesions are relatively asymmetric.

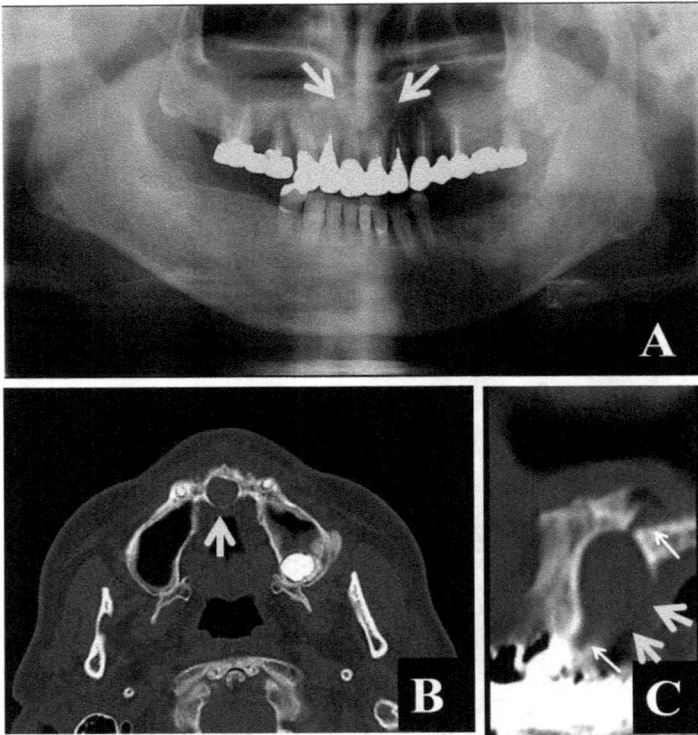

Fig. 5. Panoramic radiograph image (A), axial (B) and oblique sagittal (C) CT image of an incisive canal cyst (arrows) and incisive canals (narrow arrows).

3.2 Postoperative maxillary cysts

The postoperative maxillary cyst occurs 20 to 30 years after Caldwell-Luc surgery and is one of the non-odontogenic cysts.[14] Pathologically, the cystic lining originates from the epithelium of the maxillary sinus, based on its histologic similarity. The characteristic features of the post-Caldwell-Luc maxillary sinus are a right-angle triangular shape and an ill-defined panoramic innominate line on panoramic radiographs **(Fig. 6A)** and the contracted sinus and a thickened posterior wall on CT scans **(Fig. 6B)**. In addition, this cyst is indicated as a well-circumscribed radiolucency bounded by a thin rim of cortical bone **(Fig. 6C)** and as a water-dense mass with a well-defined margin on CT images **(Fig. 6D, E)**.

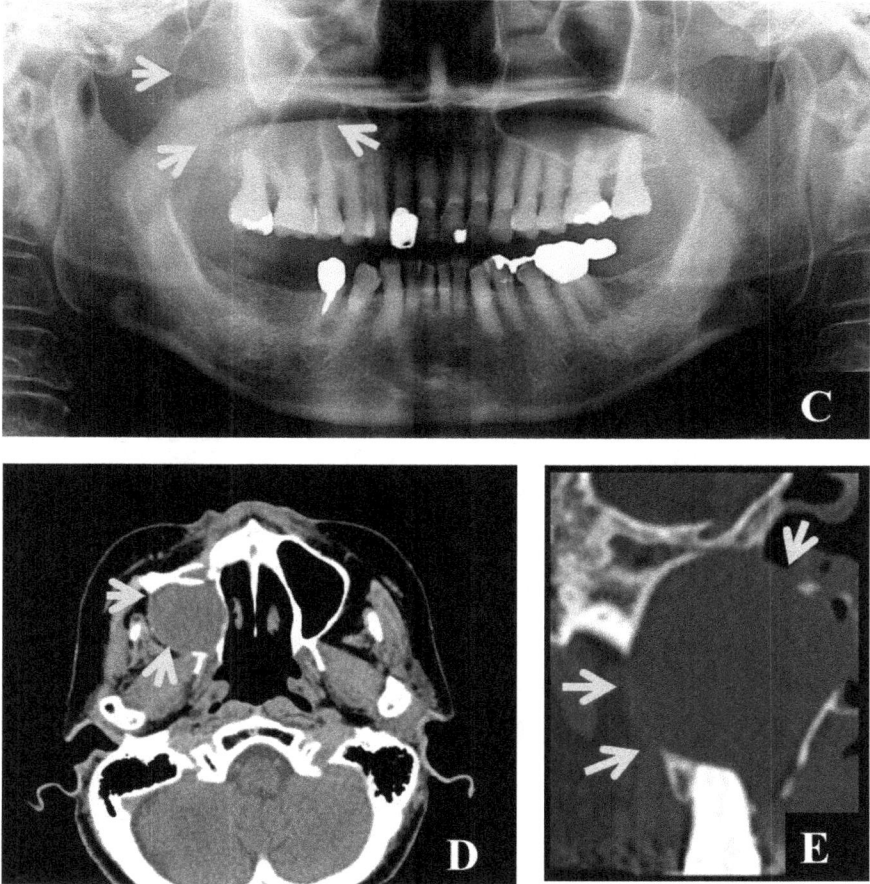

Fig. 6. Panoramic radiograph images (A, C), axial CT images (B, D), oblique coronal CT image (E) of a postoperative maxillary cyst in the right sinus region (arrows).

4. Pseudo-cysts in jaws

4.1 Simple bone cysts

A simple bone cyst is a representative pseudo-cyst, which does not have epithelium. The cyst lining consists of loose vascular connective tissue that may have areas of recent or old hemorrhage.[15] The cyst tends to occur in the mandible of young men. These cysts often are asymptomatic and most are discovered incidentally during examination of the teeth for other purposes.[16] Radiologically, the cyst is a well-circumscribed radiolucency bounded by a thin rim of cortical bone **(Fig. 7A)**. On CT images, this cyst is indicated as a water-dense mass with a well-defined margin **(Fig. 7B)**. As radiological characteristic features, the outline of the cyst between the roots of teeth has a scalloped appearance **(Fig. 7C)**.

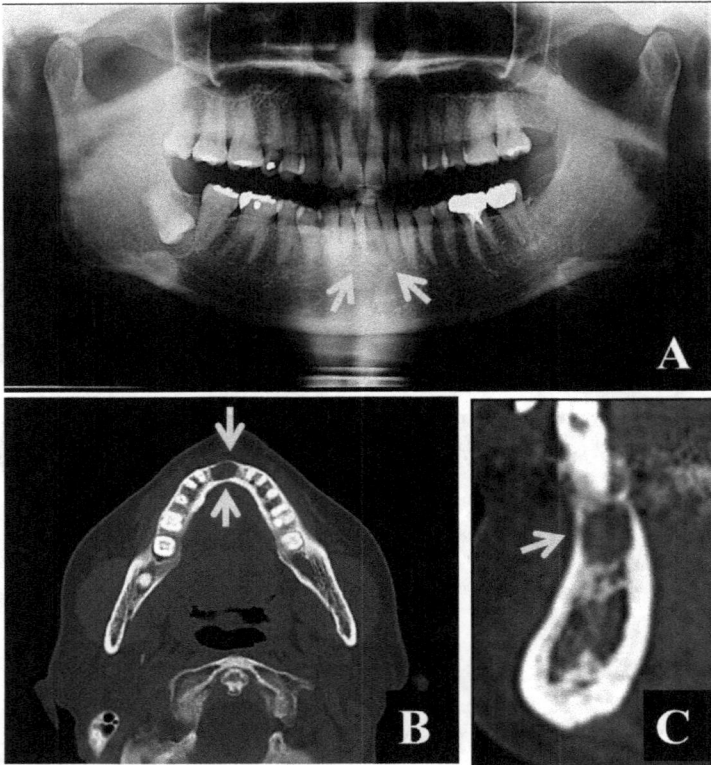

Fig. 7. Panoramic radiograph image (A), axial (B) and sagittal (C) CT image of a simple bone cyst in the mandible (arrows).

4.2 Static bone cavity

A static bone cavity incidentally appears as an ovoid or round radiolucency in the posterior mandible on X-ray radiographs completely like cysts in jaws **(Fig. 8A)**, but it is not a cyst. It is simply a bony defect on the lingual surface of the mandible that is demonstrated on CT images **(Fig. 8B)**, but not X-ray radiographs. The static bone cavity usually includes salivary gland tissues, fatty tissues, and air.[17]

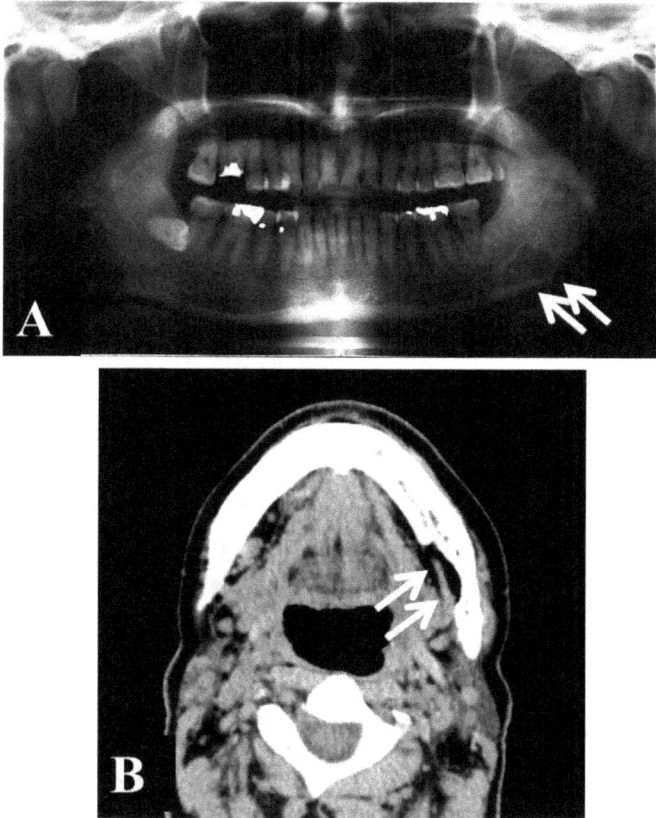

Fig. 8. Panoramic radiograph image (A) and axial CT image (B) of a static bone cavity in the left angle of the mandible (arrows).

5. Tumors in jaws

Tumors occurring in the maxilla and mandible are divided into benign and malignant types and most tumors are benign. At the same time, tumors occurring in the jaws are odontogenic, such as keratocystic odontogenic tumors (KCOT) and ameloblastomas, and some are non-odontogenic such as osteomas. Moreover, odontogenic tumors are subdivided into four categories by the World Health Organization (WHO) based on the tissue origin.[10] In addition, fibrous-osseous lesions also occur as tumor-like lesions in the jaws. In this report, the CT image findings of tumors and tumor-like lesions are shown and interpreted.

6. Benign odontogenic tumors in jaws

6.1 Keratocystic odontogenic tumors

Keratocystic odontogenic tumors (KCOT) are odontogenic tumors as classified by the WHO in 2005.[10] It is a cystic neoplasm of Category 1 (originating from odontogenic epithelium) of the WHO classification and often affects the posterior mandible. Keratocystic odontogenic tumors are thought to arise from the dental lamina and have a similar keratinized squamous epithelium without rete ridges.[10, 18] Radiologically, the cystic mass is a well-circumscribed multi-loculated radiolucency bounded by a thin rim of cortical bone with smooth or scalloped margins **(Fig. 9A)**. On CT images, the cystic mass is indicated as a water-dense mass with well-defined smooth or scalloped margins **(Fig. 9B)**. The contents of KCOT are thick due to desquamated keratinizing squamous cells. These contents can occasionally increase the radiographic attenuation of the lesion on CT scans, but this is not appreciable on panoramic radiographs.[19] In the case of multiple KCOT in the maxilla and mandible, basal cell nevus syndrome (Gorlin-Goltz syndrome), which is a genetic disorder inherited as an autosomal dominant trait with variable penetrance and expressivity, should be suspected **(Fig. 9C)**.

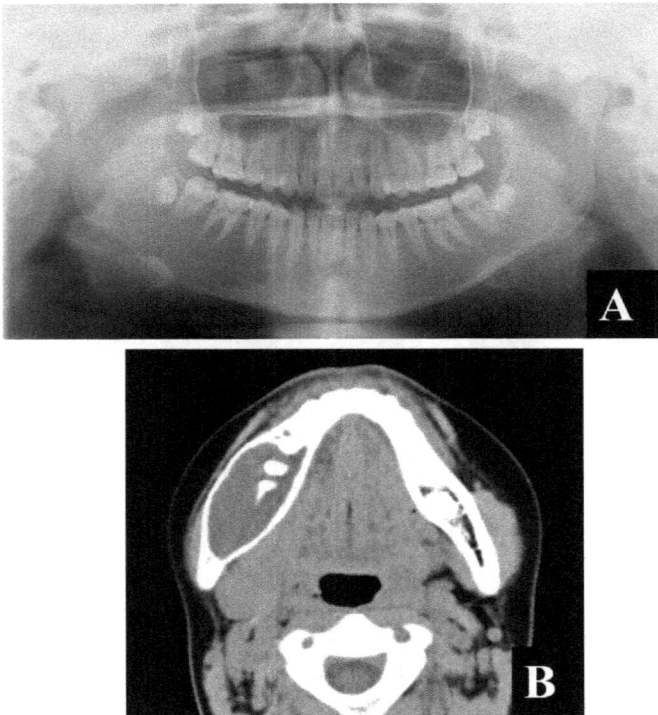

Fig. 9. Panoramic radiograph image (A), and axial CT images (B) of a keratocystic odontogenic tumor in the mandible. Axial CT image **(C)** of the keratocystic odontogenic tumor with basal cell nevus syndrome.

6.2 Ameloblastomas

An ameloblastoma is also a representative tumor of Category 1 by the WHO classification and is thought to arise from ameloblasts.[20-22] The common clinical findings of ameloblastomas are painless swelling in the posterior mandible of adults less than 40 years old. Radiologically, the tumor is a well-circumscribed multi-loculated radiolucency bounded by a thin rim of cortical bone with smooth or scalloped margins **(Fig. 10A)**. On CT images, the tumor is indicated as a soft tissue or water-dense mass with well-defined smooth or scalloped margins **(Fig. 10B)**. Therefore, it is sometimes very difficult to differentiate between ameloblastomas and KCOT by characteristic radiographic findings. However, ameloblastomas tend to replace the roots of teeth with knife-edge resorption **(Fig. 10C)**, but KCOT have relatively less resorption if the lesions are contiguous with teeth. In addition, ameloblastomas tend to expand the marked buccolingual cortical bone **(Fig. 10D)**, but KCOT do not if the lesions are contiguous with cortical bone in the maxilla and mandible. In addition, about 5% of ameloblastomas can transform into malignancy **(Fig. 10E)** and the mass should be excised appropriately.

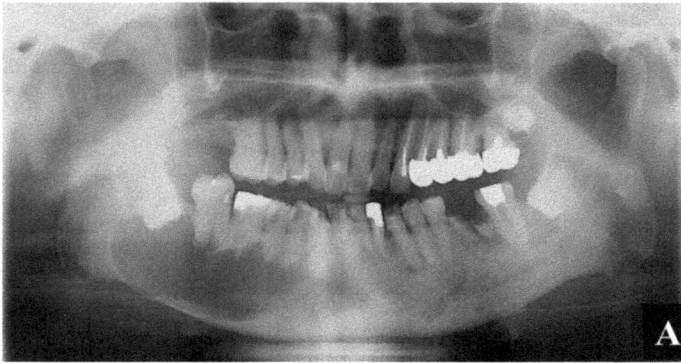

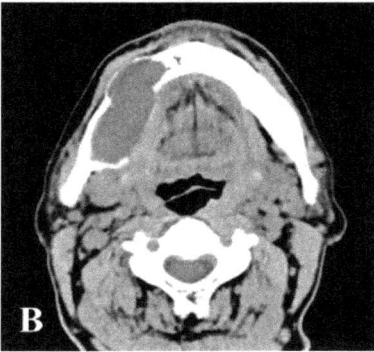

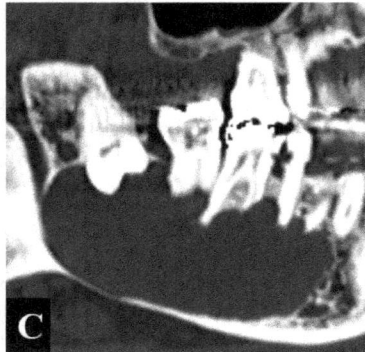

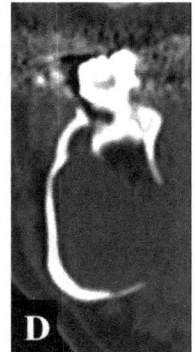

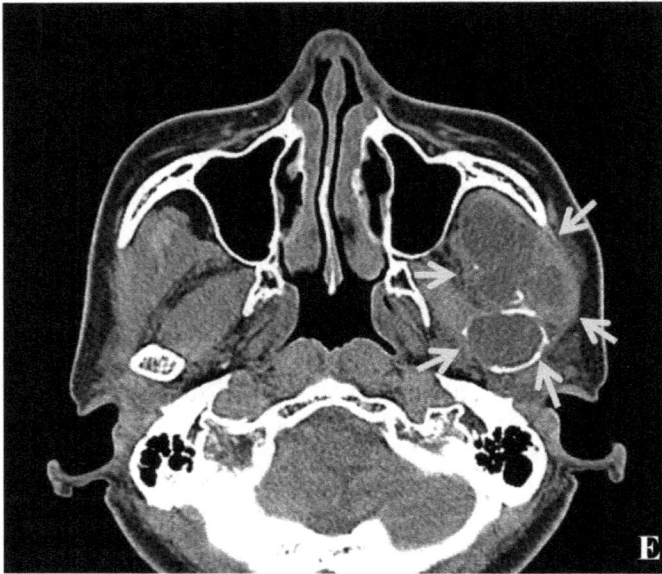

Fig. 10. Panoramic radiograph image (A) and axial (B), oblique sagittal (C), oblique coronal (D) CT images of an ameloblastoma in the right mandible. Axial CT image (E) of a malignant ameloblastoma (arrows).

6.3 Odontomas

Odontoma is a representative Category 2 tumor (originating from odontogenic epithelium and mesenchyme with hard tissue formation). By the WHO classification, odontomas are divided into two types, complex and compound.[18] Pathologically, the compound odontoma gathers and arranges in an orderly pattern such that the lesion resembles multiple normal tooth-like structures. The complex odontoma is arranged in a disorderly pattern such that the lesion does not resemble tooth-like structures. Therefore, radiologically, odontomas usually are not difficult to differentially diagnose. Both compound and complex odontomas are surrounded by a thin radiolucent area consisting of a connective tissue capsule. Compound odontomas are radiopaque masses composed of many tooth-like structures on X-ray radiographs (**Fig. 11A**) and on CT images (**Fig. 11B**). The areas of inter tooth-like structures are radiolucent and soft tissue density areas on the respective modalities (**Figs. 11A, B**). The compound odontomas are well-demarcated, radiopaque masses surrounded by narrow radiolucent zones (**Figs. 11C, D**).

6.4 Benign cementoblastomas

Benign cementoblasoma is a representative Category 3 tumor (originating from mesenchyme and/or ectomesenchyme with/without odontogenic epithelium), and is called a true cementoma.[25] Pathologically, a benign cementoblastoma is characterized by the formation of cementum or a cementum-like mass connected with a tooth root.[23, 24] Radiologically, a benign cementoblastoma has intimate involvement with the whole tooth root and has three stages: radiolucent, radiopaque, and mature radiopaque with an

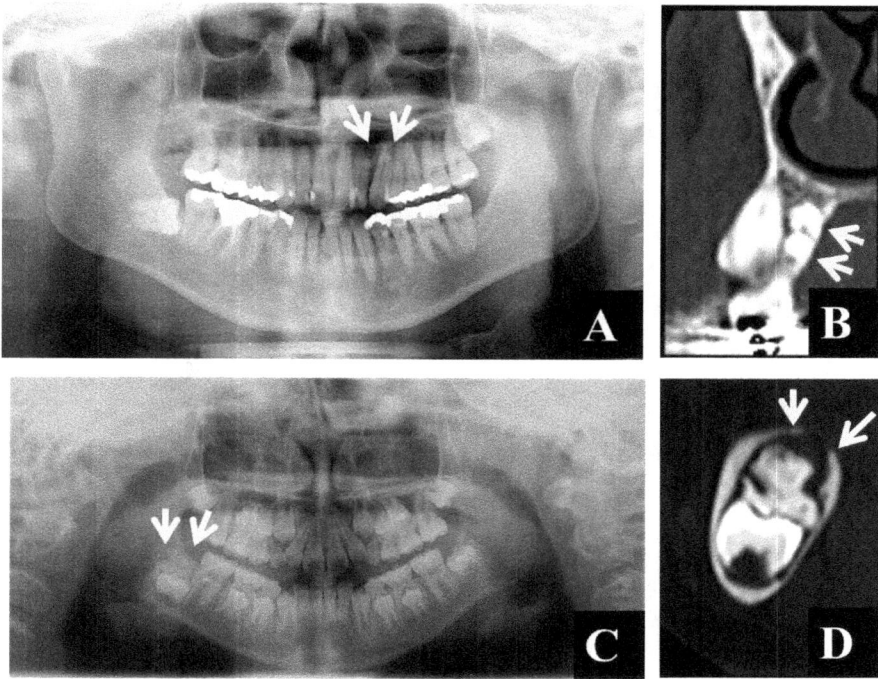

Fig. 11. Panoramic radiograph image (A) and oblique sagittal CT image (B) of compound odontoma (arrows). Panoramic radiograph image (C) and oblique coronal CT image (D) of complex odontoma (arrows).

obscured root outline within the lesion. The benign cementoblastoma is a central high-density mass attached to the tooth root surrounded by a well-defined low-density area **(Fig. 12A, B)**. Periapical cemental dysplasia involves cementomas and is a reactive disorder rather than a neoplastic process. Periapical cemental dysplasia also has three phases: ostolytic, cementoblastic, and a mature stage likely to be benign cementoblastomas. Most cases of periapical cemental dysplasia appear as radiopaque masses with well-defined radiolucent areas at multiple periapical regions **(Fig. 12C, D)**.

6.5 Fibrous dysplasia
Fibrous dysplasia is a representative tumor-like lesion classified as a Category 4 condition (bone-related lesions) by the WHO. In this category, simple bone cysts are also included.[12] Fibrous dysplasia is divided into two types.[12] Monostotic fibrous dysplasia affects only one bone and polystotic fibrous dysplasia affects multiple bones. In polystotic dysplasia, McCune-Albright's syndrome is induced by point-mutations of the GNAS1 gene[25, 26] and Lichtenstein-Jaffe syndrome is a milder form.[25, 26] Radiological changes as a result of fibrous dysplasia are sometimes related to multiple bones such as the skull, facial bones, and femur,

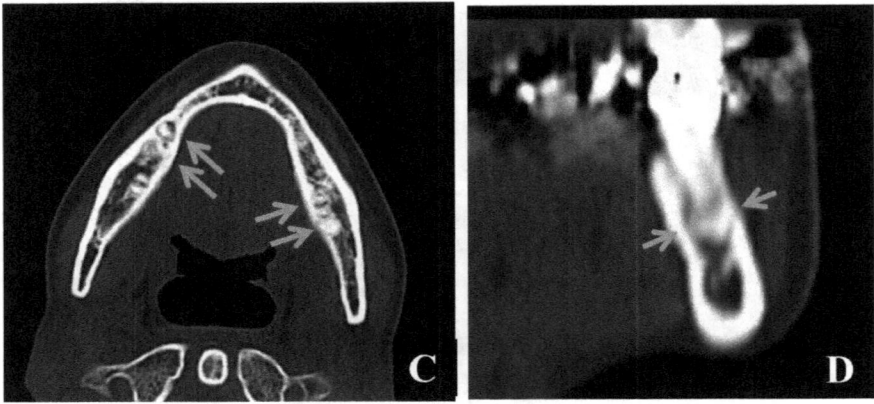

Fig. 12. CT images (A, B) of a benign cementoblastoma in the mandible (arrows). CT images (C, D) of periapical cemental dysplasia in the mandible (arrows).

in addition to the jaws. Various areas should be examined whenever one area of fibrous dysplasia is suspected. Pathologically, fibrous dysplasia is characterized by fibrous tissue alternating with trabeculae, woven bone, and less organized lamellar bone. Radiological characteristic features also vary and may be radiolucent, radiopaque, or mixed-density according to the degree of bone present within the lesion. One representative case is seen as mass-like unilocular mixed-density changes with a poorly defined margin and the other representative case is seen as radiopaque change with a poorly defined margin accompanied by bone deformity, such as the expansion of cortical bone, on X-ray radiographs **(Fig. 13A)** and on CT **(Fig. 13B, C)**.

7. Benign non-odontogenic tumors in jaws

7.1 Osteomas
An osteoma is a representative benign non-odontogenic tumor composed of compact and/or spongy bone.[27] Radiologically, an osteoma is a radiopaque mass with a well-circumscribed margin attached to the bone surface **(Fig. 14A)**. The degree of radiopacity is related to the composition within the osteoma such as compact or spongy bone.
In cases of multiple osteomas in the jaw, Gardner's syndrome should be suspected. Exostoses in the jaws are outgrowths of the bone and are similar to osteomas. A representative exostosis is a torus mandibularis, which is bilateral bone growth of the lingual surface of the mandible in the premolar regions **(Fig. 14B)**.

7.2 Osteochondromas
An osteochondroma is the most common benign tumor and occurs at the condyles of the mandible in the temporomandibular joints. Pathologically, the surface of the tumor is covered with cartilage and the inner part is composed of spongy bone. Therefore, radiopaque masses with well-defined margin are indicated as radiological features **(Fig. 15)**.

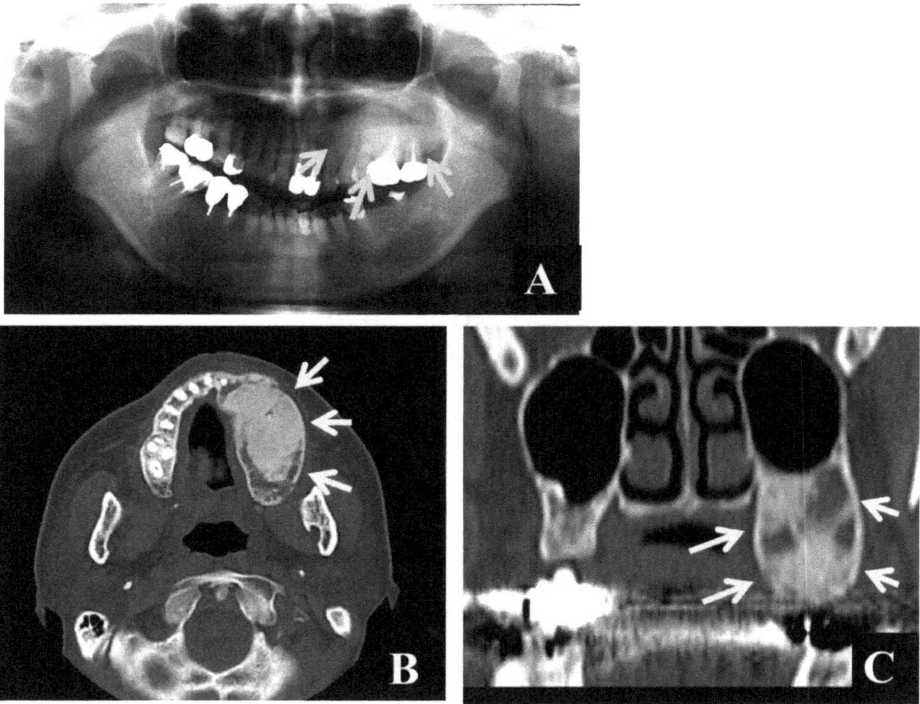

Fig. 13. Panoramic radiograph image (A) and axial (B), coronal (C) CT images of fibrous dysplasia in left maxilla (arrows).

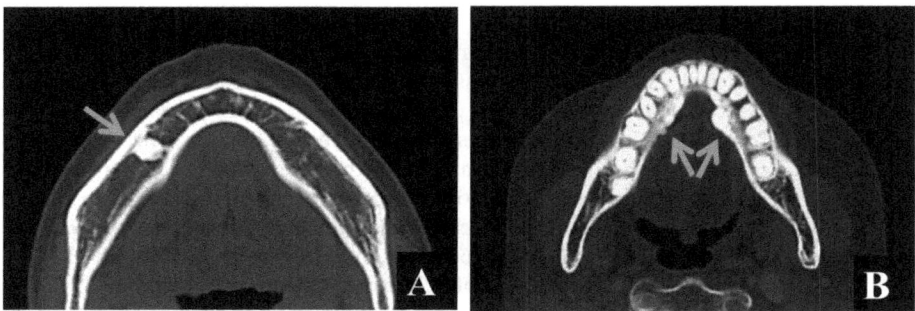

Fig. 14. Axial CT images of an osteoma in the mandible (A) and the torus mandibularis (B) (arrows).

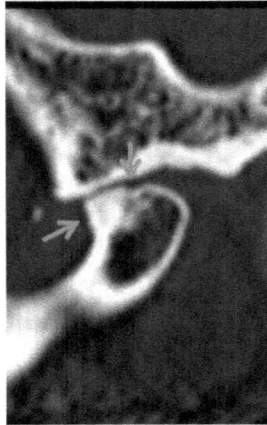

Fig. 15. Oblique sagittal CT image of an osteochondroma in the temporomandibular joint (arrows).

8. Malignant tumors in jaws

Malignant tumors occurring in the jaws are various kinds of lesions such as primary intraosseous carcinomas, lymphomas, malignant ameloblastomas, and metastatic tumors to the jaws. In particular, the lesions that attention should be paid to are oral cancers with erosive changes to the mandible and maxilla, such as gingival carcinomas and metastatic cancers to the jaws.

8.1 Oral cancers with erosive changes to the jaws

Most of the lesions encountered routinely in malignant tumors of jaws are gingival or tongue carcinomas of the mandible or maxilla. Tumors occurring in soft tissues should not be included in non-odontogenic tumors of the jaws. However, because oral and maxillofacial surgeons including dentists often have an opportunity to deal with these lesions, they should be described in this section. Their pathological cause is transformation of the epithelium and the carcinomas are derived from odontogenic cysts **(Fig. 16A)** and remnants in primary intra-osseous regions **(Fig. 16B)** in rare cases. These lesions are included in non-odontogenic malignant tumors of the jaws.

In cases where an exact evaluation of erosive changes to the mandible and maxilla is required, coronal plane views should be produced using multi-planar reconstruction techniques after the acquisition of axial planes with very thin (0.5-1 mm) slices.[28, 29] In those cases, metal dental artifacts should be minimized. Furthermore, a CT scan can encompass the area from the cavernous sinuses to the thoracic inlet to examine the primary cancer and possible lymph node metastases in the neck. Radiologically, the crestal portion of the alveolar ridge attached to lesions indicates saucerization and beneath this area, there may be a wide transition zone and a relative lack of sclerosis at the margin **(Fig. 16C, D, E)**. In addition, there may be motheaten and permeative patterns of bone destruction and floating teeth from bone loss **(Fig. 16F)**. CT images commonly include soft tissue density masses with mild contrast enhancement associated with bone destruction **(Fig. 16G, H)**. However, masses affected by dental metal streak artifacts are often undetectable on CT images. It has been reported that particular radiological findings and parameters using dynamic CT could also be useful.[30-32] Wakasa *et al.* reported that the peak height, which is the relative CT value measured from the base CT value to the point where the curve reaches its peak, is useful for distinguishing between inflammation and tumors.[31] Transit time, which is the time between two transit points on the time-density curve, has been reported to be significantly longer in benign tumors than in malignant tumors.[31]

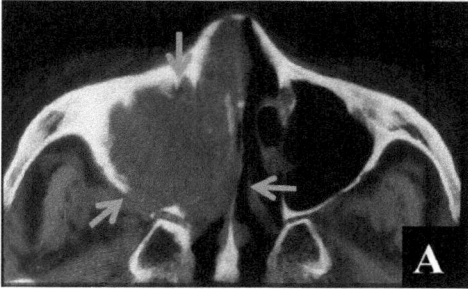

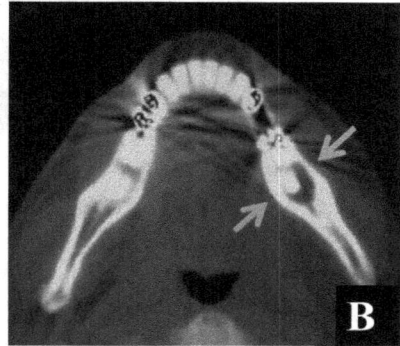

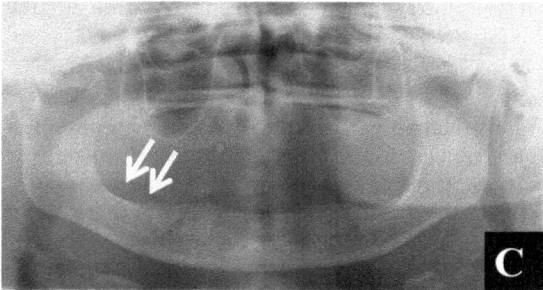

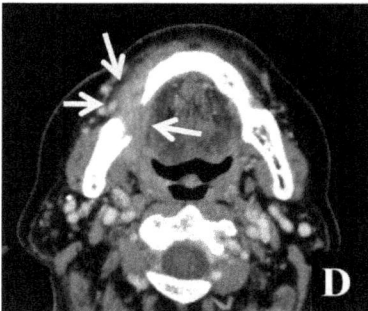

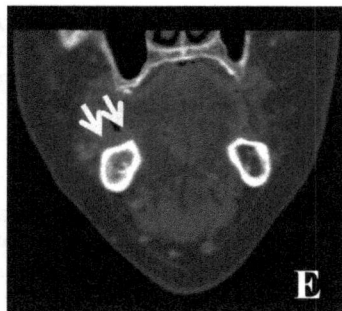

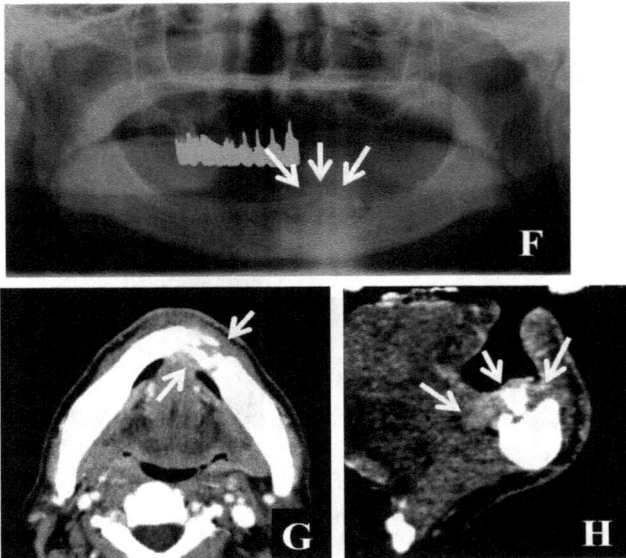

Fig. 16. Axial CT image (A) of the carcinomas derived from odontogenic cysts (arrows). Axial CT image (B) of the carcinoma in the primary intra-osseous region (arrows). Panoramic radiograph image (C), axial contrast-enhanced CT image (D) and coronal CT image (E) of the gingiva carcinoma in the molar region (arrows). Panoramic radiograph image (F), axial (G) and coronal (H) contrast-enhanced CT images of the gingiva carcinoma in the mandibular canine region (arrows).

8.2 Metastatic cancers to jaws

Metastatic cancers to the jaws are relative rare, but we should pay attention to them. In particular, if patients had primary cancers in the lung, breast, liver, prostate, or kidney, and if patients with the clinical manifestations of numb chin syndrome have known cancers, it would be important to be aware of the criteria used to judge whether the known cancers had worsened.[33] Radiologically, in most patterns, the metastatic masses with ill-defined margins destroy the bone diffusely **(Fig. 17A)**.[33] In rare case, the metastatic mass with diffuse calcification destroys the mandible and replaces it with muscle **(Fig. 17B)** .[33] The inner nature of the masses tends to be determined according to that of the primary lesions. To prevent the misdiagnosis of numb chin syndrome, dentists need to be aware of the clinical manifestations of numb chin syndrome, the need for CT imaging, and the shortcomings of panoramic radiographs.[33]

9. Infections in jaws

9.1 Osteomyelitis including bisphosphonate-related osteonecrosis of the jaws

Infections caused by dental caries, periodontitis, and pericoronitis, tend to spread into and around the jaws. When infections produce intra-osseous expansion, osteomyelitis occurs in the jaws. Osteomyelitis is divided into acute and chronic types by the period from the onset of infection. In addition, there are other kinds of osteomyelitis such as common suppuration osteomyelitis without particular infection, radiotherapy-related, and bisphosphonate-related

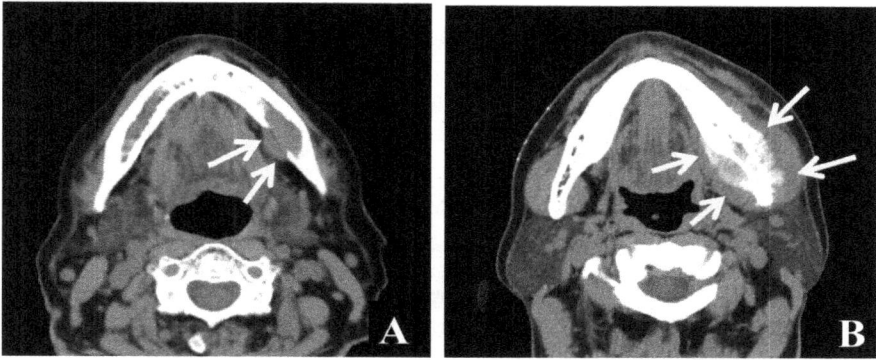

Fig. 17. Axial CT images (A, B) of a metastatic mass (arrows) in the mandible.

osteomyelitis. Basic radiological features are the same and there is little radiological change in the jaws in acute osteomyelitis **(Fig. 18A)**. In chronic osteomyelitis, osteolytic and/or osteogenic changes with ill-defined margins are demonstrated in the jaws. In osteogenic osteomyelitis, diffuse sclerosing jaws are shown and the clarity of the mandibular canal can be visualized **(Figs. 18B, C)**. In addition, in some cases, periosteal reactions are also visualized on CT images **(Fig. 18D)**. In some cases of chronic osteomyelitis, a sequestrum can be visualized **(Fig. 18E)**. Recently, bisphosphonate-related osteonecrosis of the jaws (BRONJ) has become recognized as a potentially serious complication in patients, including those with cancer and osteoporosis, who are treated with long-term administration of bisphosphonates.[34] Once BRONJ has occurred in a patient, it is difficult to completely cure the disease. Therefore, its prevention is especially important. However, the radiological findings in BRONJ are the same as those in chronic osteomyelitis, except for the prominent bone destruction **(Figs. 18F, G, H)**. If chronic multifocal recurrent osteomyelitis occurs in the jaw, we should suspect SAHPO (synovitis, acne, pustulosis, hyperostosis, osteitis) syndrome, and additional examinations should be performed.[35]

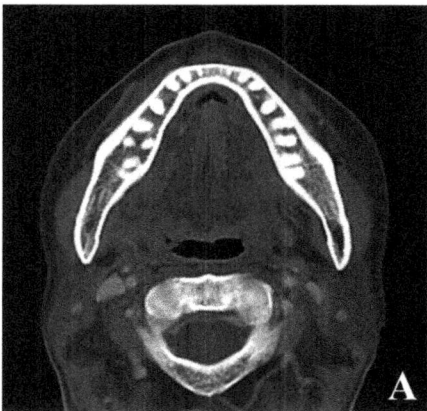

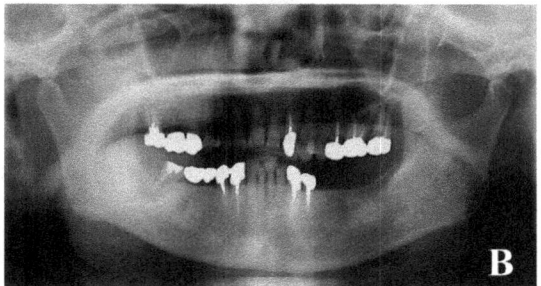

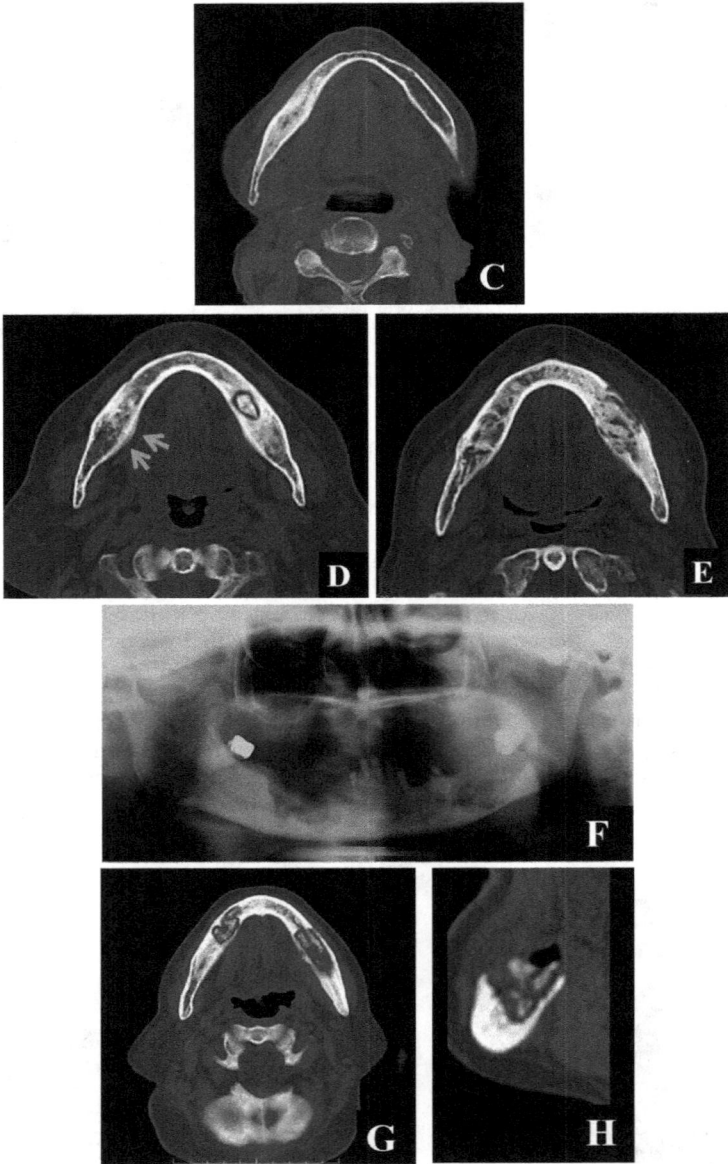

Fig. 18. Axial CT image of acute osteomyelitis in the left mandibular molar region (A). Panoramic radiograph image (B) and axial CT image (C) of chronic osteomyelitis in the right mandibular molar region. Axial CT image of periosteal reactions (arrows) in a case of chronic osteomyelitis (E). Axial CT image of a sequestrum in a case of chronic osteomyelitis (E). Panoramic radiograph image (F), axial (G) and oblique coronal (H) CT images of a sequestrum in a case of bisphosphonate-related osteonecrosis of the jaws.

10. References

[1] Weber AL, Romo L, Hashmi S. Malignant tumors of the oral cavity and oropharynx: clinical, pathologic, and radiologic evaluation. Neuroimag Clin N Am 2003; 13: 443-64.

[2] Simon LL, Rubinstein DR. Imaging of oral cancer. Otolaryngol Clin N Am 2006; 39: 307-17.

[3] Abrahams JJ. Dental CT imaging: a look at the jaw. Radiology 2001; 219: 334-345.

[4] Schuknecht B. Latest techniques in head and neck CT angiography. Neuroradiology 2004; 46: s208-13.

[5] Stuhlfaut JW, Barest G, Sakai O, Lucey B, Soto JA. Impact of MDCT angiography on the use of catheter angiography for the assessment of cervical arterial injury after blunt or penetrating trauma. AJR Am J Roentgenol 2005; 185: 1063-8.

[6] Tyndall DA and Rathore S. Cone-beam CT diagnostic applications: caries, periodontal bone assessment, and endodontic applications. Dent Clin N Am 2008; 52: 825-41.

[7] Hechler SL. Cone-beam CT: applications in orthodontics. Dent Clin N Am 2008; 52: 809-23.

[8] Peck JN, Conte GJ. Radiologic techniques using CBCT and 3-D treatment planning for implant placement. J Calif Dent Assoc. 2008; 36: 287-97.

[9] Lofthag-Hansen S, Gröndahl K, Ekestubbe A. Cone-Beam CT for Preoperative Implant Planning in the Posterior Mandible: Visibility of Anatomic Landmarks.Clin Implant Dent Relat Res. 2009;11(3):246-55.

[10] World Health Organization Classification of Tumours Pathology and Genetics of Head and Neck Tumours. Barnes L, Eveson JW, Reichart P, Sidransky D, editors. Lyon: IARC Press: 2005.

[11] Boeddinghaus R, Whyte A. Current concepts in maxillofacial imaging. Eur J Radiol. 2008; 66(3):396-418.

[12] Diagnostic Imaging of the Jaws. Langlais RP, Langland OE, Nortje CJ, 1995, Willliams&Wilkins, Chapter 7, 181-212.

[13] Ackermann G, Cohen MA, Altini M. The paradental cyst: a clinicopathologic study of 50 cases. Oral Surg Oral Med Oral Pathol.1987: 64(3): 308-312.

[14] Ohba T, Morimoto Y, Nagata Y, Tanaka T, Kito S. Comparison of the panoramic radiographic and CT features of post-Caldwell-Luc maxillary sinuses. Dentomaxillofac Radiol. 2000: 29(5):280-5.

[15] Suei Y, Tanimoto K, Wada T. Simple bone cyst. Evaluation of contents with conventional radiography and computed tomography. Oral Surg Oral Med Oral Pathol. 1994;77(3):296-301.

[16] Saito Y, Hoshina Y, Nagamine T, Nakajima T, Suzuki M, Hayashi T. Simple bone cyst. A clinical and histopathologic study of fifteen cases. Oral Surg Oral Med Oral Pathol. 1992 Oct;74(4):487-91.

[17] Morimoto Y, Tanaka T, Kito S, Fukuda J, Muraki Y, Ohba T. Posterior lingual mandibular bone depression. Dentomaxillofac Radiol.1999: 28(4):256.

[18] Oral and Maxillofacial Pathology 3th edition. Neville BW, Damm DD, Allen CM, Bouquot JE, editors: Saunders. Elsevier: 2009.

[19] Boeddinghaus R, Whyte A. Current concepts in maxillofacial imaging. European Journal of Radiology. 2008; 66: 396-418.

[20] Small IA, Waldron CA. Ameloblastoma of the jaw. Oral Surg Oral Med Oral Pathol.1955: 8(3): 281-297.

[21] Hylton RP Jr, McKean TW, Albright JE. Simple ameloblastoma: report of case. J Oral Surg. 1972;30(1):59-62.

[22] Mehlisch DR, Dahlin DC, Masson JK. Ameloblastoma: a clinicopathologic report. J Oral Surg. 1972; 30(1):9-22.

[23] Cherrick HM, King OH Jr, Lucatorto FM, Suggs DM. Benign cementoblastoma. A clinicopathologic evaluation. Oral Surg Oral Med Oral Pathol. 1974;37(1):54-63.

[24] Eversole LR, Sabes WR, Dauchess VG. Benign cementoblastoma. Oral Surg Oral Med Oral Pathol. 1973;36(6):824-30.

[25] Waldron CA, Giansanti JS. Benign fibro-osseous lesions of the jaws. I. Fibrous dysplasia of the jaws, Oral Surg Oral Med Oral Pathol. 1973;35:190-201.

[26] Cohen MMJr, Howell RE. Etiology of fibrous dysplasia and McCune-Albright's syndrome, Int J Oral Maxillofac Surg. 1999; 28:366-371.

[27] Head and neck imaging 4th edition. Som PM, Curtin HD, editors: Mosby. 2003.

[28] Weber AL, Romo L, Hashmi S. Malignant tumors of the oral cavity and oropharynx: clinical, pathologic, and radiologic evaluation. Neuroimag Clin N Am 2003; 13: 443-464.

[29] Harnsberger, editors. Diagnostic imaging head and neck, 1st Edition. Salt Lake City, Utah, Amirsys 2004.

[30] Michael AS Michael AS, Mafee MF, Valvassori GE, Tan WS. Dynamic computed tomography of the head and neck: differential diagnostic value. Radiology 1985; 154: 413-419.

[31] Wakasa Wakasa T, Higuchi Y, Hisatomi M, Aiga H, Honda Y, Kishi K. Application of dynamic CT for various diseases in the oral and maxillofacial region Eur J Radiol 2002; 44: 10-15.

[32] Yerli H, Teksam M, Aydin E, Coskun M, Ozdemir H, Agidere AM. Basal cell adenoma of the parotid gland: dynamic CT and MRI findings. Br J Radiol 2005; 78: 642-645.

[33] Yoshioka I, Shiiba S, Tanaka T, Nishikawa T, Sakamoto E, Kito S, Oda M, Wakasugi-Sato N, Matsumoto-Takeda S, Kagawa S, Nakanishi O, Tominaga K, Morimoto Y. The importance of clinical features and computed tomographic findings in numb chin syndrome: a report of two cases. J Am Dent Assoc. 2009; 140(5): 550-554.

[34] Marx RE, Sawatari Y, Fortin M, Broumand V. Bisphosphonate-induced exposed bone (osteonecrosis/osteopetrosis) of the jaws: risk factors, recognition, prevention, and treatment. J Oral Maxillofac Surg. 2005;63(11):1567-75.

[35] Lazarovici TS, Yarom N. Risk factors for bisphosphonate-related osteonecrosis of the jaws. J Oral Maxillofac Surg. 2011;69(4):959-60.

2

Estimated Specific Gravity with Quantitative CT Scan in Traumatic Brain Injury

Vincent Degos, Thomas Lescot and Louis Puybasset

Neuro-ICU Unit, Department of Anesthesiology and Critical Care
Groupe Hospitalier Pitié-Salpêtrière, APHP, Université Pierre et Marie Curie, Paris
France

1. Introduction

An uncontrolled increase in intracranial pressure (ICP), often due to cerebral oedema, is the most common cause of death in traumatic brain injury (TBI) patients. Different types of oedema coexist in TBI patients: vasogenic oedema and cytotoxic oedema. Vasogenic oedema occurs with the extravasation of fluid into the extracellular space following blood brain barrier (BBB) disruption. Cytotoxic oedema results from a shift of water from the extracellular compartment into the intracellular compartment due in part to alterations in normal ionic gradients. The description of the localisation, and the knowledge of the chronology, the determinants, and the kinetics of the BBB disruption are necessary to adapt therapeutic strategy.

Although nuclear magnetic resonance is not advisable during the acute phase of human TBI, especially in unstable TBI patients, this imaging is one of the most accurate for the study of brain oedema. Diffusion-weighted imaging provides a useful and non-invasive method for visualizing and quantifying diffusion of water in the brain associated with oedema. Apparent diffusion coefficients (ADC) can be calculated and used to assess the magnitude of water diffusion in tissues. For example, a high ADC value indicates more freely diffusible water which is considered as a marker of vasogenic oedema. On the other hand, cytotoxic oedema restricts water movement and results in decreased signal intensities in the ADC map. In a rat model of diffuse TBI, an early increase in ADC values during the first 60 minutes was observed, followed by a decrease in ADC values reaching a minimum at one week [1]. This result suggests a biphasic oedema formation following diffuse TBI without contusion, with a rapid and short disruption of the BBB during the first hour post injury, leading to an early formation of vasogenic edema. Contrary to the non-contused areas, there are numerous arguments in favour of a profound and prolonged alteration of the BBB in traumatic areas of contusion appearing on CT [2-7]. Several methods have been used to study oedema formation and the BBB changes following animal and human TBI, however its underlying mechanisms are still not well understood. For these reasons, it might be interesting to investigate a new and more accessible technique to study the oedema formation at the acute phase of human TBI, particularly to compare the non-contused and the contused areas and to follow the BBB state in these areas with time.

Computed Tomography (CT) scan, the iconographic gold standard to describe acute brain lesions, is widespread and accessible. CT scan image acquisitions are prompt and reproducible with high quality. With specific software, volume, weight and an estimation of specific gravity (eSG) can be quantified from CT DICOM image and can be used to study different anatomic areas at different periods after injury. The goal of this review is to describe the use of quantitative CT scan results in non-contused and contused areas in TBI patients.

2. Quantitative computed tomography

Since its development in the 1970's, CT scan has become the radiological examination of choice in the acute assessment of patients with acute brain lesions and especially TBI. CT maps the way in which different tissues attenuate or absorb the beam of X-ray. A crucial point is that the radiological attenuation is linearly correlated with the physical density in the range of human tissue densities [8, 9]. For example, blood clot has relatively little water content and absorbs X-rays more than the normal brain. It is displayed as hyperdense area. On the other hand, ischemia and liquid collection are displayed in dark areas because there is an increase in water content.

BrainView, a recent software package developed for Windows workstations, provides semi-automatic tools for brain analysis and quantification from DICOM images obtained from cerebral CT scan. For each exam, BrainView inputs series of continuous axial scans of the brain. It then automatically excludes extracranial compartments on each section (**Figure 1**).

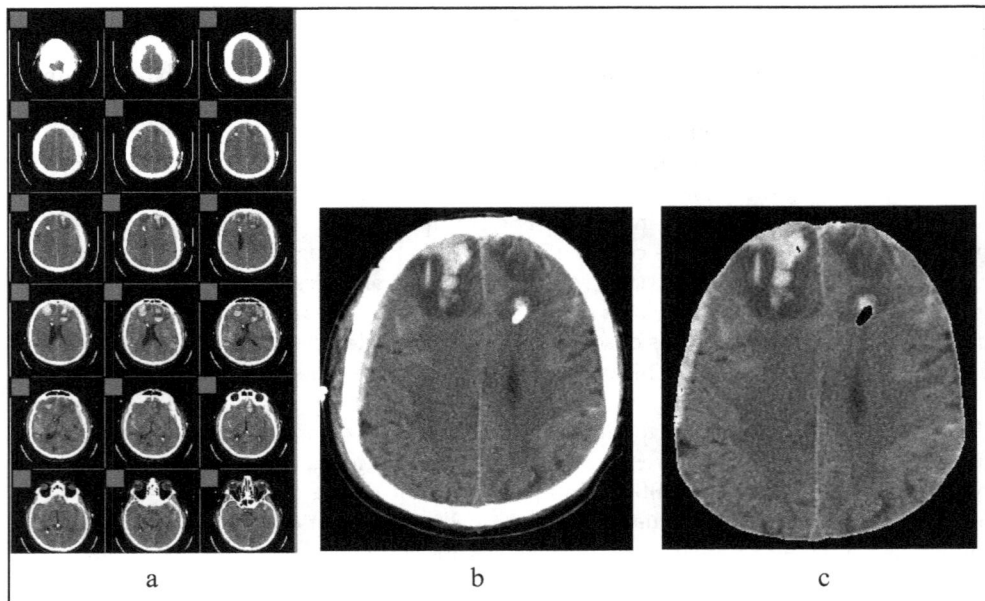

Fig. 1. Brainview software working window. CT DICOM image imports (a, b), automatic exclusion of extracranial compartments (c).

Interactive slice-by-slice segmentation allows the user to select different anatomical territories indexed throughout the whole sequence. The software is an upgrade of Lungview, another software previously developed by the same institution (Institut National des Télécommunications) and used for lung and heart weight, volume and density analysis by our group [10-12]. For each compartment of a known number of voxels, the volume, weight and eSG are computed using the following equations:

1. Volume of the voxel = surface x section thickness.
2. Weight of the voxel = (1 + CT / 1000) x Volume of the voxel where CT is the attenuation coefficient (expressed in Hounsfield Unit).
3. Volume of the compartment = number of voxels x volume of the voxel.
4. Weight of the compartment = summation of the weight of each individual voxel included in the compartment.
5. Estimated specific gravity (eSG) of the compartment = Weight of the compartment / Volume of the compartment. The eSG is expressed as a physical density in g/mL.

Brainview technology was first validated *ex vivo*. We measured the specific gravity of different solutes by determining the weight of one litter of these solutes (**Figure 2**). The eSG of the same solutes was then computed using BrainView. The two values were linearly correlated especially in the range of densities in human brain tissue [13]. Using the correlation between the specific density and the radiological attenuation, Brainview allowed

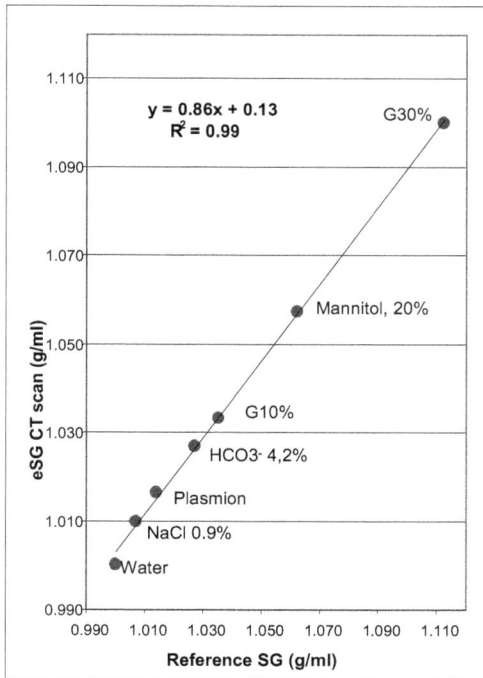

Fig. 2. Comparison of the specific gravity (SG) of the different solutes measured by the electronic scale method (weight/volume) and the estimated specific gravity (eSG) with quantitative CT scan [13].

us to assess the weight, volume and eSG of different anatomical parts of the brain (the two hemispheres, the cerebellum, the brainstem and the intraventricular and subarachnoid cerebrospinal fluid, the white and grey matters, contused and non-contused hemispheric areas). The technology also allows the comparison of different populations (TBI patients, subarachnoid haemorrhage patients, controls) or the same population at different periods (first hours after injury, CT controls at 1 week, before or after a treatment etc.).

In theory, eSG measurement is a good reflection of the density variations. When studying the consequence of BBB disruption in TBI, a complete disruption of the BBB with leakage of water, electrolytes, proteins and cells would increases the brain eSG since the added volume (exsudat) has a density greater than the brain. However, a partial disruption of the BBB with leakage of water and electrolytes would decrease the density since the added volume (transudat) has a density lower than the brain (**Figure 3**).

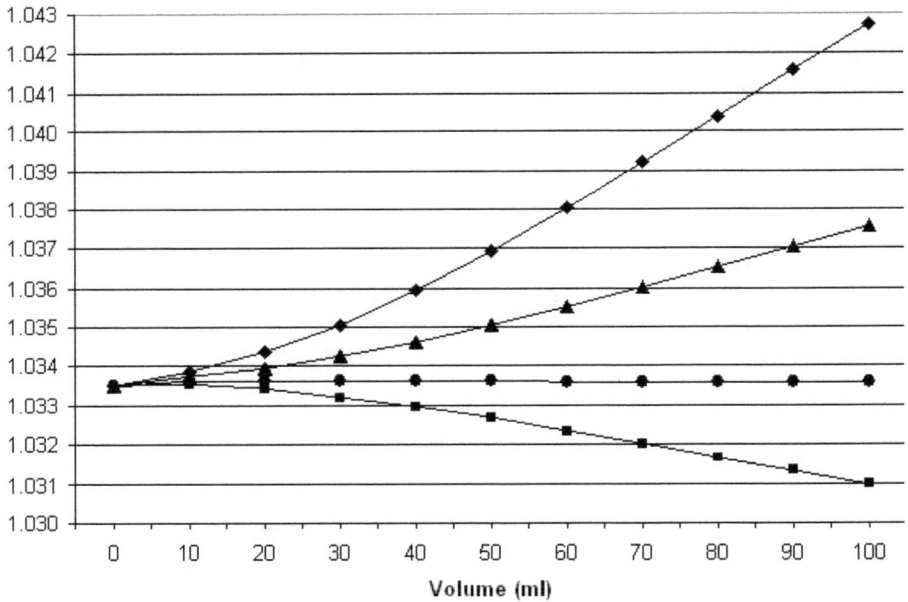

Fig. 3. Computation of the resulting specific gravity after adding a given volume (x axis) of a solute with a density of 1.026 g/mL (square), 1.0335 (round), 1.045 (triangle) and 1.060 (diamond) in hemispheres having a volume of 1041 mL, a weight of 1076 g and a SG of 1.0335 g/mL (mean values of controls). 1.026 g/mL is the density of plasma. 1.060 g/mL is the density of blood. 1.045 g/mL is the density of a solute explaining an increase in the hemispheric volume of 85 mL combined with a raise in SG from 1.0335 up to 1.0367 g/mL (mean value of controls and TBI patients [13].

3. Quantative CT study of non-contused hemispheric areas

Using the methodology of Brainview, weight, volume and eSG of the brain were measured in 15 TBI patients, 3±2 days after the trauma and in 15 controls. For similar age and overall intracranial volume, TBI patients had an overall brain weight 82g heavier, and hemispheres weight 91g heavier, than controls [13]. Volume of intraventricular and subarachnoid CSF was reduced in TBI patients. In this first series of measurements in 15 TBI patients, eSG of hemispheres, brainstem and cerebellum was significantly higher in TBI patients as compared to controls (all $P<0.0001$). The increase in eSG was statistically similar in these three anatomical compartments, and in white and grey matter. Furthermore, there was no correlation between the hemispheric eSG and age, natremia at computed tomography time, presence of a traumatic subarachnoid hemorrhage, or presence of intraparenchymal blood [13].

To confirm these results, a second study was performed in a larger cohort of 120 severe TBI patients. The measurement of eSG from the initial CT scan performed in the first 5 hours after trauma was also increased. eSG increase was present in the overall intracranial content and in the non-contused hemispheric areas [14]. The follow up changes in eSG of the overall intracranial content showed that it takes more than ten days to return to a normal value of eSG (**Figure 4**). The same cohort was divided into two groups according to the initial eSG of the non-contused hemispheric areas. The normal specific gravity (NSG) group was defined as patients having an eSG less than 1.96 SD above controls. In the increased specific gravity (ISG) group, patients had an eSG higher than 1.96 SD above controls. Patients in the ISG group had a lower Glasgow coma scale (GCS) and more often had a mydriasis at the scene of the accident, more frequently received osmotherapy in the initial phase, more frequently had an extra-ventricular drainage implanted for ICP monitoring and CSF drainage, more frequently received barbiturates as a second line therapy and more frequently had a CT classified in the third category of the Marshall score. In this cohort, the initial GCS, the velocity, the occurrence of mydriasis at the scene and the use of osmotherapy were

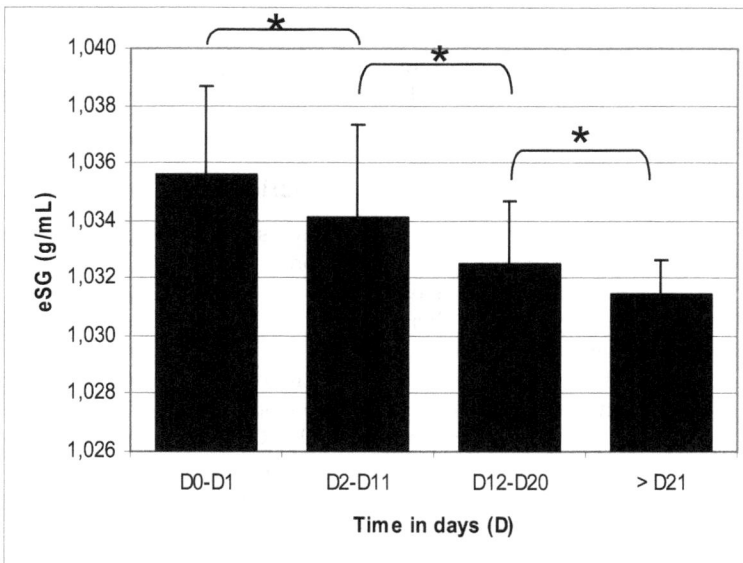

Fig. 4. Follow-up changes in estimated specific gravity (eSG) of the overall intracranial content (n=15) [14].

predictors of outcome at ICU discharge and at one year. eSG of the overall intracranial content or of the non-contused areas were also predictors of outcome (**Table 1**). This study indicated also that eSG was strongly correlated with the intensity of therapeutics to maintain ICP below 20 mmHg. To understand the relationship between eSG and brain swelling, we compared eSG values of TBI patients and high grade subarachnoid haemorrhage (SAH) patients with a similar severity of brain swelling. The increase of eSG was only highlighted in the TBI group [15]; it was not observed in the high grade SAH group. In a fourth study, we compared eSG value of the non-contused hemispheric areas before and after an hypertonic saline bolus administration, and we observed an increase of eSG associated with a decrease in the volume, corresponding to a correct permeability of the BBB in these areas [16].

	ICU discharge		1 yr	
	GOS 1–3 ($n = 46$)	GOS 4–5 ($n = 74$)	GOS 1–3 ($n = 37$)	GOS 4–5 ($n = 83$)
Age (yr)	37 ± 15	33 ± 14	39 ± 15	33 ± 14
Initial GCS	6 ± 3	8 ± 3†	6 ± 3	8 ± 3†
SAPS 2	50 ± 11	40 ± 9†	51 ± 12	41 ± 10†
Mechanisms				
Assault	6 (13)	5 (7)	6 (16)	5 (6)
Fall	13 (28)	20 (27)	10 (27)	23 (28)
MVA	22 (48)	38 (51)	16 (43)	44 (53)
Pedestrian	5 (11)	11 (15)	5 (14)	11 (13)
Velocity				
Low	15 (32)	7 (10)*	14 (38)	8 (10)†
Mydriasis on scene				
Yes	21 (46)	17 (23)*	17 (46)	21 (25)*
Use of osmotherapy on scene				
Yes	24 (52)	17 (23)*	19 (51)	24 (29)*
eSG overall intracranial content	1.0352 ± 0.0034	1.0338 ± 0.0026*	1.0348 ± 0.0032	1.0341 ± 0.0029
eSG noncontused areas	1.0355 ± 0.0033	1.0340 ± 0.0027*	1.0351 ± 0.0032	1.0343 ± 0.0029

Table 1. Predicting factors of outcome at Intensive Care Unit (ICU) and 1 year later in patients with severe TBI. GOS: Glasgow outcome scale; SAPS: simplified acute physiological score; MVA: motor vehicle accident; * $p<0.01$; † $p<0.001$ [14] .

4. Quantitative CT study of contused hemispheric areas

In TBI, osmotherapy such as hypertonic saline has been shown to decrease ICP; therefore it is used in an emergency to control ICP augmentation. From a theoretical point of view, it can be expected that hypertonic saline is effective only in the areas of the brain where the BBB is still functional after trauma. As there seem to be BBB alterations in contusion areas, the patient population that is most likely to respond to hypertonic saline needs to be further defined. A prospective study was designed to evaluate, using quantitative CT scan, the regional effects of hypertonic saline on contused and non-contused brain tissue after TBI [16]. Global and regional brain volumes, weights and eSGs were compared with Brainview before and after hypertonic saline bolus administration in a prospective series of 14 patients 3±2 days after severe TBI. Hypertonic saline presented opposite effects on non-contused and contused hemispheric areas (**Figure 5**). Hypertonic saline decreased the volume of the non-contused hemispheric tissue by 14 ± 9 mL while increasing the eSG by 0.029 ± 0.027 %. The volume of the contused tissue ranged from 3 mL to 157 mL (50 ± 55 mL). Hypertonic saline increased the volume of contused hemispheric tissue by 6 ± 4 mL without any concomitant change in density. The increase of the contusion's volume with hypertonic saline injection was significantly related to baseline contusion volume expressed in percentage (r^2= 0.62, P = 0.01, **Figure 6**). Hypertonic saline consistently decreased the weight of the non-contused areas while increasing the eSG, indicating a decrease in water content and, consequently, a functional BBB. On the other hand, hypertonic saline always increased the weight of the contused area. By using quantitative CT scan, this study was able to describe in human TBI the BBB permeability selectively in contused and non-contused areas. The BBB is still permeable in the contused areas 3 days after TBI, and thus hypertonic saline should be given with caution in TBI patients with large contusions after the immediate resuscitation period while the patient is in the ICU.

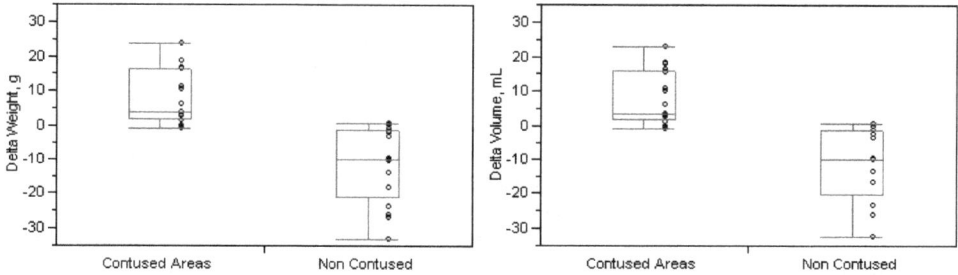

Fig. 5. Mean effect of hypertonic saline on the weight and volume of contused and non-contused areas. The box plots summarize the distribution (25th and 75th quartiles). The line across the middle of the box identifies the median sample value. The whiskers extend from the ends from the sides of the box to the outermost data point that falls within the distances computed [16].

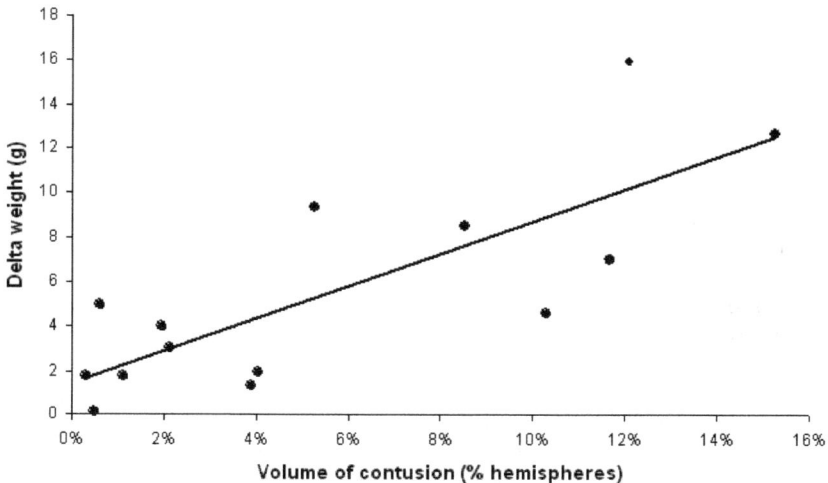

Fig. 6. Change in the weight of contusion according to its initial volume assessed in percentage of the hemispheres [16].

5. Interpretation of estimated specific gravity variations

As quantitative brain CT studies have shown, contused and non-contused hemispheric areas show opposite behaviour concerning eSG variation. In the non-contused areas, a large part of the TBI patients presented an early increase of eSG (5 hours after trauma). This increased eSG in TBI was diffuse, present in the white and grey matters, and required more than 10 days to become normal. The value of eSG was also correlated with the therapeutic intensity level in ICU and the outcome at ICU discharge. Contrary to the contused hemispheric areas, the BBB of the non-contused areas was sufficiently semi-permeable to lead to decreased water content after osmotherapy.

The observation of increased eSG in patients with TBI is in opposition with some experimental literature. Studies performed in murine models of head trauma report a decrease in eSG with a rise in the cerebral water content [17, 18]. However, and as in our three different studies [14-16], Bullock at al. observed an increased SG with severe TBI in the same proportion [19]. In another human TBI study, specific gravity determined on small pieces of subcortical tissue using a graduated specific-gravity column was also increased [20].

In our studies, eSG increase was concomitant to a gain of weight. One might argue that the increased eSG could be due exclusively to hyperemia caused by vascular dilation. However, there are some strong experimental [21] and human data against this hypothesis. Recently, Marmarou et al demonstrated, using MRI, that brain oedema is the major fluid component contributing to traumatic brain swelling following TBI in humans [22]. These authors observed a reduction in cerebral blood volume in proportion to cerebral blood flow following severe brain injury. As shown on the abacus presented in **Figure 3**, since blood has an eSG of 1.060 g/mL [23], theoretically an increase in cerebral blood volume of 45 mL would be necessary to increase hemispheric eSG from the mean value of controls to the mean value of TBI patients. Considering that normal cerebral blood volume is about 5% of the overall intracranial volume, this would mean a 65 % increase in cerebral blood volume. Together, the mean change of hemispheric volume that we observed was 85 mL, a value much higher that what could be explained by the change in cerebral blood volume alone.

Another hypothesis to explain eSG increase could be the presence of traumatic macro-haemorrhagic lesions. We first reported that the eSG value was increased in the white matter, excluding the subarachnoid space and thus subarachnoid haemorrhage [13]. Also, eSG values of the total intracranial content and of the non-contused hemispheric areas were similarly elevated [14], a finding that argues against a major role for visible macro-hemorrhagic lesions in eSG elevation.

The last hypothesis to explain eSG increase is the very early BBB disruption already described in different experimental models of TBI [24, 25]. There are many experimental arguments showing that the BBB disruption is early and brief. Time window studies indicate that the barrier seals within a few hours following severe head injury [26]. In the experimental model of Barzo et al, permeability of the BBB returned to control values as soon as 30 min after the head trauma [1]. Tanno et al also observed a pronounced abnormal permeability to IgG and horseradish peroxidase occurring within the first hour after injury that was widespread throughout both hemispheres after a lateral, fluid percussive brain injury in the rat [27]. In that study, maximal permeability occurred at 1 hr after injury. This was confirmed by Baldwin et al [2]. In humans, this early, transient and diffuse opening of the BBB might be directly or indirectly involved in the increase of eSG. Theoretically, a leak of plasma decreases the overall hemispheric eSG since the SG of plasma (between 1.0245 and 1.0285 g/mL) is lower than that of the brain. According to **Figure 3**, the volume added in hemispheres of TBI patients should have a mean density of 1.045 g/mL to explain eSG increase. This value cannot be explained by plasma leakage alone and must also involve cells. Thus, it can be hypothesized that BBB opening occurs immediately after TBI in some patients, leading to extravasation of cells and proteins into the extracellular space. This extravasation could also be associated with leucocyte infiltration and microglia proliferation already described in TBI [27]. Immune cells' proliferation increase tissue specific gravity and they also correlate with brain injuries severity, exacerbating the oedema and leading to prolonged ICP elevation and to higher treatment intensity. Thus, eSG may reflect the early BBB disruption and consequences specifically associated with TBI [15] and may explain why it is correlated with TBI outcome.

Regarding the contused areas, experimental data suggest that BBB remains open for a prolonged period of time after trauma [2, 3]. Our quantitative CT scan study of contused areas suggested that this is true in human TBI, since hypertonic saline consistently increased the weight and volume of contused areas. In the experiment performed by Tanno and al, at 24 hr after injury, abnormal permeability was restricted to the impact site and this area remained permeable up to 72 hr after trauma [28]. Experimentally, Beaumont et al demonstrated using an intravenous bolus of Gd-DTPA with serial T1 MR images that BBB permeability was the greatest in the site of contusion [29]. Gd-DTPA accumulation was greatly enhanced by secondary insult such as hypoxia and hypotension. **Figure 7** represents an illustration of BBB regional and chronological modifications and CT scan observation after TBI in contused and non-contused areas.

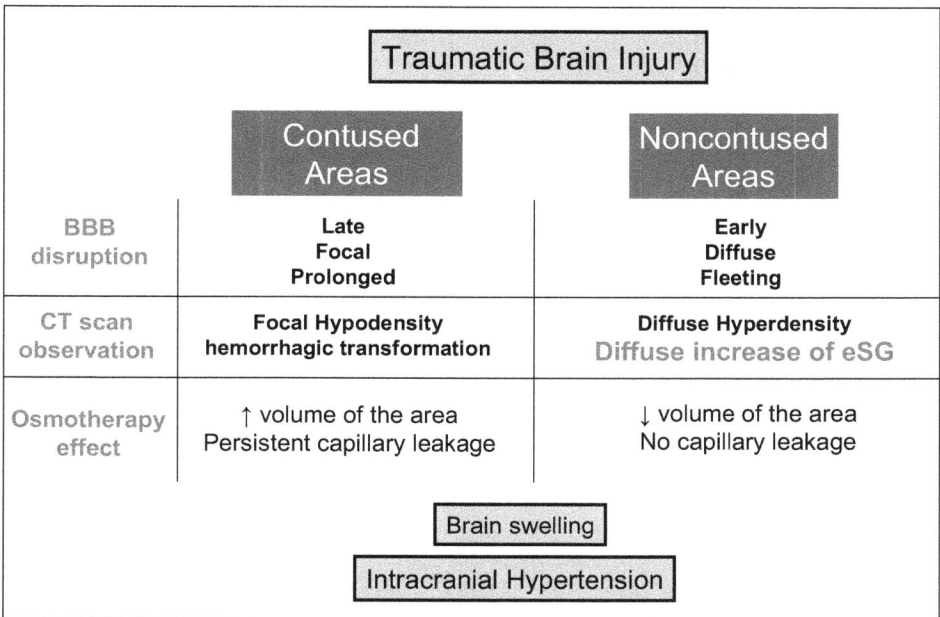

	Traumatic Brain Injury	
	Contused Areas	Noncontused Areas
BBB disruption	Late Focal Prolonged	Early Diffuse Fleeting
CT scan observation	Focal Hypodensity hemorrhagic transformation	Diffuse Hyperdensity Diffuse increase of eSG
Osmotherapy effect	↑ volume of the area Persistent capillary leakage	↓ volume of the area No capillary leakage

Brain swelling

Intracranial Hypertension

Fig. 7. Illustration of BBB modification after TBI in contused and non-contused areas

6. Conclusion

Quantitative CT scan is validated for brain imaging and may help to better characterize the regional differences (contused and non-contused areas) in TBI and the BBB disruption time-course. These studies argue for a distinction between the contused and non-contused area and also for a consideration of the change of the lesions over time.

The clinical usefulness of the automatic determination of eSG in human TBI to characterize the BBB state or to establish outcome information's will have to be addressed in a large prospective study.

7. Acknowledgement

This study was supported by the non-profit organizations "Fondation des Gueules Cassées" and the Société Française d'Anesthésie Réanimation Paris, France. None of the authors have any conflicts of interest regarding this work.

8. References

[1] Barzo P, Marmarou A, Fatouros P, Corwin F, Dunbar J.(1996) Magnetic resonance imaging-monitored acute blood-brain barrier changes in experimental traumatic brain injury. J Neurosurg;85(6):1113-1121.

[2] Baldwin SA, Fugaccia I, Brown DR, Brown LV, Scheff SW.(1996) Blood-brain barrier breach following cortical contusion in the rat. J Neurosurg;85(3):476-481.

[3] McLaughlin MR, Marion DW.(1996) Cerebral blood flow and vasoresponsivity within and around cerebral contusions. J Neurosurg;85(5):871-876.

[4] Daneyemez M.(1999) Microangiographic changes following cerebral contusion in rats. Neuroscience;92(2):783-790.

[5] Furuya Y, Hlatky R, Valadka AB, Diaz P, Robertson CS.(2003) Comparison of cerebral blood flow in computed tomographic hypodense areas of the brain in head-injured patients. Neurosurgery;52(2):340-345; discussion 345-346.

[6] Hoelper BM, Soldner F, Chone L, Wallenfang T.(2000) Effect of intracerebral lesions detected in early MRI on outcome after acute brain injury. Acta Neurochir Suppl;76:265-267.

[7] von Oettingen G, Bergholt B, Gyldensted C, Astrup J.(2002) Blood flow and ischemia within traumatic cerebral contusions. Neurosurgery;50(4):781-788; discussion 788-790.

[8] Phelps ME, Gado MH, Hoffman EJ.(1975) Correlation of effective atomic number and electron density with attenuation coefficients measured with polychromatic x rays. Radiology;117(3 Pt 1):585-588.

[9] Mull RT.(1984) Mass estimates by computed tomography: Physical density from CT numbers. Am J Radiol;143:1101-1104.

[10] Puybasset L, Cluzel P, Gusman P, et al.(2000) Regional distribution of gas and tissue in acute respiratory distress syndrome. I. Consequences for lung morphology. CT Scan ARDS Study Group. Intensive Care Med;26(7):857-869.

[11] Rouby JJ, Puybasset L, Cluzel P, et al.(2000) Regional distribution of gas and tissue in acute respiratory distress syndrome. II. Physiological correlations and definition of

an ARDS Severity Score. CT Scan ARDS Study Group. Intensive Care Med;26(8):1046-1056.

[12] Rouby JJ, Puybasset L, Nieszkowska A, Lu Q.(2003) Acute respiratory distress syndrome: lessons from computed tomography of the whole lung. Crit Care Med;31(4 Suppl):S285-295.

[13] Lescot T, Bonnet MP, Zouaoui A, et al.(2005) A quantitative computed tomography assessment of brain weight, volume, and specific gravity in severe head trauma. Intensive Care Med;31(8):1042-1050.

[14] Degos V, Lescot T, Zouaoui A, et al.(2006) Computed tomography-estimated specific gravity of noncontused brain areas as a marker of severity in human traumatic brain injury. Anesth Analg;103(5):1229-1236.

[15] Degos V, Pereira AR, Lescot T, et al.(2008) Does brain swelling increase estimated specific gravity? Neurocrit Care;9(3):338-343.

[16] Lescot T, Degos V, Zouaoui A, et al.(2006) Opposed effects of hypertonic saline on contusions and noncontused brain tissue in patients with severe traumatic brain injury. Crit Care Med;34(12):3029-3033.

[17] Gardenfors A, Nilsson F, Skagerberg G, Ungerstedt U, Nordstrom CH.(2002) Cerebral physiological and biochemical changes during vasogenic brain oedema induced by intrathecal injection of bacterial lipopolysaccharides in piglets. Acta Neurochir (Wien);144(6):601-608; discussion 608-609.

[18] Talmor D, Roytblat L, Artru AA, et al.(1998) Phenylephrine-induced hypertension does not improve outcome after closed head trauma in rats. Anesth Analg;87(3):574-578.

[19] Bullock R, Smith R, Favier J, du Trevou M, Blake G.(1985) Brain specific gravity and CT scan density measurements after human head injury. J Neurosurg;63(1):64-68.

[20] Nath F, Galbraith S.(1986) The effect of mannitol on cerebral white matter water content. J Neurosurg;65(1):41-43.

[21] Kita H, Marmarou A.(1994) The cause of acute brain swelling after the closed head injury in rats. Acta Neurochir Suppl (Wien);60:452-455.

[22] Marmarou A, Portella G, Barzo P, et al.(2000) Distinguishing between cellular and vasogenic edema in head injured patients with focal lesions using magnetic resonance imaging. Acta Neurochir Suppl;76:349-351.

[23] Blacque-Belair A, Mathieu de Fossey B, Fourestier M. Dictionnaire des constantes biologiques et physiques. In. 4th edition ed. Paris: Maloine; 1965.

[24] Habgood MD, Bye N, Dziegielewska KM, et al.(2007) Changes in blood-brain barrier permeability to large and small molecules following traumatic brain injury in mice. Eur J Neurosci;25(1):231-238.

[25] Chen Y, Constantini S, Trembovler V, Weinstock M, Shohami E.(1996) An experimental model of closed head injury in mice: pathophysiology, histopathology, and cognitive deficits. J Neurotrauma;13(10):557-568.

[26] van den Brink WA, Santos BO, Marmarou A, Avezaat CJ.(1994) Quantitative analysis of blood-brain barrier damage in two models of experimental head injury in the rat. Acta Neurochir Suppl (Wien);60:456-458.

[27] Israelsson C, Wang Y, Kylberg A, Pick CG, Hoffer BJ, Ebendal T: Closed head injury in a mouse model results in molecular changes indicating inflammatory responses. J Neurotrauma 2009; 26: 1307-14

[28] Tanno H, Nockels RP, Pitts LH, Noble LJ.(1992) Breakdown of the blood-brain barrier after fluid percussive brain injury in the rat. Part 1: Distribution and time course of protein extravasation. J Neurotrauma;9(1):21-32.

[29] Beaumont A, Marmarou A, Fatouros P, Corwin F.(2002) Secondary insults worsen blood brain barrier dysfunction assessed by MRI in cerebral contusion. Acta Neurochir Suppl;81:217-219.

3

CT Scanning in Archaeology

Stephen Hughes

Department of Physics, Queensland University of Technology, Brisbane, Queensland
Australia

1. Introduction

In this chapter we will review the use of x-ray computed tomography (CT) scanning in the field of archaeology. The story will be told in roughly chronological order, starting with the first reported use of a CT scanner in the field of archaeology and then look at some some possibilities for the future. Since the introduction of the x-ray CT scanner in the 1970's the quality of the images has steadily improved enabling the role of the CT scanner to expand into the field of archaeology. In the context of this chapter, archaeology will be deemed to include the study of ancient human remains and artefacts but exclude remains from pre-history, which normally comes under the heading of palaeontology. (It would perhaps be appropriate to note that CT scanners have been successfully applied in the study of fossils). CT scans have mostly been used to study mummies but have also been used to examine other archaeological artefacts such as clay tablets, scrolls, pottery, bronze statues and swords.

2. Use of plain x-rays in archaeology

Before reviewing the use of CT scanning in the field of archaeology it would perhaps be useful to briefly review the role of conventional plain x-rays in archaeology to set the scene. X-rays were first used to look inside a mummy in 1898, just three years after the discovery of x-rays by Wilhelm Roentgen in 1895. In the same year, a scientist by the name of Konig x-rayed a mummified child and cat in Frankfurt, Germany, followed by Thurstan Holland in Liverpool, England, who x-rayed a mummified bird. In 1898, the famous archaeologist, Sir Flinders Petrie used x-rays to examine Egyptian mummies, followed by Elliot Smith and Howard Carter in 1904, and two French journalists, C. Leleux and M. Gouineau, in 1926.

During the 1960's a British radiologist of the name of Gray (Dawson and Gray, 1968) carried out the most comprehensive x-ray examination of Egyptian mummies. Gray studied 133 mummies and found that osteoarthritis of the spinal column was common and that 30% of all the mummies had lines of arrested growth, most likely caused by periods of famine. Many post-mortem fractures and dislocations were also found. On plain x-rays, post-mortem fractures can be distinguished from ante-mortem fractures as post-mortem fractures show no evidence of healing. The presence of post-mortem fractures in mummies suggests that occasionally embalmers could be rough, which was likely to happen when there was a backlog of bodies stacked on top of each other waiting to be mummified, which might occur for example in an epidemic.

Gray found that dental disease and attrition were very common, hardly surprising in view of the unavoidably sandy diet of the Egyptians. However, he found no evidence of bone cancer, tuberculosis, syphilis, leprosy or rickets. The dry atmosphere of Egypt would tend to inhibit the tuberculosis bacillus, which survives best in damp conditions. The abundance of sunlight, essential for the conversion of vitamin D from the inactive to active state, may have been a large contributing factor in the absence of rickets. Osteoarthritis is part of the ageing process, but can occur in the spine by middle age as a result of hard labour, which suggests a large fraction of the Egyptian population was engaged in hard labour – hardly surprising since prior the Industrial Revolution the majority of the populations of all societies worked in agriculture.

3. Physical autopsies

Another subject we should touch on before discussing the use of CT in archaeology is the use of autopsies. The word autopsy is usually applied to the technique of examining a dead body to determine the cause of death. In some cases autopsies have been used to determine the cause of the death of a mummified person several millennia after death. However, in archaeology the term "autopsy" is used in a wider sense and includes determining the type and quality of the mummification process and ascertaining the age of the body at death and wear and tear on the body that occurred during life.

Various research groups around the world have carried out autopsies on mummies, most notably at Manchester University in the UK (David et al, 1979, 1992) and Pennsylvania University in America (Cockburn et al, 1975). In most cases, autopsies involve the physical destruction of a mummy in the sense that the body is unwrapped and broken open. In view of this, the highest quality mummies tend not to be subjected to this form of examination. Autopsies are sometimes used to examine the contents of burial urns, also destructive in the sense that it would be extremely difficult, if not impossible, to reassemble the contents of the urn exactly as before the examination. CT scans make it possible to perform virtual autopsies on mummies and burial urns without disturbing internal structure.

4. A brief history of the CT scanner

The first clinical x-ray CT scanner entered operation in the early 1970's (Beckmann 2006) and was a quantum leap in diagnostic imaging. The CT scanner was the first time that 3D images of the body could be produced, initially just the head, and then the rest of the body as the aperture of later generations of scanners increased. Another factor vital in the introduction of the CT scanner in clinical medicine was the development of the mini computer.

In essence, an x-ray CT scanner comprises an x-ray source, similar to that in an ordinary x-ray machine, and a group of x-ray detectors opposite the x-ray source arranged in an arc. A fan-shaped x-ray beam shines through the patient or archaeological artefact and is absorbed differently depending on the material between the x-ray source and detector. The greater the density of material the greater the attenuation of the x-ray beam. (For more information on the workings of an x-ray CT scanner please see Michael (2001)). Generally, the x-ray source and detectors move on a ring so that each detector is in the same position relative to the source. In first generation of scanners, the x-ray source rotated around a stationary patient and the x-ray absorption pattern recorded by the detectors used to generate a 2D cross-sectional image - a process known as back projection. The couch was then moved a set distance ready for the next image to be acquired.

In 1989 a new generation of CT scanner was introduced, the spiral CT scanner (sometimes known as a helical scanner). In a spiral CT scanner the couch moves continuously as the x-ray source and detectors rotate around the patient. The advantage of this approach is that CT images are acquired much quicker. For example it might take 20 minutes to acquire 20 images on a first generation CT scanner but only 20 seconds on a spiral scanner. The next step in the development of the CT scanner was the MSCT – the Multi-detector Spiral CT. In a MSCT, the one dimensional arc of detectors is replaced by multiple arcs side by side. In the year 2000, MSCTs were available with four rows of detectors capable of acquiring four slices simultaneously every half a second. In 2011, MSCTs were available capable of acquiring 256 slices simultaneously every 0.27 of a second. These scanners are so fast that they are able to capture high resolution 3D images of the beating heart.

A large number of calculations are required to produce a single CT image. If minicomputers had not been invented at the same time as CT scanners the introduction of the CT scanner into routine clinical use would have been delayed. It would have been necessary for CT data to be stored on magnetic tape and transported to a main frame computer remote from the hospital. The processed CT images data would then need to have been transported on magnetic tape back to the hospital for viewing and diagnosis. This would obviously reduce the number of patients that could be scanned each day. (Remember that at this time the internet was 20 years in the future).

The invention of the minicomputer enabled CT data to be processed locally increasing patient throughput. Also, the development of the MSCT would not have been possible without the huge increases in computer processing power and memory that have occurred since the invention of the mini computer.

A major advantage of x-ray CT scans over other forms of investigation is that the technique is able to show the internal structure of an object in a non-destructive way thus preserving the artefact for posterity. A good example is the study of mummies. Prior to the advent of the CT scanner the only way of finding out about the internal structure of a mummy was to unwrap and dissect it. However, CT scanning can be used to effectively unwrap a mummy electronically without disturbing the body, wrappings or coffin – a kind of virtual dissection. The x-ray dose is low enough not to damage the artefact and images have sub-mm spatial resolution with very little spatial distortion over the entire field of view.

In some ways, CT scanning is actually superior to physical examination of an artefact as it gives information about the internal composition as well as the overall shape. In this regard CT scanners have a distinct advantage over plain x-rays. When a plain x-ray is taken of the body it is not obvious at what depth various structures lie, although of course in the case of a medical image it is known that the heart lies between the ribs. However, in the case of a plain x-ray of a mummy it may not be obvious whether a piece of jewellery is on the surface, or inside the body between the wrappings. CT is also able to provide information on the internal structure of bones, organ packs, amulets etc. that could not otherwise be acquired without cutting open the object.

CT images of mummies can be clearer than CT images of live patients as it is easier for x-rays to pass through the dehydrated tissues of a mummy with less scatter resulting in images with a higher signal to noise ratio and therefore better spatial contrast and resolution. In the case of scanning mummies there are no movement artefacts, as there are for a live patient.

When it comes to imaging archaeological artefacts CT has no real competition as there are serious difficulties that prevent other 3D imaging modalities being used in archaeology. For example, ultrasound imaging depends on high frequency sound waves being propagated through contiguous material of fairly uniform density. Since mummies contain a lot of air between wrappings, ultrasound will be strongly reflected at linen/air interfaces making ultrasound images impossible to form.

Magnetic Resonance Imaging (MRI) is also generally unsuitable for use in archaeology as MRI relies on the scanned object having significant moisture content, which is generally not the case for archaeological artefacts. Notman *et al* (1986) attempted a MR scan of an Egyptian mummy but were unable to acquire enough signal to produce an image. However, one group (Rühli *et al* 2007) has been able to successfully use MR to image an Egyptian mummy and Peruvian corpse using an ultra short pulse sequence not possible on earlier generations of MR scanners.

In 2009 terahertz (THz) imaging was performed on parts of a mummy in conjunction with CT and was found to provide more soft tissue information than CT, although at lower spatial resolution (Ohrstrom et al, 2009). THz rays have a wavelength between light and microwaves and so have properties midway between light and microwaves. THz waves are more penetrating than light waves and can produce images with a higher resolution than microwaves. THz waves are strongly absorbed by water, and therefore are capable of penetrating deep into dehydrated mummified tissue. THz waves are also non-ionizing and therefore safer to use than x-rays and the small amount of heat produced is not damaging. THz imaging may find an increasing role in archaeological imaging. THz will probably never replace CT scanning in archaeology but rather will be a complimentary imaging modality.

5. CT scans of mummies in North America

The first CT scan of a mummy was performed in 1977 by Derek Harwood-Nash in Toronto, Canada only about four years after the clinical introduction of the CT scanner (Harwood-Nash, 1979). Harwood-Nash performed a CT scan on the desiccated brain of a boy and the mummy of a young woman, demonstrating that x-ray CT scanning was a useful tool in archaeology.

In 1983, four mummies from the 18th and 25th Egyptian dynasties were x-rayed in Minnesota (Notman 1986). Scans showed the remains of the heart within the chest. The group also carried out the first ever MRI scan of an Egyptian mummy to check for residual moisture. The mummy given this distinction was Lady Tashat from the 25th dynasty, a resident of the Minneapolis Museum of Art. What little moisture still retained within the body was too low for an MR image to be produced.

Between 1983 and 1987, 15 mummies from the Museum of Fine Arts in Boston, MA, USA were CT scanned at the Brigham and Womens' Hospital in Boston (part of the Harvard group of hospitals). The images showed soft tissue packing material, schmorl's nodes (herniations of vertebral discs) and aortic calcification. The images assisted curators to plan a mummy restoration program (Marx and D'Auria 1986). A 3D reconstruction performed on one of the mummies called Tabes, a songstress of Amun who lived in c.950 BC in the 22nd dynasty, showed sunken eyes caused by the embalming process and a metal heart scarab in the region of the xiphoid (Marx and D'Auria 1988). It appears that Tabes died in her thirties.

A 21st dynasty male and female mummy on display in the Albany Institute of History and Art, Albany, New York, which were originally bought from the Cairo museum in 1909, underwent a series of CT scans and plain X-rays (Wagle 1994). The X-rays showed that the female mummy was given a two-component foot prosthesis by the embalmers, an indication of the importance the Egyptians placed on the body being complete in order for the soul to exist in the afterlife.

In 2001, Cessarini *et al* performed CT scans on 13 mummies from the Egyptian Museum in Torino, Italy using a multi-dector CT scanner. An advantage of using this type of scanner is that whole body can be scanned quickly in a single session without the need to re-position the body between scans and register different sets of images. The group used a computer to perform virtual endoscopy on the mummies, i.e. the computer was used to display views from inside the body as if an actual endoscope had been placed inside the body.

A group at the Orthopaedic University Hospital Balgrist, Zurich, performed a CT guided biopsy on the mummy of an Egyptian child from the Museum für Völkerkunde in Burgdorf, Switzerland (Rühli 2002). The mummy had been previously x-rayed in the 1920s and researchers had concluded that the child had died from spinal tuberculosis. However, a sample of lumbar vertebral bone showed that the bone had disintegrated after death and therefore TB was not the cause of death.

In 2008, Chan *et al* published a paper describing a CT study of a female mummy from the Egyptian city of Akhmim (about 470 km south of Cairo on the east bank of the Nile) dating from the Ptolemaic period (305 – 200 BC). The mummy is in the collection of the Academy of Natural Sciences in Philadelphia, Pennsylvania. The mummy was x-rayed at the Hahnemann University Hospital, Philadelphia using a GE Medical Systems 16-detector row helical CT scanner. The main purpose of the study was to determine the social status of the mummy on the basis of the embalming technique used.

The CT scans showed that the quality of embalming was good, although the body showed signs of decomposition prior to embalming. There was no obvious physical cause of death. Scans showed that the brain had been removed through the nose and only one of the four molars had erupted indicating the mummy was probably 17 – 25 years old at death. The CT scans showed an unusual dislocation of two of the two cervical vertebrae at the top of the spinal column (C1 and C2). The authors suggest that this dislocation occurred as a result of the body lying in the river Nile after death. According to Herodotus, if the people of a town found someone dead in the Nile they embalmed them as if they were of high social status. Therefore it is possible that the young girl was found floating in the river near Akhmim and given a top quality embalming even although she was unknown to the inhabitants of the city.

An interesting CT study was performed on 22 mummies from the Egyptian National Museum of Antiquities in Cairo in February 2009 (Allam et al, 2009). The mummies were dated as being from 1981 BC – AD 334. Seven out of eight mummies who were over 45 years old when they died showed evidence of arteriosclerosis, whereas only two out of eight mummies younger than 45 showed evidence of ateriosclerosis. This study demonstrates that in ancient Egypt people suffered from arteriosclerosis and therefore arteriosclerosis is not exclusively a disease of modern society related to diet and sedentary life style. Potentially, this finding could lead to new approaches to finding a cure for arteriosclerosis.

6. The Ice Man

The Ice Man (Otzi) is probably the most famous mummy of recent times. Otzi's head and upper torso were found protruding out of the ice in the Austrian Alps by German hikers in

September 1991. There was no evidence of decay, which suggests that Otzi had only recently been uncovered. If the body had been regularly thawed and refrozen in the intervening millennia significant decay would be expected. In view of the fact that Otzi was discovered in September, i.e. the end of summer in the northern hemisphere this may have been an early sign of global warming.

Otzi was transported to the anatomy department of the University of Innsbruck in Austria for extensive analysis that included taking plain x-rays and CT scans. An initial set of CT scans were acquired in September 1991 (Nedden 1994) and three sets of spiral CT scans acquired over the following 10 years (Murphy et al 2003). In total 2,190 CT scans of Otzi were acquired. Artefacts recovered from the ground where Otzi was discovered and carbon 14 dating indicate that Otzi lived about 5,300 years ago.

The CT scans revealed an arrowhead lodged in Otzi's shoulder, which was probably the cause of death, and evidence of calcification was discovered in the region of the carotid artery and abdominal aorta indicating the presence of arteriosclerosis (hardening of the arteries). His brain, although generally well preserved, was shrunken during the natural freeze-drying mummification process. Subsequently it was discovered that Otzi had in fact been found just inside the Italian border and so was later moved from Austria to the South Tyolean Archaeological Museum in Italy[1].

7. CT scanning of an Egyptian mummy: A case study

A case study of the use of CT scanning a mummy will now be presented including some examples of the x-ray CT images and 3D reconstructions. The study was performed at the end of 1991 and beginning of 1992 by the author of this chapter and associates at St. Thomas' Hospital (STH), London and the Department of Egyptian Antiquities of the British Museum (BM), London (Hughes 2010). It is interesting to note that this appears to be the first time an Egyptian mummy was CT scanned outside North America.

The mummy in question was an Egyptian priestess/temple singer who lived at Karnak (modern day Luxor) during the 22nd dynasty ((c. 945-715 BC). The mummies name is Tjenmutengebtiu but will be contracted to *Jeni* in this chapter. Jeni was selected for scanning by the staff of the BM, as the art/science of embalming is considered to have peaked in 22nd dynasty.

The purpose in performing the scan was to find out more about Jeni than had been discovered from plain x-rays. Some questions were: where were amulets placed on the body, how was the brain removed from the skull? The Egyptians embalmed their dead in order to preserve the body over a long period of time. Jeni was scanned about 2,700 years after she died and open arteries can still be seen in her legs and the remains of her spinal cord, confirming that her embalmers were experts in their field. Jeni was brought over to STH from the BM on five occasions at night when the scanner was not being used for patients. Software developed to produce 3D images of the head from CT scans for planning brain surgery was used to produce 3D images of Jeni. The head and neck were scanned with 2mm slices, the teeth with 1mm slices and the rest of the body with 4 mm slices. In each case a 512 × 512 matrix was used. The 2D CT images, and 3D surface reconstructions, demonstrate many features of the embalming techniques and funerary customs of the 22nd dynasty. Figure 1 shows Jeni on the CT couch and figure 2a shows a CT image of Jeni's head

---

[1] http://www.bolzano.net/english/museum-archaeology.html

showing the presence of artificial glass eyes inserted into Jeni's shrunken sockets after her body was dried in the embalming process.

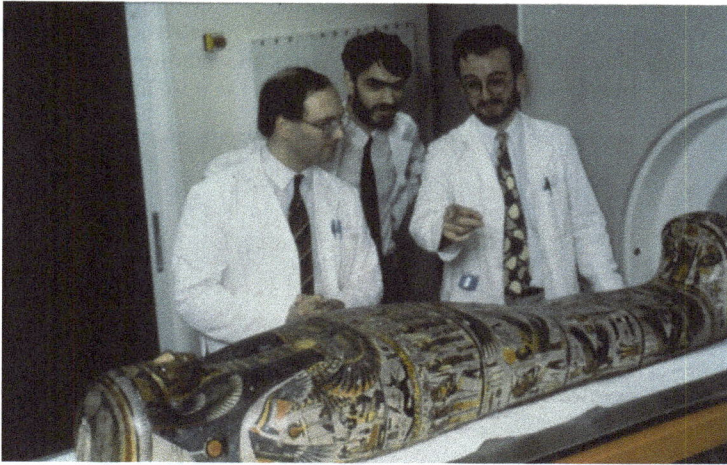

Fig. 1. Jeni on the CT scanning couch in the radiology department of St. Thomas' Hospital, London. (The author is on the left).

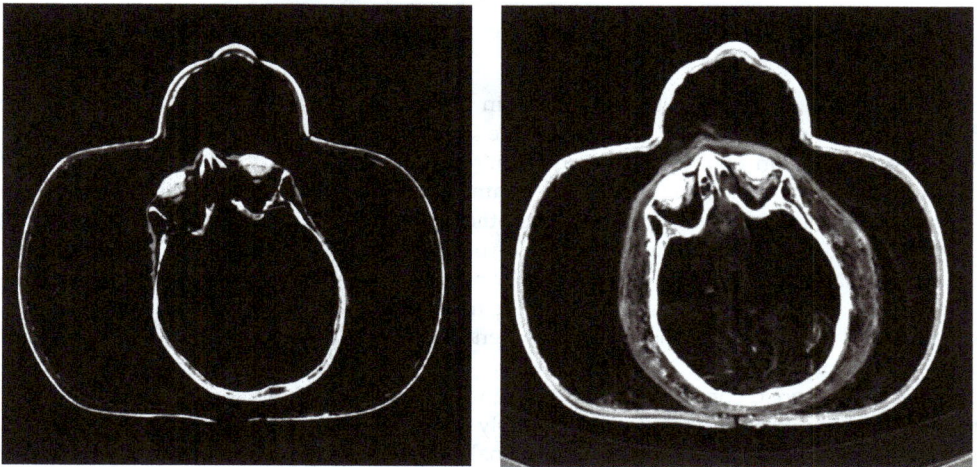

Fig. 2. CT scan through Jeni's head before (a) and after (b) adjustment of the range of the pixel values displayed in the image enabling different features to be seen.

Figure 2b shows the same scan as in figure 2a but with a different range of CT numbers used to display the image. This exemplifies the power of digital CT over CT images stored on film. Digital images can be manipulated in various ways to bring out particular features. For example in the images above it can be seen that the artificial eyes have two components –a denser outer eye, and a less dense inner eye and Jeni's head appears to be empty. Both versions of the image show that the nasal septum and ethmoid bone have been broken.

However, when the image is adjusted (a process known as *windowing*) it is apparent that Jeni's head is not empty but is filled with some kind of low density material, most probably linen that appears to converge on the nasal cavity. A 3D reconstruction of the lower half of the head confirms that linen passes through from the cranium into the nasal cavity indicating that the embalmers inserted the linen through the nose into the cranium.

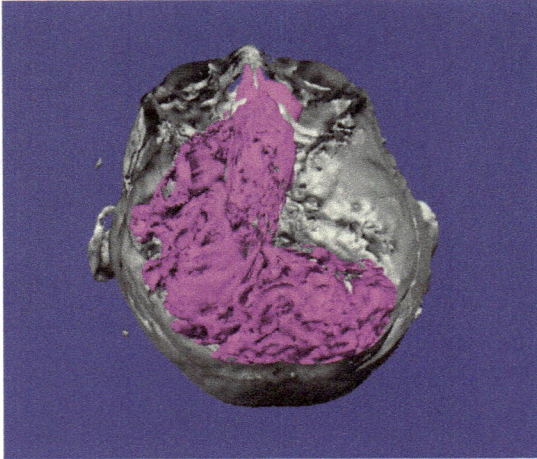

Fig. 3. 3D reconstruction of the lower half of Jeni's head showing the linen (in false colour) converging on the nasal cavity.

Sometimes the embalmers extracted the brain through the foramen magnum which is the hole in the base of the skull through which the spinal cord enters the cranium.

A 3D reconstruction of the linen inside Jeni's head reveals that the brain was extracted through the nose rather than through the foramen magnum. The reconstruction shows cloth protruding from the nasal cavities into the otherwise empty cranial cavity. This would not have happened if the cloth was pushed through the foramen magnum. This is a good example of the advantage of CT over plain x-rays. The remains of the heart can be seen as well as four organ packs corresponding to the mummified and repackaged lungs, intestines, stomach and liver. Each of the organ packs encloses a wax figurine representing of one of the four sons of Horus.

The teeth are in good condition with little signs of wear, which, in view of the gritty diet of the Egyptians, indicates that Jeni was probably between 19 and 23 years old when she died. A young age of death is also suggested by analysis of the shape of the molar teeth. Neither the plain x-rays nor CT scans reveal an obvious cause of death. The plain x-rays reveal that three of Jeni's back ribs on the right side, as well as the right side of the pelvis have been fractured, possibly indicating a fall or some kind of collision with an animal or chariot as the cause of death. An image of 3D skull was used by an artist to draw a picture of what the mummy may have looked like during life (figure 4). Morphological analysis of the skull revealed that Jeni was most likely an Egyptian female (Hughes, 2005). Other researchers have also used CT scans to reconstruct faces (Hill 1993, Manly 2002).

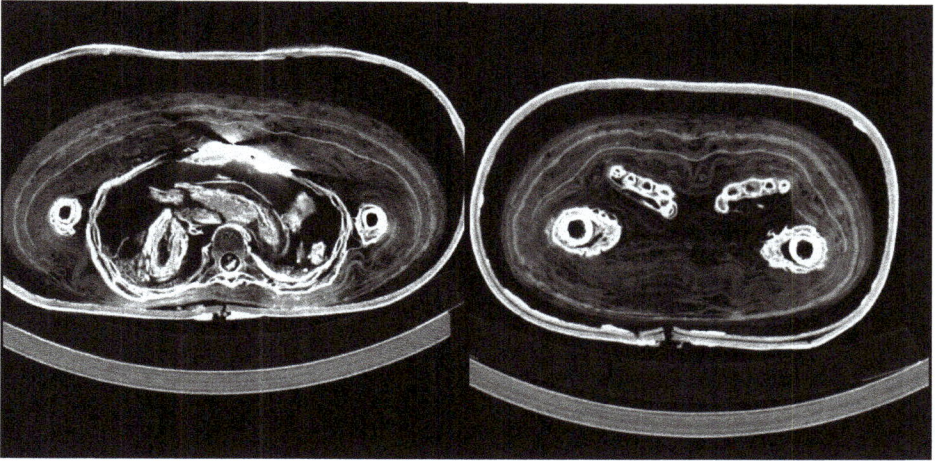

Fig. 3. (a) CT scan through Jeni's abdomen showing the remains on the heart and spinal cord. (b) CT scan through Jeni's legs showing the femoral arteries.

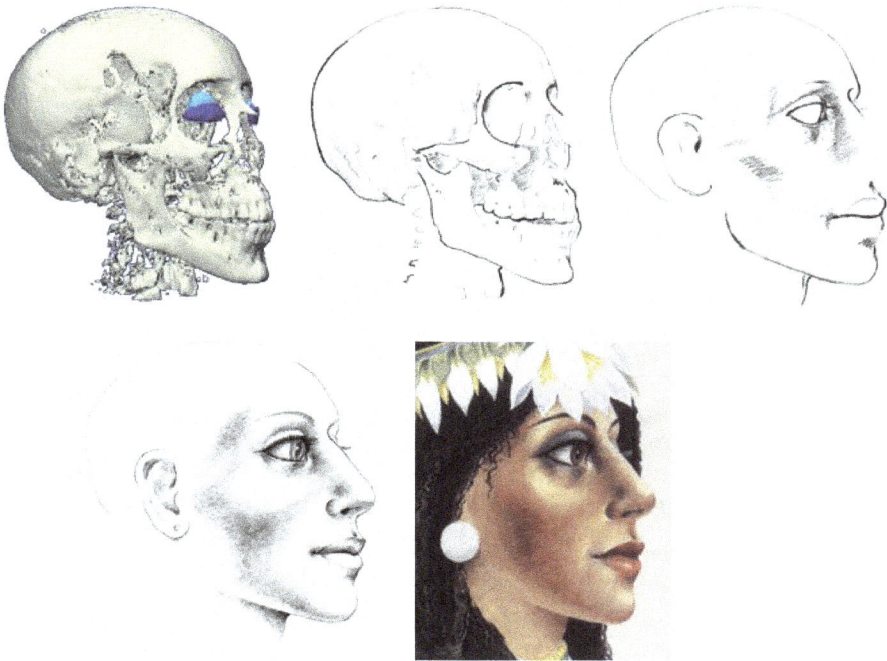

Fig. 4. The steps involved in constructing a picture of what a mummy may have looked like during life, starting from a frontal oblique view of a 3D reconstruction of a skull.

In total about 700 CT scans were taken for this project taking several hours spread over five nights.

8. Non-Egyptian mummies

The majority of CT scan studies have been performed on Egyptian mummies, however CT scans have also been performed on other types of mummies, for example 'environmentally' mummified bodies and bodies buried in peat bogs. The acidic environment of peat bogs increases the density of soft tissue and softens the bones so they become flexible. CT imaging has been used to examine bog bodies (Lynnerup, 2009). Bodies have been discovered in the high Andes in Peru that have been naturally mummified by freeze drying. For example, Appelboom and Struyven (1999) performed a CT scan on an Incan Peruvian mummy dating from the 13th century. The mummy is on display in the Royal Museum of Ancient Art in Brussels and was transported to the University Hospital Erasme for scanning. The researchers found the mummy in a very good state of preservation with no foreign objects hidden within the mummy.

9. Reading the writing in clay tablets and scrolls

An Israeli team have used CT scanning to read the cuneiform writing on clay tablets enclosed in a clay envelopes (Applbaum and Applbaum 2004). A group at the University of Kentucky, USA have developed an algorithm for extracting writing from CT scans of scrolls (Lin 2005). This technique is particularly valuable in situations where unravelling the scroll would cause extensive damage.

10. Bronze artefacts

The physics department of the University of Bologna, Italy developed a cone beam CT system for the study of the numerous bronze artefacts of archaeological and artistic significance in Italy (Rossi 1999). In a cone beam CT system, a cone-shaped x-ray beam encompasses the object and falls on a 2D digital detection system. A major advantage of this technique is that the data can be acquired much faster than in conventional CT scanners in which the object is translated axially as the x-ray source and detectors are rotated about the object. The object being scanned is placed on a turntable and images taken as the object is rotated. A CT reconstruction technique known as back projection is used to produce cross-sectional x-ray images. Since bronze is highly absorbing of x-rays the system is optimised for scanning bronze objects, for example the system has a tube that produces higher energy x-rays than a medical scanner so that the x-rays are more penetrating.
A team at the Laboratory of Palaeopathology[2] at the University of Pisa have used CT to analyse 35 Etruscan cremation urns prior to physical examination. One advantage of performing CT scans on cremation urns is that it is possible to see the outlines of rusted metal artefacts that have long since disintegrated.

11. The future of CT scanning in archaeology

In the nearly 40 years since the introduction of the CT scanner there has been a great improvement in image quality and speed of acquisition brought about by technological

---

[2] The study of disease in ancient populations

advances in scanner design and computer speed. The increase in computer speed has also led to improvements in the quality and speed of generation of 3D x-ray images.

The internet now enables data to be transported around the world in increasing amounts and decreasing cost. This opens up the possibility for researchers and the public to gain access to the large data sets generated by CT scanners. An example of this is the data available associated with the scanning of a mummy in the British Museum. A complete sequence of CT images and 3D reconstructions can be downloaded from http://eprints.qut.edu.au/31522/.

Over the last few years, 3D computer and TV displays have fallen in cost opening up the possibility for 3D reconstructions to be viewed in 3D. An example of this is shown in figure 5 where a researcher is viewing Jeni's skull using stereoscopic spectacles at the University of Queensland in Brisbane.

Access to CT scanners for archaeological research will continue to be a problem. Clinical CT scanners tend to be too expensive for exclusive archaeological use – the initial purchase cost is high and there is the issue of the cost of on-going maintenance and repair. Also mummies have to be transported to a scanner, usually located in a hospital, and it is more difficult to recover costs in archaeology compared to medicine. However, the increase in scanner speed means more scope for out-of-hours use of CT scanners for archaeology.

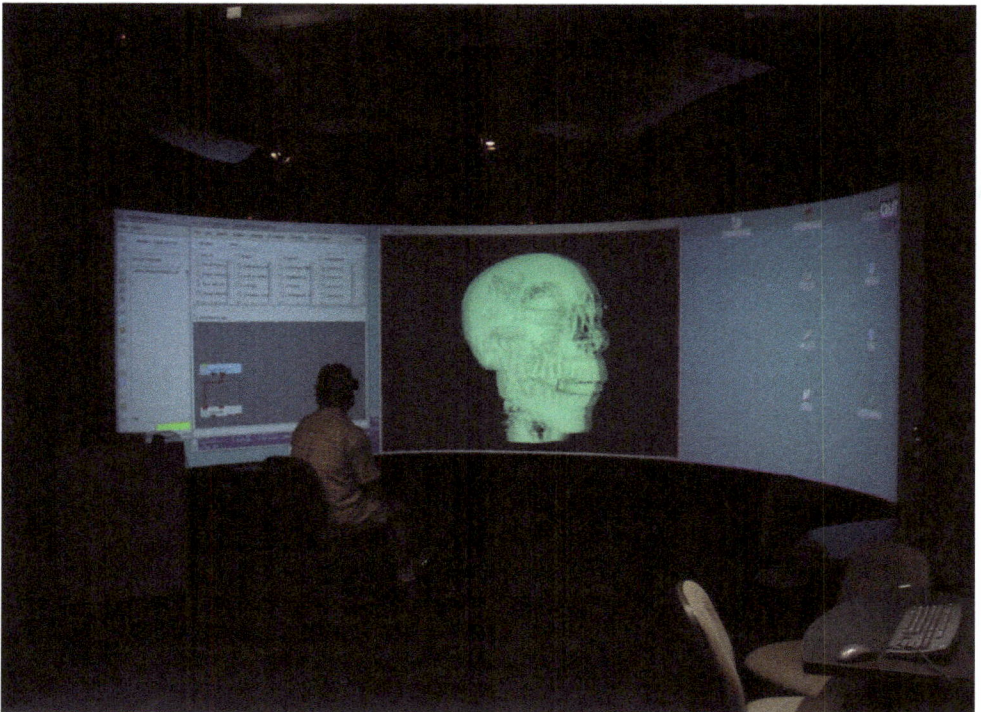

Fig. 5. Mark Barry of the High Performance Computing unit of QUT viewing a 3D rendering of Jeni's skull through stereoscopic glasses at the University of Queensland Silicon Graphics Reality Centre.

A major issue in the world at the moment is security of archaeological artefacts, i.e. the danger of artefacts being lost to theft, fire, earthquake, tsunami or war. An example of this occurred February 2011 when two mummies were destroyed in the Cairo Museum during the anti-government protests[3]. X-ray CT scans combined with photography are the best way of 'saving' archaeological artefacts for posterity.

Such a scheme would be expensive and could run into several tens of millions of dollars but the cost would be a tiny fraction of the amount of money spent on the wars leading to the destruction of artefacts.

One possible scenario would be for money to be obtained to perform scans of the highest quality currently possible on most of the significant archaeological artefacts in the world – mummies, clay tablets, scrolls, pottery, statues etc - and make the data publicly available. Transportable CT scanners now exist – these are scanners that are housed in a truck and can be taken to remote locations to scan patients. One of these could be parked in the grounds of a museum to improve access to artefacts. The data would then be available for researchers to perform 'digital autopsies'. At the same time of scanning, a high resolution digital camera attached to a robot could take photographs of the object from all directions and map the photos onto the 3D surface of the artefact generated from the 3D reconstructions.

The data could be deposited in a Virtual Museum – maybe in a way similar the Virtual Observatory project in astronomy (http://en.wikipedia.org/wiki/Virtual_Observatory). An advantage of this approach is that artefacts preserved in digital form will still be available in cases where the body has decayed.

12. References

Allam, A.H; Thompspon, R.C; Wann, L. S; Miyamoto, M.I; Thomas, G.S 2009 Computed tomographic assessment of atherosclerosis in ancient Egyptian mummies, *Journal of the American Medical Association* 18:2091-2094.

Applbaum, N; and Y. H. Applbaum, Y,H The use of medical computed tomography (ct) imaging in the study of ceramic and clay artifacts from the ancient near east. In *X-rays and Archaeology*. Kluwer, 2004.

Appelboom, T; Struyven, J 1999 Medical imaging of the Peruvian mummy Rascar Capac, *The Lancet* 354:2153-2155.

Beckmann, E. C. 2006 CT scanning the early days. *The British Journal of Radiology*, 79:5-8 doi:10.1259/bjr/29444122

Cesarani, F; Martina, M.C; Farraris, A; Grilletto, R; Boano, R; Marochetti; E.F; Donadoni, A.M; Gandini, G 2003 Whole-body three-dimensional multidetector CT of 13 Egyptian human mummies, *American Journal of Roentgenology* 180:597-606.

Chan, S.S; Elias, J.P; Hysell, M.E; Hallowell, M.J. 2008 CT of a Ptolemaic period mummy from the ancient Egyptian city of Akhmim, *RadioGraphics* 28:2023-2032, doi: 10.1148/rg.287085039

Cockburn, A; Barraco, R, A; Reyman, T, A; Peck, W, H. 1975. *Autopsy of an Egyptian mummy*, Science 187:1155-60.

David, A.R., ed., 1979. *The Mystery of the Mummies, The Manchester Mummy Project*, Manchester.

---

[3] http://www.telegraph.co.uk/news/worldnews/africaandindianocean/egypt/8291526/Egypt-crisis-Looters-destroy-mummies-in-Cairo-museum.html

David, A.R. and Tapp, E., eds., 1992. *The Mummy's Tale*, Michael O'Mara Books Ltd, London.

Dawson, W.R. and Gray, P.H.K., 1968. *Catalogue of Egyptian antiquities in the British Museum: 1 mummies and human remains*, British Museum Press, London.

Harwood-Nash, D.F.C, 1979. Computed tomography of ancient Egyptian mummies, *Journal of Computer Assisted Tomography* 3:768-773.

Hill, B. et al., 1993. Facial reconstruction of a 3500-year-old Egyptian mummy using axial computed tomography *Journal of Audiovisual Media in Medicine* 16:11-3

Hughes, S.W. 2010 Unwrapping an ancient Egyptian mummy using x-rays, *Physics Education* 45:235-242, doi:10.1088/0031-9120/45/3/002

Hughes, S.W; Wright, R; Barry, M 2005 Virtual reconstruction and morphological analysis of the cranium of an ancient Egyptian mummy. *Physics Education* 28:122-127

Lin, Y (2005). "Opaque document imaging: Building images of inaccessible texts". *Computer Vision (ICCV), International Conference on* , 1, p. 662

Lynnerup, N (2009) Medical imaging of mummies and bog bodies – a mini-review, *Gerontology* 56:441-448 doi:10.1159/000266031

Manly, B; Eremin, K; Shortland, A; Wilkinson, C 2002 The facial reconstruction of an ancient Egyptian queen, *Journal of Audiovisual Media in Medicine* 25:155-159 doi: 10.1080/0140511021000051144

Marx, M; D'Auria, S.H 1986 CT examination of eleven Egyptian mummies, *Radiographics* 6:321-330.

Marx, M; D'Auria, S.D. 1988 Three dimensional CT reconstruction of an ancient Egyptian mummy. *American Journal of Radiology* 150:147-149.

Michael, G. 2001 X-ray computed tomography, *Physics Education* 36:442-451, doi: 10.1088/0031-9120/36/6/301 (http://eprints.qut.edu.au/31012).

Murphy, William A., Jr.; zur Nedden, Dieter; Gostner, Paul; Knapp, Rudolf; Recheis, Wolfgang; Seidler, Horst (24 January 2003), "The Iceman: Discovery and imaging", *Radiology* (Oak Brook, Il.: Radiology) 226 (3): 614–629, doi:10.1148/radiol.2263020338, issn = 0033-8419, PMID 12601185. On-line pre-publication version.

Nedden, D; Knapp, R; Wicke, K; Judmaier, W; Murphy, WA, Seidler, H; Platzer, W; Skull of a 5,300 year old mummy: reproduction and investigation with CT guided stereolithography, *Radiology* 193:269-272, 1994.

Notman, 1986 Modern imaging and endoscopic biopsy techniques in Egyptian mummies, *American Journal of Roentgenology* 146:93-96.

Öhrström, L; Bitzer, A; Walther, M; Rühl, F. J. 2009 Technical note: terahertz imaging of ancient mummies and bone, *American Journal of Physical Anthropology* 142:497-500, doi: 10.1002/ajpa.21292

Rossi, M; Casali, F; Chirco, P; Morigi, M.P; Nava, E; Querzola, E; Zanarini, M 1999 X-ray 3D computed tomography of bronze archaeological samples *IEEE Transactions on Nuclear Science* 46:897-903. doi: 10.1109/23.790700

Rühli, F.J; von Waldburg, H; Nielles-Vallespin, S. Böni, T; Speier, P 2007 Clinical magnetic resonance imaging of ancient dry human mummies without rehydration *Journal of the American Medical Association* 298: 2618 – 2620.

Rühli, F.J; Hodler, J; Böni, T 2002 Technical Note: CT-guided biopsy: a new diagnostic method for the paleopathological research. *American Journal of Physical Anthropology* 117:272-275, doi: 10.1002/ajpa.20003

Wagle, W.A. 1976 Toe prosthesis in an Egyptian human mummy, *American Journal of Roentgenology*, 164:999.

4

Adrenal Imaging Methods: Comparison of Mean CT Attenuation, CT Histogram Analysis and Chemical Shift Magnetic Resonance Imaging for Adrenal Mass Characterization and Review of the Literature

Ahmet Mesrur Halefoglu

Sisli Etfal Training and Research Hospital Radiology Department, Sisli, Istanbul
Turkey

1. Introduction

Adrenal masses are commonly incidentally discovered on abdominal computed tomography (CT), occuring in up to 5 % of patients (1). Most of these adrenal masses turn out to be adenomas. In a patient with a known history of primary extra-adrenal neoplasm especially lung carcinoma, diagnosis or exclusion of an adrenal metastasis is mandatory. Because it requires appropriate therapy of the primary tumor in metastasis cases and imaging follow-up is a suitable strategy for adenomas. The presence of intracellular lipid in adenomas has been proven to be useful for distinguishing these lesions from nonadenomas.

In the routine work-flow, a 10 Hounsfield unit (HU) attenuation value is used as a threshold for the diagnosis adrenal adenomas on unenhanced CT examinations (2). Although it is regarded as a very useful method in many adenoma cases, it in fact has limited value because approximately 29 % of these adenomas have an attenuation value of more than 10 HU due to their poor lipid content and therefore can be classified as indeterminate masses (3).

The delayed contrast-enhanced CT attenuation or washout CT method has been shown to be very sensitive for adrenal mass characterization. It makes the distinction between adenoma and metastases on the basis of physiological temporal differences in the enhancement and exit iodinated contrast from the adrenal lesion. Adrenal adenomas show a percentage enhancement washout of at least 60 % or greater or a relative percentage washout of 50 % on delayed contrast-enhanced CT (4). Although it is regarded as a very sensitive diagnostic method, also holds some disadvantages. In a busy clinical practice, monitoring every CT scan performed is not feasible. Hence a separate patient visit may be needed after an indeterminate finding on an unenhanced CT scan. The patients are also subjected to multiphasic scanning and injection of intravenous contrast material. There has also been a recently heightened concern about radiation relating to use of CT with adrenal washout CT, including 3 passes through the upper abdomen. Even though complications are infrequent, risks related to IV contrast material remain. Certainly, one can agree that a test avoiding both radiation and intravenous contrast would have better patient acceptance. An additional work-flow related issue is the need to obtain a delayed scan at 15 minutes following contrast material administration.

The other method for diagnosis of an adenoma is percutaneous biopsy. But due to its invasive nature and inherent risk, it should be considered as a last procedure when all other noninvasive methods were inconclusive.

Mean CT attenuation method which is widely used in clinical practice results in averaging of tissue density over the CT pixels. Tissue heterogeneity therefore may result in inadequate information being obtained about densities that present a smaller volume from a region of interest (ROI) where the mean CT attenuation is measured.

Recently the use of CT histogram analysis to evaluate adrenal masses has been proposed by Bae et al (5). CT histogram analysis provides objective insight into the varying CT densities and the number of pixels with these densities and therefore is more likely to be sensitive for lipid detection, represented as pixels with negative attenuation, particularly in lipid poor adenomas, which are likely to have a mean CT attenuation of more than 10 HU. This technique has the advantage of involving no additional tests, radiation or repeat trips to the hospital by the patient if an adenoma is confirmed. Obviously, if the CT histogram analysis is indeterminate, other imaging tests such as adrenal washout CT will be necessary and will require an additional patient visit.

Magnetic resonance imaging (MRI) using in-phase and opposed-phase images, known as chemical-shift MRI, has been proposed as an effective alternative to CT for characterization of adrenal masses. (6, 7). Quantitative analysis of the signal intensity of adrenal lesions compared with that of the liver, fat, muscle and image background was subsequently shown to improve characterization of adrenal masses compared with qualitative analysis of signal intensity variations. (6, 7 ,8).

The purpose of this chapter is to discuss mean attenuation method using 10 HU threshold value on unenhanced CT, CT histogram analysis method both on unenhanced and contrast enhanced CT and chemical shift MRI method using quantitative analysis with adrenal to spleen chemical shift ratio and adrenal signal intensity index formulas based on our recently published prospective research studies. We also reviewed the literature in terms of comparing our results in order to lightening this topic.

2. Materials and methods

Both of these studies were approved by our hospital's institutional research ethics board and informed consents were obtained from all patients. These studies were performed between March 2007 and November 2008. During this period, patients who exhibited adrenal masses on either CT or MRI examinations were routinely detected in the daily work-flow and then evaluated as to whether or not they were appropriate for our studies. The inclusion criterion was mass size, where a 1- cm cut-off value was used in order to eliminate possible partial volume effects. Adrenal cysts, adrenal masses that contain large amount of macroscopic fat visible to the naked eye with a high probability of myelolipomas were also excluded from the study. Adrenal masses that contained large necrotic, calcified, cystic and hemorrhagic areas were also not included.

Patients with adrenal masses showing consistency with the inclusion criterion were prospectively evaluated with the mean attenuation method using 10 HU threshold value on unenhanced CT images and CT histogram analysis method on unenhanced and contrast enhanced CT images in the first study. CT histogram analysis method on unenhanced CT images and chemical-shift MRI using in-phase and opposed-phase gradient-echo images were compared in the second study. All of the patients who had adrenal masses were evaluated by at least two experienced abdominal radiologists.

In the first study, 94 patients (46 males, 48 females, age range : 30-79 years) with 113 adrenal masses were included. These adrenal masses ranged from 1.07 to 8.02 cm in a diameter with a mean average of 3.03 ± 1.91 cm. These masses consisted of 66 adenomas, 45 metastases and 2 pheochromocytomas. Nine patients had bilateral adenomas and 10 patients had bilateral metastases.

In the second study, 93 patients (45 males, 48 females, mean age : 56.7 ± 11.4 years , age range 22-85 years) with 109 adrenal masses were included. The mass size ranged from 1.52 cm to 13.22 cm in a diameter with a mean of 3.02 ± 1.83 cm. These masses were 67 adenomas, 42 metastases. Nine patients had bilateral adenomas and 7 patients had bilateral metastases.

In both studies, final diagnoses of these adrenal masses were based on available clinical, imaging and pathological data. The first reference standard for the diagnosis of an adenoma was established on the basis of stable mass size for at least 6 months during imaging follow-up. If the mass conformed with this criterion, we regarded it as benign. In our first study, 34 of 66 adenomas and in the second study 39 of 67 adenomas had previous imaging studies and showed no interval change during this time period, and therefore were regarded as benign masses. In the first study two patients and in the second study only one patient were subjected to a biopsy procedure which revealed lipid- poor adenomas. In the remaining 30 patients of the first group and 27 patients of the second group who did not have a previous imaging study, an adrenal washout study was performed in order to have a reference standard for the adenoma diagnosis. This required at least a 60 % absolute percentage enhancement washout on delayed contrast enhanced images. Absolute enhancement washout AEW) was calculated as follows :

$$AEW = \frac{\text{Enhanced attenuation value - Unenhanced attenuation value}}{\text{Enhanced attenuation value - Delayed enhanced value}}$$

In the 45 and 42 metastases in our research studies respectively, the following reference standards were used : pathological data obtained either by biopsy or during operation, rapid growth of a mass or identification of a new mass in less than 6 months in a patient with a known primary malignant tumor, or regression in the size of the mass subsequent chemotherapy. In the 45 metastases ; the diagnoses were based on biopsy in 5 patients, operation results in 2 patients, reduction of mass size following chemotherapy in 2 patients, increase of mass size during follow up in 31 patients and identification of a new mass in 5 patients. In the second group consisting of 42 metastases, the reference standards were biopsy in 5 patients, reduction of mass size following chemotherapy in 2 patients, increase of mass size during follow up in 32 patients and identification of a new mass in 3 patients.

In the first group the primary malignant tumors were lung carcinoma in 26 patients, cervix carcinoma in 1 patient, testis carcinoma in 4 patients, gastric carcinoma in 2 patients, colon carcinoma in 3 patients, breast carcinoma in 1 patient, Hodkgin lymphoma in 1 patient, neuroendocrine tumor in 1 patient, larynx carcinoma in 1 patient, renal cell carcinoma in 1 patient, bladder carcinoma in 1 patient, and malignant melanoma in 3 patients. In the second group, lung carcinoma in 23 patients, unknown primary tumor in 4 patients, malignant melanoma in 2 patients, gastric carcinoma in 2 patients, colon carcinoma in 2 patients, testicular carcinoma in 2 patients, breast carcinoma in 1 patient, Hodkgin lymphoma in 1 patient, neuroendocrine tumor in 1 patient, larynx carcinoma in 1 patient, renal cell carcinoma in 1 patient, cervix carcinoma in 1 patient and metastatic sarcoma in 1 patient.

In the two pheochromocytoma cases included in the first study, the reference standards were the clinical, laboratory and MRI findings. These patients had hypertension attacks, showed elevated urine normetanephrine and vanillymandelic ascites levels and exhibited characteristic MRI findings for these tumors.

3. CT technique

All CT examinations were performed either by using a dual-detector row helical CT scanner (Somatom Emotion Duo / Emotion 6, Siemens Medical Systems, Erlangen, Germany) or a multi-detector row helical CT scanner (Somatom Sensation 16, Siemens Medical Systems, Erlangen, Germany). We performed both unenhanced and contrast-enhanced CT examinations for all of the patients with the following imaging parameters : 10 mm collimation and 5 mm reconstructed section thickness for dual-detector row CT scanner and 5 mm collimation and 5 mm section thickness for multi-detector row CT scanner, no overlap reconstruction and 130 kVp for each scanner, 1 : 1 pitch for both dual-detector row scanner and multi-detector row scanner, 180 mA for dual-detector row scanner and 135-160 mA for multi-detector row scanner. The images were reconstructed with a standard soft-tissue-kernel algorithm. Contrast-enhanced CT images were obtained following 150 mL of contrast material (Ultravist 370, Schering, Germany) administration by using a power injector at a rate of 2-4 mL / sec. Adrenal washout CT protocol included unenhanced CT and following the two-phase contrast-enhanced CT in which images were obtained at 60 seconds (early contrast-enhanced) and 15 minutes (delayed contrast-enhanced) following bolus contrast material injection.

4. CT histogram analysis

CT histogram measurements were performed on a postprocessing Workstation (Magic View 1000, Siemens Medical Solutions). A commercially avaliable software (CT Perfusion, Siemens Medical Systems) was used to obtain the histograms. For each adrenal mass, the image showing the maximal cross-sectional area was chosen. The long-axis and short-axis diameters of the mass were measured on that image. A circular ROI was placed on the adrenal mass to include as much as the mass possible but avoiding the outermost portion of edges to prevent partial volume effects. If possible, approximately two thirds of the mass was measured.The mean attenuation over the ROI was recorded. A CT histogram was obtained from the ROI using software application on the workstation. A graph of the number of pixels on the y-axis versus the pixel attenuation on the x-axis was obtained from the ROI (Figure 1). Histogram analysis included recording the total number of pixels, number of negative pixels (pixels with attenuation less than 0 HU), and the resultant percentage of negative pixels in each ROI.

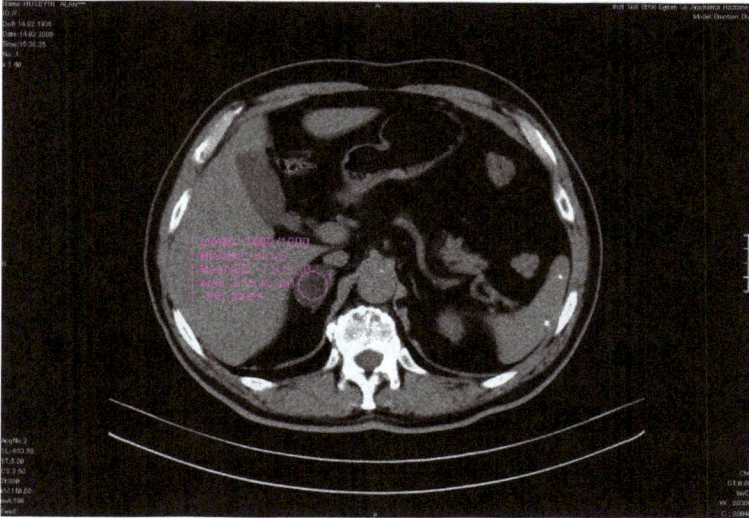

(a)

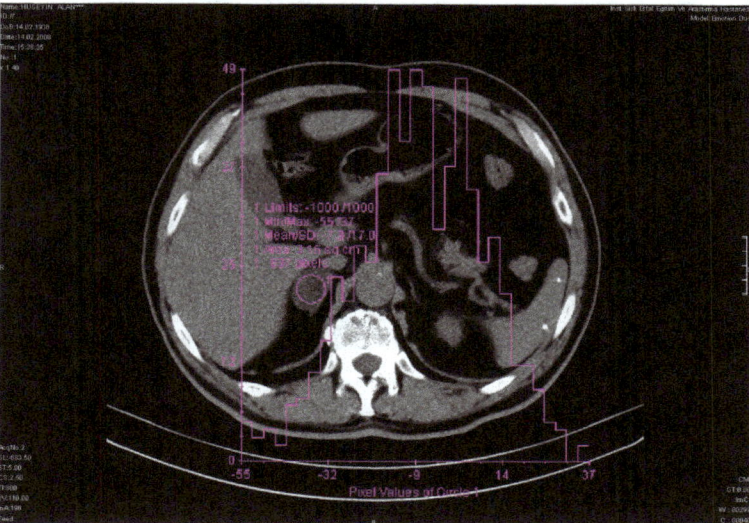

(b)

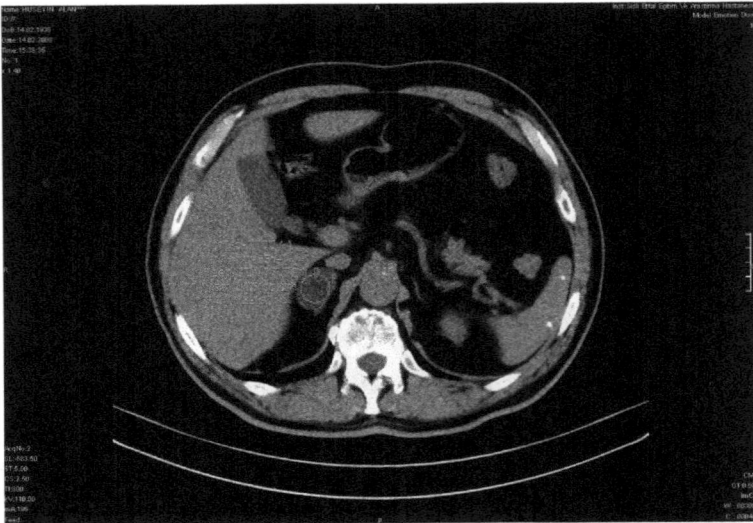

(c)

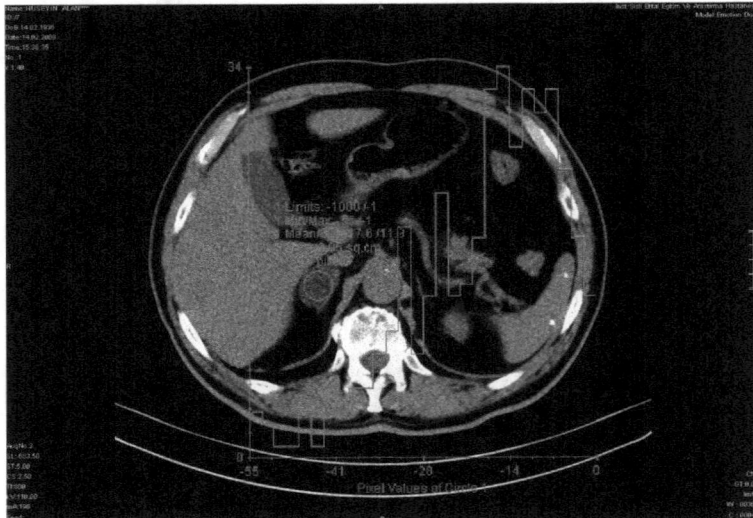

(d)

(a) Unenhanced CT scan using ROI demonstrates 637 pixels with a mean attenuation of – 7.9 HU. The upper and lower limits of pixel attenuation are + 1000 and - 1000, respectively.

(b) Corresponding histogram analysis shows pixel attenuation ranging from - 55 to 37 HU.

(c) Unenhanced CT scan using ROI shows that the mass containing 414 negative pixels. The upper and lower limits of pixel attenuation are – 1 and - 1000, respectively.

(d) Corresponding histogram analysis reveals that 65 % of the mass contains negative pixels.

Fig. 1. 72 year-old man with a right adrenal adenoma

5. Data analysis

The percentage of negative pixels were calculated from the total number of pixels and the number of negative pixels in each ROI. The percentage of adrenal masses showing a mean attenuation value of 10 HU or less were calculated for unenhanced and contrast-enhanced CT images of adenomas, metastases and pheochromocytomas. Also percentage of adrenal masses that show a mean attenuation value of more than 10 HU were calculated for unenhanced and enhanced CT images of all adrenal masses. We also investigated the percentage of each type of adrenal mass in terms of containing any negative pixel and at the threshold values of 5 % and 10 % negative pixel on both unenhanced and contrast-enhanced CT images. All the reviews and calculations were performed by at least two experienced abdominal radiologists and final results were achieved by a consensus for each evaluation.

6. MR technique

MR examination was performed by means of a 1.5 tesla superconducting magnet (Signa, GE Medical Systems, Milwaukee, Wisconsin, USA). In all cases, a torso multi-channel phased-array coil was used. All patients underwent axial breath-hold dual-echo T 1- weighted 2D spoiled gradient-echo in- and opposed-phase imaging using the following parameters ; TR : 175 msec., TE : 4.4 (in-phase) / 2.2 (opposed-phase) msec., 80° flip angle, 256 x 160 matrix, 48 cm field of view, 0.60 phase FOV, 0.75 Nex, 6 mm slice thickness, 1.5 mm interslice gap, and 62.5 kHz bandwidth.

7. MR evaluation

Two experienced abdominal radiologists performed the quantitative MR measurements by reaching a consensus. An ellipsoid ROI was placed on the center of the adrenal mass and spleen on both in-phase and opposed-phase MR images to obtain signal intensity values. ROIs were placed on each adrenal mass covering as much as the mass possible while avoiding to contain the outermost portions in order to eliminate chemical shift artifact. We calculated the adrenal-to-spleen chemical shift ratio and adrenal signal intensity index for each adrenal mass. The adrenal-to-spleen chemical shift ratio was calculated as the adrenal mass-to-spleen signal intensity ratio on the opposed-phase images divided by the adrenal mass-to-spleen signal intensity ratio on the in-phase images. The signal intensity index was calculated as the adrenal mass signal intensity on the in-phase images minus the adrenal mass signal intensity on the opposed-phase images divided by the adrenal mass signal intensity on the in-phase images multiplied by 100.

8. Results for first research

Adrenal adenomas at unenhanced CT

The mean attenuation of 66 adenomas at unenhanced CT ranged from – 83.1 to 48.8 HU (mean : 0.5 HU ± 18.1). Of the 66 adenomas, 51 (77.3 %) had a mean attenuation value of ≤ 10 HU and 15 (22.7 %) showed a mean attenuation value of more than 10 HU. All of these adenomas contained negative pixels on unenhanced CT. Overall, the percentage of negative pixels for adenomas on unenhanced CT ranged from 0-96 %, with a mean value of 50.4 ±

30.2. The number of adenomas when we used a negative pixel percentage threshold of 10 % was 60 (90.9 %) (Figure 1).There was no adenoma containing negative pixel between % 5 and 10 %. We found only 6 adenomas containing less than 5 % negative pixel among which two cases were diagnosed as lipid poor adenomas following biopsy, two cases showed no interval change in size during follow-up and the remaining two cases demonstrated more than 60 % absolute percentage enhancement washout. An increase in the percentage of negative pixels was correlated with a decrease in mean attenuation (p < 0.001). We obtained a 90.9 % sensitivity for 10 % negative pixel percentage threshold compared to 77.2 % sensitivity for ≤ 10 HU mean attenuation threshold value for unenhanced CT. Both methods resulted in a 100 % specificity for the diagnosis of adenoma (Figure 2).

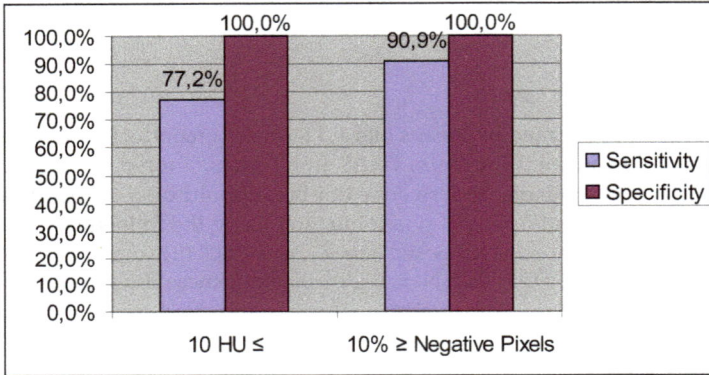

Fig. 2. Bar chart comparing sensitivity values of CT histogram analysis method to mean attenuation method at a threshold of 10 % negative pixel on unenhanced CT.

Adrenal adenomas at contrast-enhanced CT

The mean attenuation of 66 adenomas at contrast-enhanced CT ranged from 0.5 to 97.3 HU (mean : 32.5 HU ± 19.8). Of the 66 adenomas at contrast-enhanced CT, 58 (87.9 %) showed a mean attenuation value of more than 10 HU and only 8 (12.1 %) had a mean attenuation value of ≤ 10 HU. The lowest percentage of negative pixels regarding these adenomas with a mean attenuation value of ≤ 10 HU, was 25 % (mean attenuation of this mass was 8.7 HU). 45 in 66 adenomas (68.2 %) which demonstrated negative pixels at contrast-enhanced CT (Figure 3). All of the 8 adenomas with a mean attenuation value of ≤ 10 HU contained negative pixels and the percentage range of negative pixels was between 25-47 % (mean : 34.4 ± 6.6 HU). 37 of the 58 adenomas (63.8 %) with a mean attenuation value of more than 10 HU had negative pixels and the percentage range of negative pixels was between 1-35 % (mean : 8.0 ± 9.2 HU). The overall percentage range of negative pixels for adenomas at contrast-enhanced CT was 0-47 % with a mean value of 12.7 ± 13.4. The highest mean attenuation value of an adenoma containing negative pixels (0.14 %) was found to be as 62.2 HU at contrast-enhanced CT. only found 6 adenomas (9.1 %)containing between 5-10 % negative pixel on contrast-enhanced CT. 20 adenomas (30.3 %) had negative pixels less than 5 %. But when we used a more than 10 % negative pixel threshold 19 adenomas (28.8 %) were detected. Increase in the percentage of negative pixels was again correlated well with a decrease in mean attenuation (p < 0.001). We obtained a 37.9 % sensitivity for 5

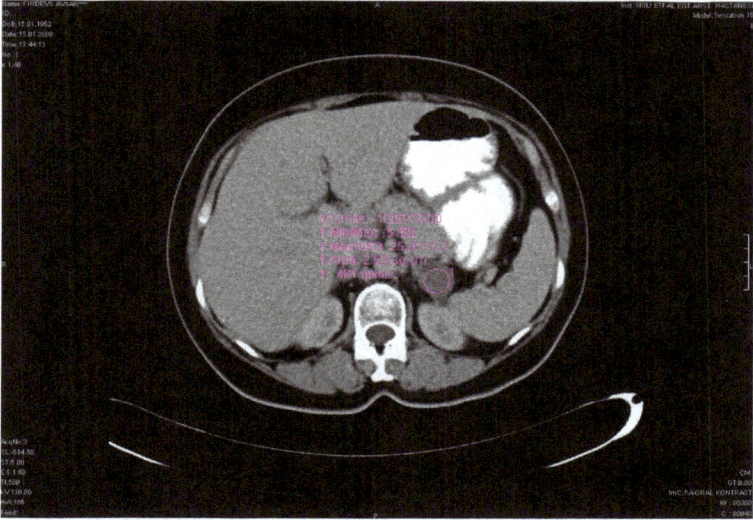

(a)

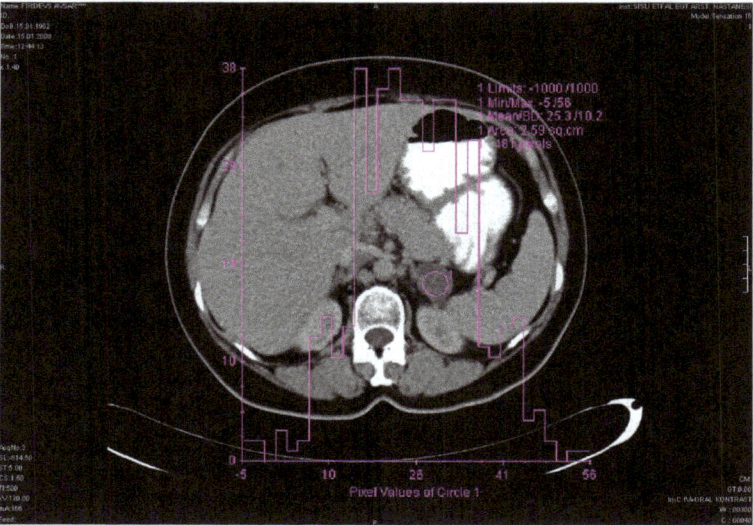

(b)

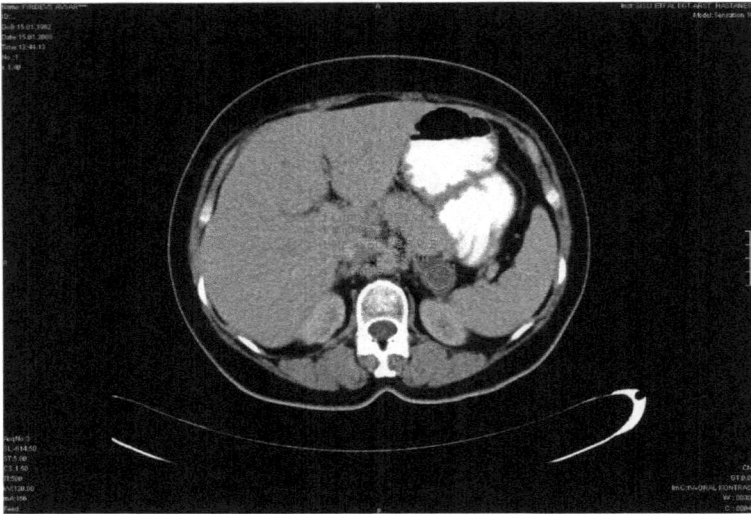

(c)

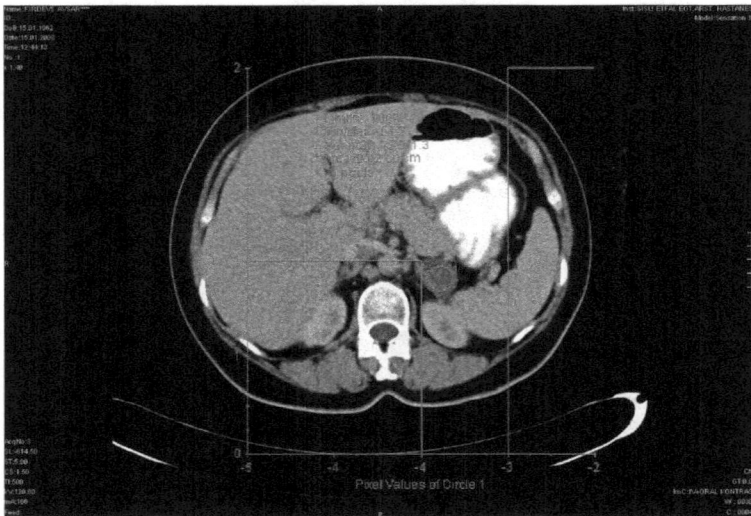

(d)

(a) Contrast- enhanced CT scan using ROI demonstrates 481 pixels with a mean attenuation of 25.3 HU. The upper and lower limits of pixel attenuation are + 1000 and - 1000, respectively.

(b) Corresponding histogram analysis shows pixel attenuation ranging from - 5 to 56 HU.

(c) Contrast- enhanced CT scan using ROI shows that the mass containing 4 negative pixels. The upper and lower limits of pixel attenuation are – 1 and - 1000, respectively.

(d) Corresponding histogram analysis reveals approximately 1 % of the mass contains negative pixels on contrast- enhanced CT.

Fig. 3. 46 year-old woman with a left adrenal adenoma.

Adrenal Imaging Methods: Comparison of Mean CT Attenuation, CT Histogram Analysis and Chemical
Shift Magnetic Resonance Imaging for Adrenal Mass Characterization and Review of the Literature

61

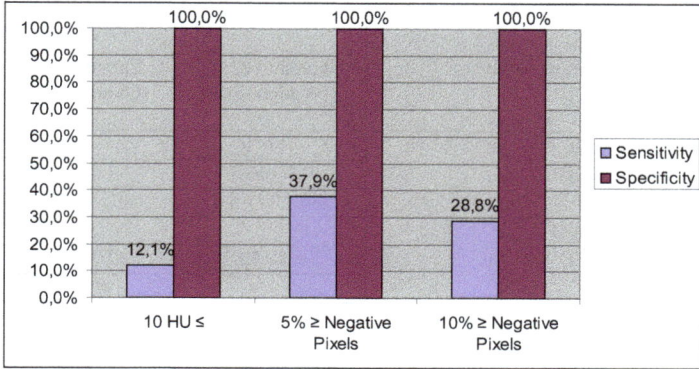

Fig. 4. Bar chart comparing sensitivity values of CT histogram analysis method to mean attenuation method at thresholds of 5 % and 10 % negative pixels on contrast- enhanced CT.

% negative pixel threshold and 28.8 % sensitivity for 10 % negative pixel threshold compared to 12.1 % sensitivity for ≤ 10 HU mean attenuation threshold value for contrast-enhanced CT. Both methods yielded a 100 % specificity for the diagnosis of adenoma (Figure 4). If we use a mean attenuation threshold value of ≤ 30 HU, our sensitivity increases to 51.5 % while 100 % specificity is being maintained. But with a more increase of mean attenuation threshold value of ≤ 40 HU, although a 75.7 % sensitivity is achieved, our specificity decreases to 90 %.

Adrenal adenomas at unenhanced and contrast-enhanced CT

All of the 66 adrenal adenomas demonsrated an increase in mean attenuation values (mean increase : 26.6 ± 20.3) and a decrease in the percentage of negative pixels (mean decrease : 24.5 ± 22.4) following contrast media administration. Although 51 of 66 (77.3 %) adenomas had a mean attenuation of ≤ 10 HU on unenhanced CT images, only 8 of the adenomas (12.1 %) demonstrated a mean attenuation value of ≤ 10 HU on contrast-enhanced images. While all 66 of the adenomas (100 %) had negative pixels on unenhanced CT images, only 45 adenomas (68.2 %) persisted to show negative pixels on contrast-enhanced CT images (Table 1).

Adrenal metastases at unenhanced CT

The mean attenuation of 45 metastases on unenhanced CT ranged from 23.2 to 44.5 HU mean : 33.8 HU ± 5.3). None of the adrenal metastases had a mean attenuation value of ≤ 10 HU on unenhanced CT images (Figure 5). Of the 45 metastases 21 (46.6 %) contained negative pixels. The mean percentage of negative pixels was found to be 0-3 % on unenhanced CT images (Table 2).

Adrenal metastases at contrast-enhanced CT

The mean attenuation of 45 metastases on contrast-enhanced CT ranged from 31.5 to 83.2 HU (mean : 53.3 HU ± 12.9). None of the adrenal metastases had a mean attenuation value of ≤ 10 HU on contrast-enhanced CT images (Figure 5). Of the 45 metastases only 7 (15.5 %) contained negative pixels. The percentage of negative pixels was 0-1 % for these metastases (Table 2).

Histogram Analysis	Adrenal Adenomas	
	Unenhanced CT (66 adenomas)	Enhanced CT (66 adenomas)
Atenuation (HU)		
Average ± SD	0,5 ±18,1	32,5 ±19,8
Range	-83,1 to 48,8	0,5 to 97,3
Negative Pixels %		
Average ± SD	50,4 ±30,2	12,7 ±13,4
Range	0 - 96	0 - 47
Number of Cases with Negative Pixels	66 (100%)	45 (68,1%)
Negative Pixels more than 5%	60 (90,9%)	25 (37,8%)
Negative Pixels more than 10%	60 (90,9%)	19 (28,7%)
Average Atenuation ≤ 10 HU	51 (77,2%)	8 (12,1%)
Negative Pixels more than 5%	51	8
Negative Pixels more than 10%	51	8
Average Atenuation 10-20 HU	7 (10,6%)	10(15,1%)
Negative Pixels more than 5%	7	8
Negative Pixels more than 10%	7	8
Average Atenuation ≥ 20 HU	8 (12,1%)	48 (72,7%)
Negative Pixels more than 5%	2	9
Negative Pixels more than 10%	2	4

Table 1. Histogram analysis results for adrenal adenomas with unenhanced and enhanced CT.

Histogram Analysis	Adrenal Metastases	
	Unenhanced CT (45 metastases)	Enhanced CT (45 metastases)
Atenuation (HU)		
Average ± SD	33,8 ±5,3	53,3 ±12,9
Range	23,2 - 44,5	31,5 - 83,2
Negative Pixel %		
Average ± SD	0,4 ±0,8	0
Range	0 - 3	0
Number of Cases with Negative Pixels	21(46,6%)	7 (15,5%)
Negative Pixels more than 5%	0	0
Negative Pixels more than 10%	0	0
Average Atenuation ≤ 10 HU	0	0
Number of Cases with Negative Pixels	0	0

Table 2. Histogram analysis results for metastases with unenhanced and enhanced CT.

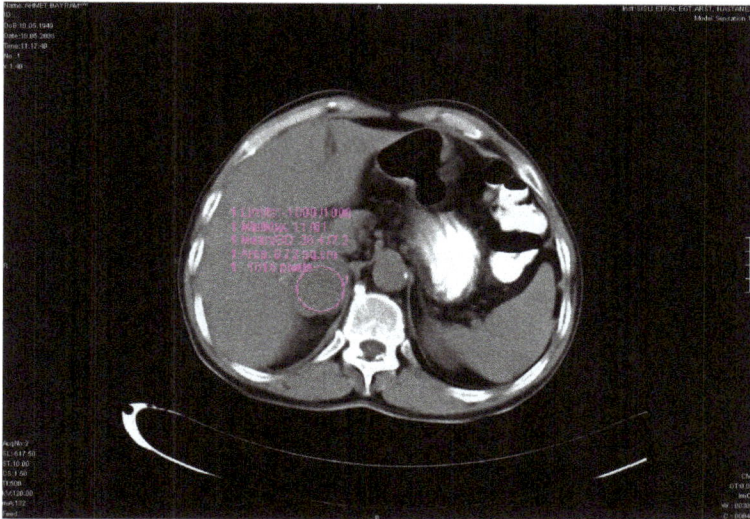

(a)

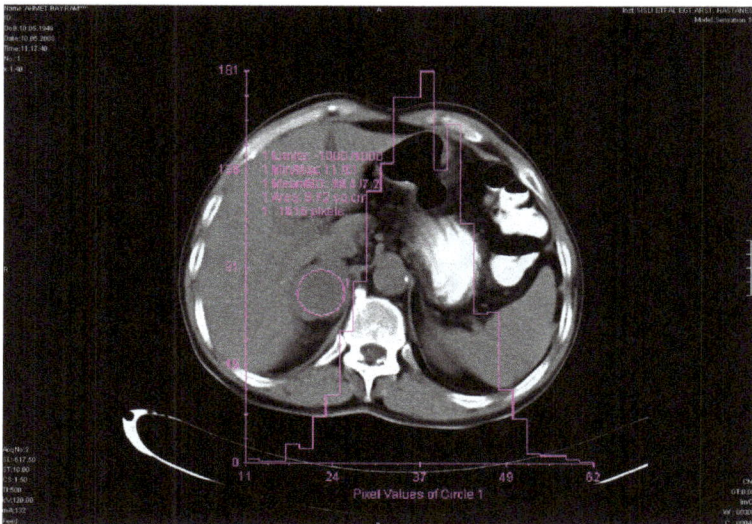

(b)

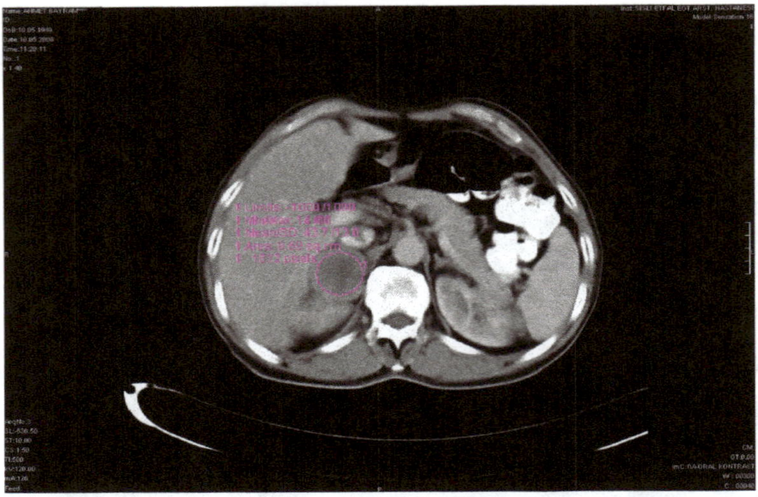

(c)

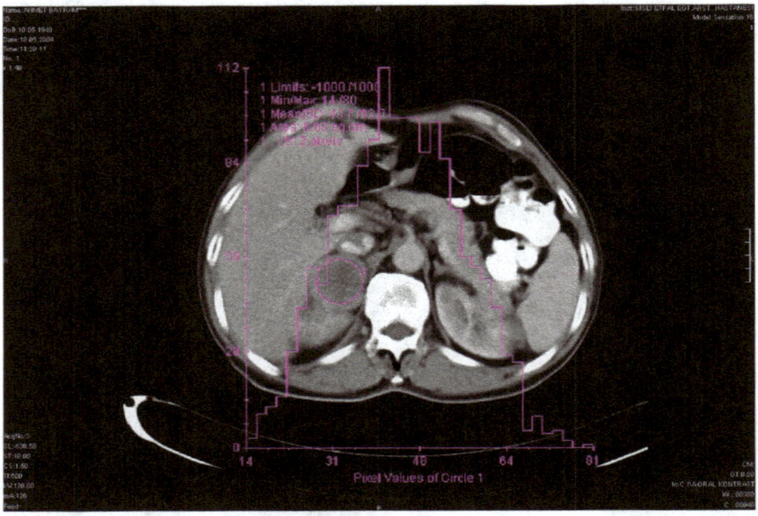

(d)

(a) Unenhanced CT scan using ROI demonstrates 1616 pixels with a mean attenuation of 36.4 HU. The upper and lower limits of pixel attenuation are + 1000 and - 1000, respectively.

(b) Corresponding histogram analysis shows pixel attenuation ranging from 11 to 61 HU without any negative pixels.

(c) Contrast- enhanced CT scan using ROI demonstrates 1612 pixels with a mean attenuation increases to 43.7 HU. The upper and lower limits of pixel attenuation are + 1000 and - 1000, respectively.

(d) Corresponding histogram analysis shows pixel attenuation range increases to 14 – 80 HU.

Fig. 5. 59 year-old man with a right adrenal metastasis who had a history of primary lung carcinoma.

Pheochromocytomas at unenhanced CT

The mean attenuation of 2 pheochromocytomas on unenhanced CT ranged from 38.1 to 39.3 HU (mean : 38.7 HU ± 0.6). None of the pheochromocytomas had a mean attenuation value of ≤ 10 HU on unenhanced CT images. Both of these pheochromocytomas had negative pixels.

Pheochromocytomas at contrast-enhanced CT

The mean attenuation of 2 pheochromocytomas on contrast-enhanced CT ranged from 38.6 to 55.9 HU (mean : 47.3 HU ± 8.7). None of the pheochromocytomas had a mean attenuation value of ≤ 10 HU on contrast-enhanced CT images. Both of these pheochromocytomas persisted to contain negative pixels on contrast-enhanced CT images (Figure 6).

Thus a mean attenuation threshold value of ≤ 10 HU and 5 % and 10 % negative pixel threshold values obtained with CT histogram analysis method yielded a 100 % specificity for the diagnosis of adrenal adenoma on both unenhanced and contrast-enhanced CT images. Our sensitivity values of unenhanced CT were found to be 77.2 % for ≤ 10 HU mean attenuation threshold value and 90.9 % for 10 % negative pixel threshold value. But at contrast-enhanced CT, our sensitivities decreased to 12.1 % for ≤ 10 HU mean attenuation value with 37.9 % for 5 % negative pixel and 28.8 % for 10 % negative pixel threshold values, respectively.

9. Results for second research

The mean CT attenuation of 67 adenomas at unenhanced CT ranged from – 83.1 to 40.8 HU (mean : - 0.2 HU ± 17.5). Of the 67 adenomas, 53 (79.1 %) had a mean attenuation value of ≤ 10 HU and 14 (20.9 %) showed a mean attenuation value of more than 10 HU. The mean attenuation of 42 metastases on unenhanced CT ranged from 20.7 to 44.5 HU (mean : 34.3 HU ± 5.1). None of the adrenal metastases had a mean attenuation value of ≤ 10 HU on unenhanced CT images. All of the adenomas contained negative pixels on unenhanced CT. Overall, the percentage of negative pixels for adenomas on unenhanced CT ranged from 0-96 %, with a mean value of 51.2 ± 29.9. Of the 42 metastases, 21(50 %) contained negative pixels on unenhanced CT. The percentage of negative pixels for metastases was found to be between 0-3 %, with a mean value of 0.5 ± 0.8 on unenhanced CT images (Table 3). When we used a more than 10 % negative pixel threshold, 61 out of 67 adenomas could be detected (Figure 7). However, none of the metastases demonstrated negative pixels reaching out to that level (Figure 8). 6 out of 67 adenomas demonstrated less than % 10 negative pixel with CT histogram analysis method resulting in indeterminate masses. Therefore CT histogram analysis method using a 10 % negative pixel threshold on unenhanced CT yielded a 91 % sensitivity and a 100 % specificity for the diagnosis of adenoma (Figure 9).

An increase in the percentage of negative pixels was correlated well with a decrease in mean attenuation (p < 0.001).

65 out of 67 adenomas demonstrated an adrenal-to-spleen chemical shift ratio of less than 0.71 and a signal intensity index of greater than 16.5 % (Figure 10). However, two adenomas in this group showed an adrenal-to-spleen chemical shift ratio of more than 0.71 and also had a signal intensity index of less than 16.5 %. Both of these adenomas were also classified in the indeterminate group containing less than 10 % negative pixel with CT histogram analysis method. One of these adenomas was diagnosed with imaging follow-up which

revealed no interval change in size during more than two years and the other one was subjected to a biopsy procedure and diagnosed as lipid-poor adenoma. On the other hand, although two adenomas could not be determined with both CT histogram analysis and chemical shift MRI methods, the 4 adenomas which were classified as indeterminate by CT histogram analysis method, MRI was able to characterize these masses. These 4 adenomas, in spite of containing less than 10 % negative pixel with CT histogram analysis method, exhibited a less than 0.71 chemical shift ratio and demonstrated a more than 16.5 % signal intensity index by MRI (Table 4). Hence, we characterized these masses as adenomas by chemical shift MRI. For these 4 adenomas, we used adrenal washout study (n = 2) and imaging follow-up (n = 2) as reference standards.

Histogram Analysis	Unenhanced CT	
	67 adrenal adenomas	42 adrenal metastases
Attenuation (HU)		
Average ± SD	-0,2 ±17,5	34,3±5,1
Range	-83,1 to 40,8	20,7 to 44,5
Negative Pixels %		
Average ± SD	51,2 ±29,9	0,5 ±0,8
Range	0 - 96	0 - 3
Number of Cases with Negative Pixels	67 (100%)	21(50%)
Negative Pixels more than 5%	61 (91%)	0
Negative Pixels more than 10%	61 (91%)	0

Table 3. a. Histogram analysis on unenhanced CT results for adrenal adenomas and metastases.

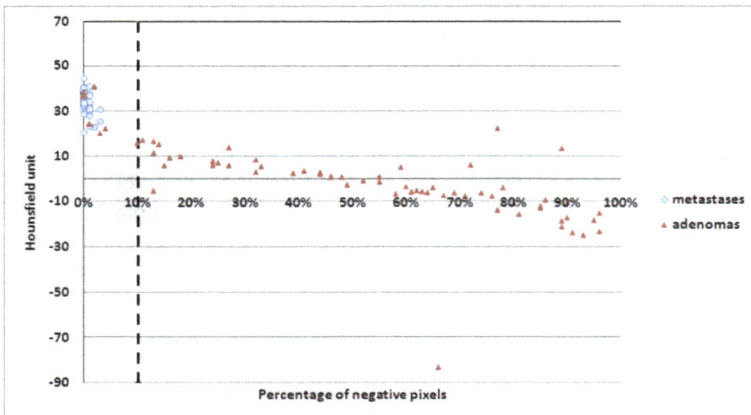

Table 3. b. Scatterplot illustrates correlation betweeen mean CT attenuation and negative pixel percentage of adenomas and metastases. Note that all of the metastases demonstrate less than 10 % negative pixels on this graph.

42 out of 42 metastases showed an adrenal-to-spleen chemical shift ratio of more than 0.71 and 39 out of 42 of them demonstrated an adrenal-to-spleen signal intensity index of less

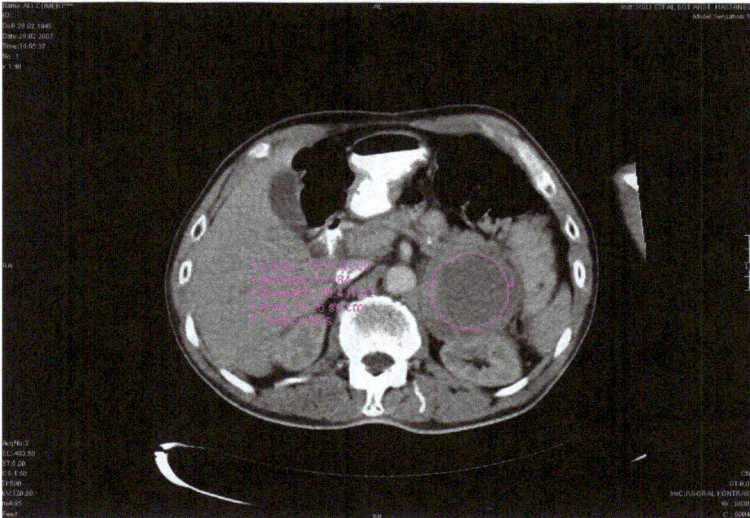

(a)

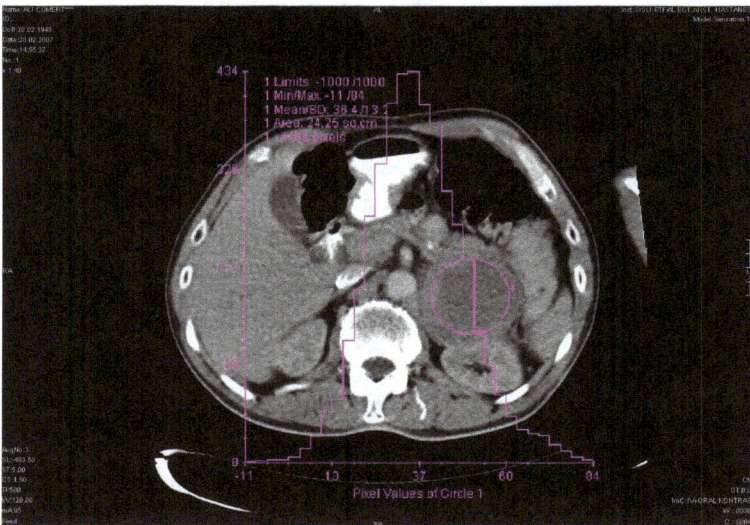

(b)

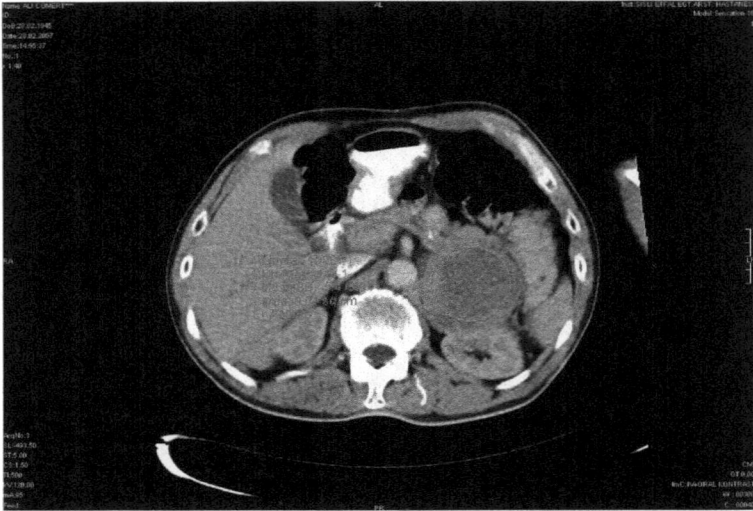

(c)

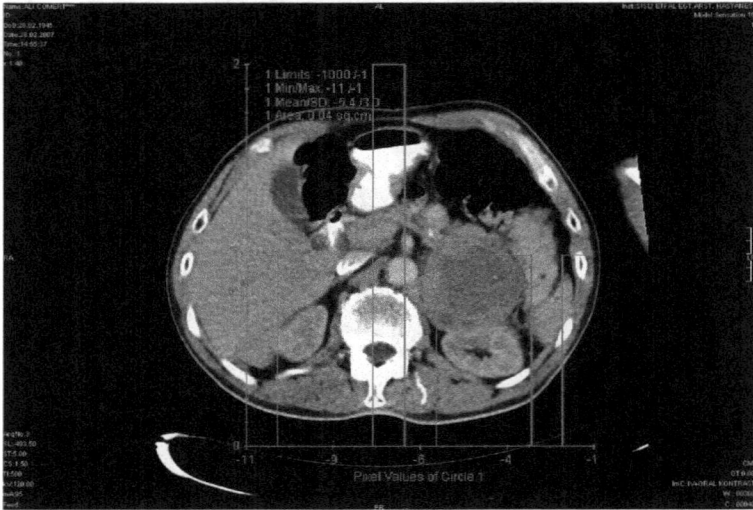

(d)

(a) Contrast- enhanced CT scan using ROI demonstrates 4496 pixels with a mean attenuation of 36.4 HU. The upper and lower limits of pixel attenuation are + 1000 and - 1000, respectively.
(b) Corresponding histogram analysis shows pixel attenuation ranging from - 11 to 84 HU.
(c) Contrast- enhanced CT scan using ROI shows that the mass containing 7 negative pixels. The upper and lower limits of pixel attenuation are – 1 and - 1000, respectively.
(d) Corresponding histogram analysis reveals approximately 0.15 % of the mass contains negative pixels on contrast- enhanced CT.

Fig. 6. 63 year-old man with a left adrenal pheochromocytoma

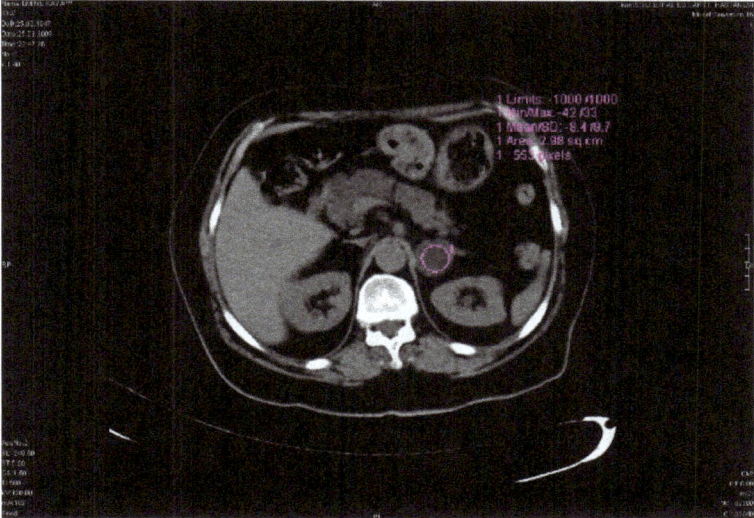

(a)

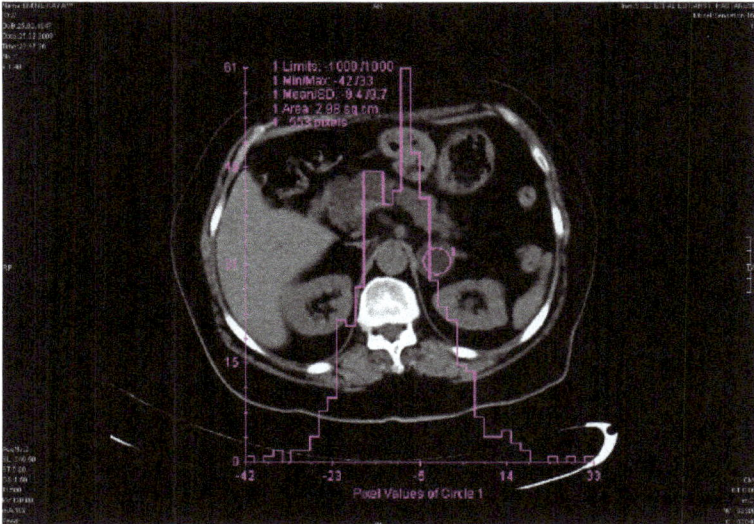

(b)

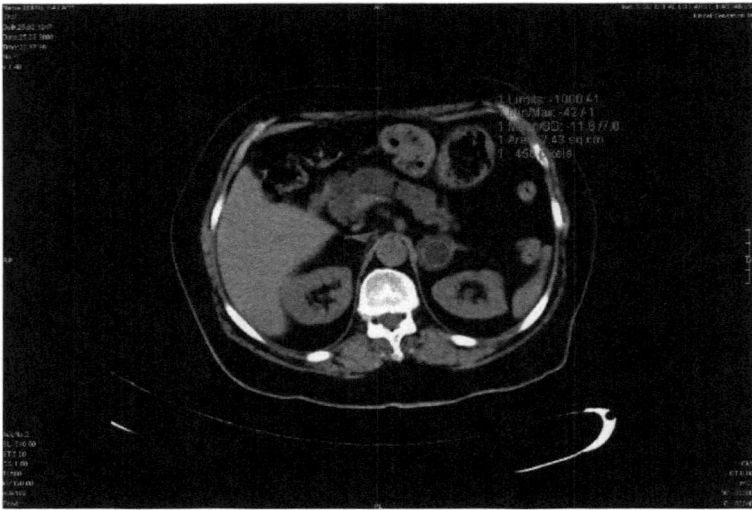

(c)

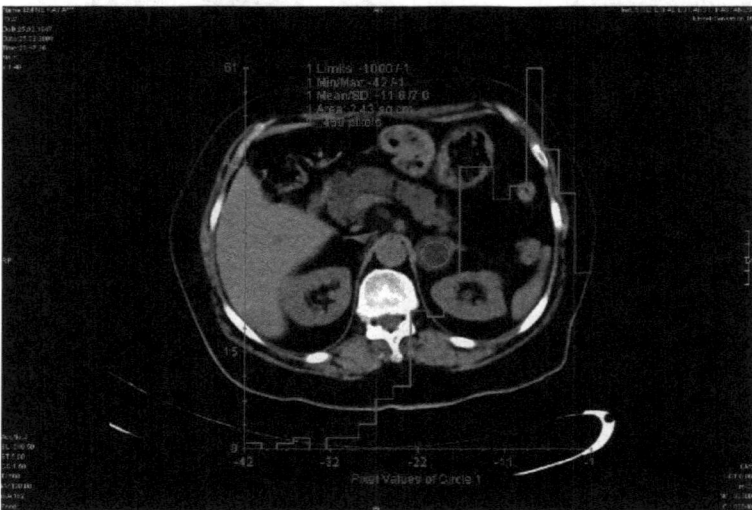

(d)

(a) Unenhanced CT scan applying ROI reveals 553 pixels and demonstrates a mean attenuation of - 8.4 HU. The upper and lower limits of pixel attenuation are + 1000 and - 1000, respectively.
(b) Corresponding histogram analysis shows pixel attenuation ranging from - 42 to 33 HU.
(c) Unenhanced CT scan applying ROI reveals that the incidentaloma containing 450 negative pixels. The upper and lower limits of pixel attenuation are – 1 and - 1000, respectively.
(d) Corresponding histogram analysis shows that incidentaloma contains 81 % negative pixels and therefore can be regarded as adenoma.

Fig. 7. 61 year-old woman with a left adrenal incidentaloma

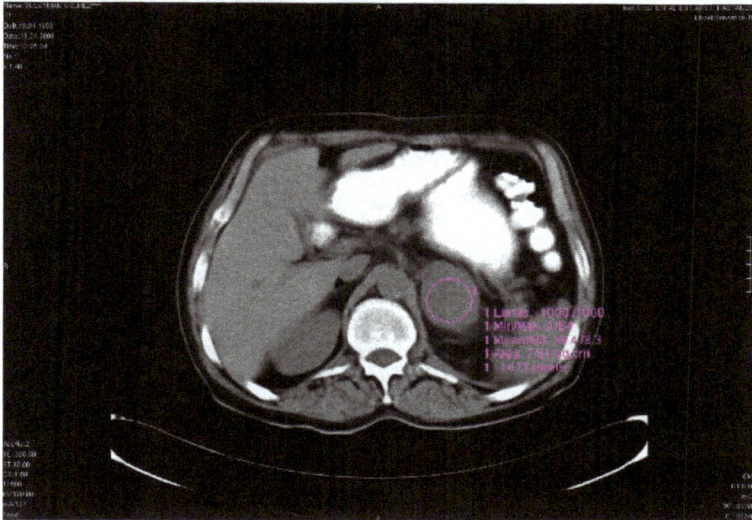

(a)

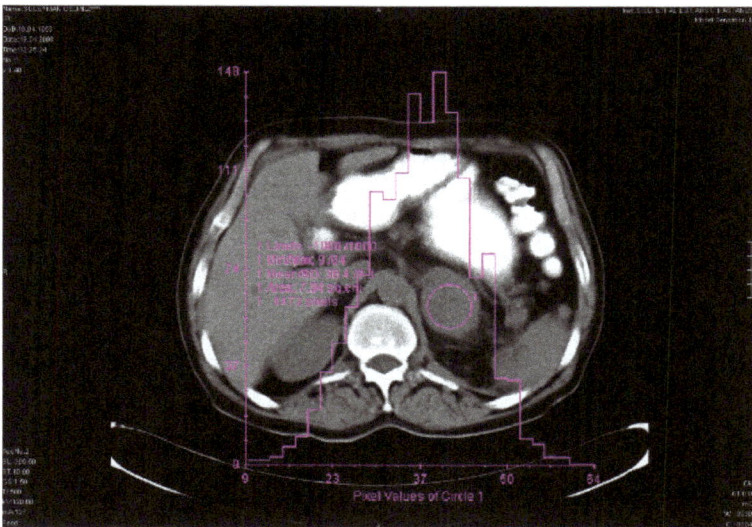

(b)

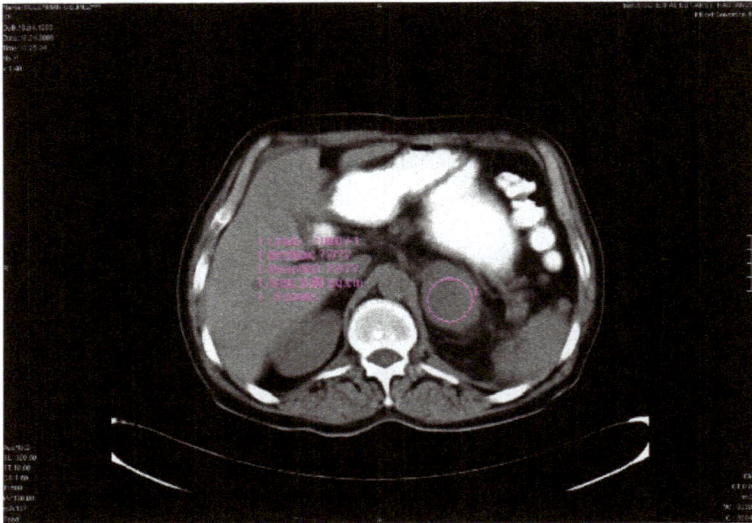

(c)

(a) Unenhanced CT scan applying ROI reveals 1472 pixels and demonstrates a mean attenuation of 36.4 HU. The upper and lower limits of pixel attenuation are + 1000 and - 1000, respectively.

(b) Corresponding histogram analysis shows pixel attenuation ranging from 9 to 64 HU without any negative pixels.

(c) Unenhanced CT scan applying ROI reveals that the mass contains no negative pixels and therefore can be regarded as metastasis. The upper and lower limits of pixel attenuation are – 1 and - 1000, respectively.

Fig. 8. 55 year-old man with known testicular carcinoma history presenting **with a left** adrenal mass

Gender	Age	Mean Attenuation (HU)	Number of Pixels	Number of Negative Pixels	Percentage of Negative Pixels (%)	SI Index	SI Ratio	Clinical Presentation	Referans Standard
M	50	38.4	684	1	0	0	0.99	Incidentaloma	Biopsy
F	24	36.7	516	0	0	8.9	0.84	Incidentaloma	Imaging follow-up
F	67	40.8	125	2	2	61	0.38	Incidentaloma	Washout study
F	51	22.3	216	8	4	31.5	0.66	Breast cancer	Washout Study
F	53	24.5	1226	17	1	45.2	0.53	Hypertension	Imaging follow-up
F	65	20.2	177	6	3	81.6	0.18	Incidentaloma	Imaging follow-up

Table 4. Indeterminate masses with CT histogram analysis (n = 6) and both CT istogram analysis and chemical shift MRI (n = 2).

GENDER	AGE	SI INDEX (%)	CS RATIO	PRIMER TUMOR
Male	78	22.6	0.72	Lung cancer
Female	79	18.6	O.87	Insulinoma
Male	37	17.2	0.76	Lung cancer

Table 5. Metastases showing more than 16.5 % signal intensity index leading to false-positive adenoma results.

than 16.5 % (Figure 11). Three metastases, even though they had a chemical shift ratio of more than 0.71, demonstrated a signal intensity index of greater than 16.5 % leading to false positive cases for adenoma diagnosis (Table 5).
When we used an adrenal-to-spleen chemical shift ratio of less than 0.71 and an adrenal-to-spleen signal intensity index of more than 16.5 % formulas, a 97 % sensitivity was obtained for both methods. However, although a 100 % specificity value was achieved for chemical shift ratio, this dropped to 93 % for signal intensity index in adenoma diagnosis (Figure 9).

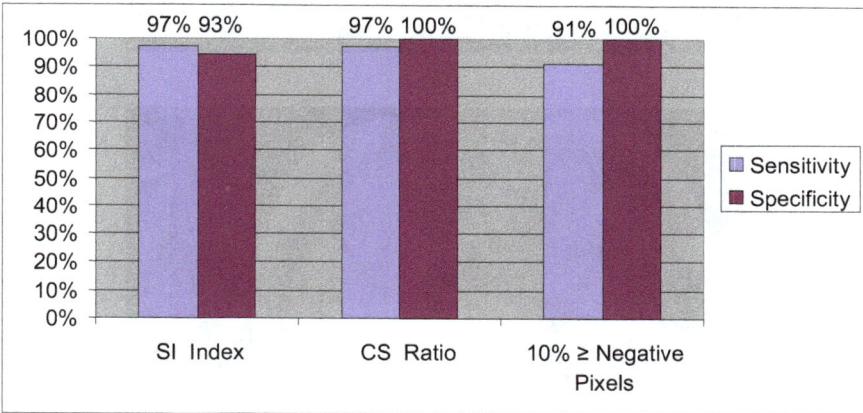

Fig. 9. Bar chart comparing sensitivity values of SI index and CS ratio formulas of chemical shift MRI to % 10 negative pixel threshold of CT histogram analysis on unenhanced CT for adenoma diagnosis.

10. Discussion

The currently used 10 HU threshold mean attenuation method is proved to be useful for differentiating adenomas from metastases at unenhanced CT and has a 71 % sensitivity for diagnosis of adrenal adenomas (3). However, this method is not sensitive in the differentiation of adenomas from nonadenomas at contrast enhanced CT because there is too much overlap in the mean attenuation between two groups (2, 9). Unfortunately, the majority of clinical CT examinations performed in daily routine practice are contrast enhanced. In this case, especially with cancer patients in whom characterization of adrenal masses is important in terms of prognosis and management, this leads to a difficult problem. In the absence of previous comparative CT scans or unenhanced CT studies, patients may be required to undergo an unenhanced CT scan or MRI for further characterization of these adrenal masses.

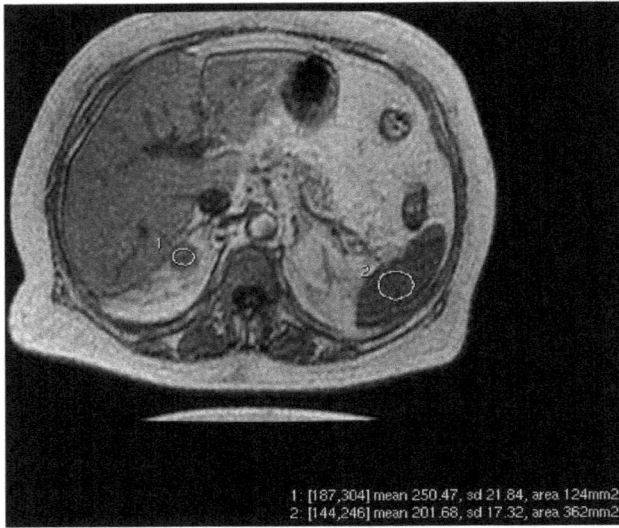

1: [187,304] mean 250.47, sd 21.84, area 124mm2
2: [144,246] mean 201.68, sd 17.32, area 362mm2

(a)

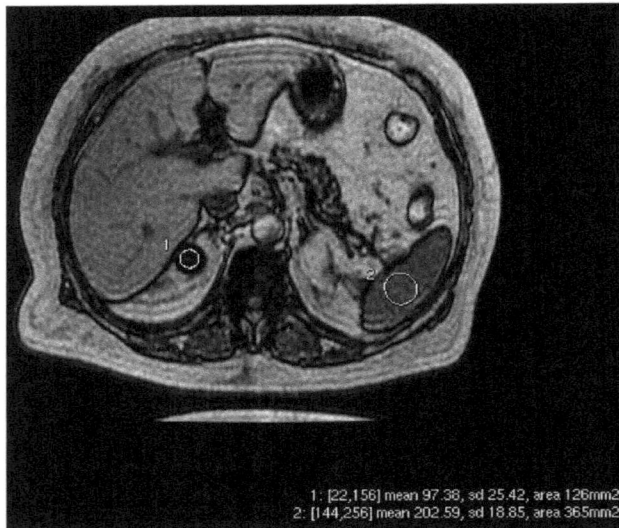

1: [22,156] mean 97.38, sd 25.42, area 126mm2
2: [144,256] mean 202.59, sd 18.85, area 365mm2

(b)

(a) Axial in-phase gradient-echo MR image shows a right adrenal mass demonstrating slight hiperintensity compared to spleen.
(b) Axial opposed-phase gradient-echo MR image demonstrates that the mass showing obvious signal intensity loss with respect to spleen. For this mass adrenal-to-spleen chemical shift ratio and adrenal-to-spleen signal intensity index were calculated as 0.34 and 61 % respectively and

Fig. 10. 72 year-old woman who has a colon carcinoma history presenting with a right adrenal mass

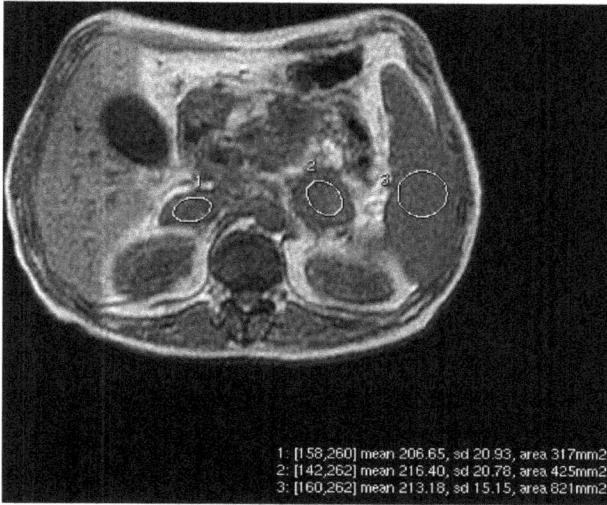

1: [158,260] mean 206.65, sd 20.93, area 317mm2
2: [142,262] mean 216.40, sd 20.78, area 425mm2
3: [160,262] mean 213.18, sd 15.15, area 821mm2

(a)

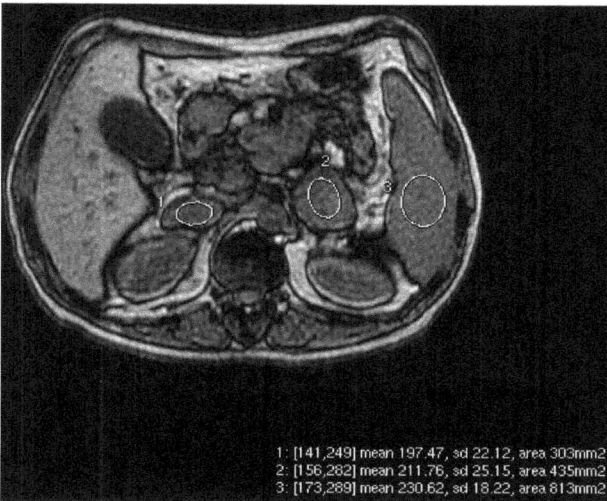

1: [141,249] mean 197.47, sd 22.12, area 303mm2
2: [156,282] mean 211.76, sd 25.15, area 435mm2
3: [173,289] mean 230.62, sd 18.22, area 813mm2

(b)

(a) Axial in-phase gradient-echo MR image reveals bilateral adrenal masses showing isointense signal intensity with spleen on this image.

(b) Axial opposed-phase gradient-echo MR image showing that these masses demonstrating no signal intensity loss with respect to spleen. For the right adrenal mass adrenal-to-spleen chemical shift ratio and adrenal-to-spleen signal intensity index were calculated as 0.88 and 4.3 % and for the left adrenal mass these values were found as 0.90 and 2.3 %, respectively. Given the results, these masses were regarded as bilateral metastases.

Fig. 11. 46 year-old man with a known history of lung carcinoma having bilateral adrenal masses

On the other hand, despite the fact that the currently used 10 HU threshold mean attenuation method on unenhanced CT is useful, this method may result in a categorization of approximately 29 % of adenomas as being indeterminate (3). In this situation, further investigations such as MRI, adrenal washout study or biopsy may be necessary for the definite characterization of the adrenal mass (10). Currently, there is little doubt that, adrenal washout CT has excellent diagnostic performance for the characterization of adrenal nodules of more than 10 HU on unenhanced CT (4, 10). However, adrenal washout CT has some disadvantages such as the need of multiphasic scanning, resulting in a small amount of added radiation burden, and the use of IV contrast material. Biopsy is an invasive procedure and MRI requires an additional visit with extra burden on the resources.

Bae et al (5) described a histogram analysis method with the goal of improving sensitivity in distinguishing between adenomas and metastases on standard contrast enhanced studies. The histogram analysis method uses a ROI within the adrenal mass and determines if pixels measuring less than 0 HU are present.

CT histogram analysis is a potentially interesting concept that, if successful, is a simple postprocessing technique that does not need additional patient visits, multiphasic scanning, intravenous contrast, or additional imaging investigations.

Bae et al (5) concluded that sensitivity in the diagnosis of an adenoma at contrast-enhanced CT was higher when used CT histogram analysis method compared with the mean attenuation value method. In this study, although only 10.9 % (20 out of 184) of adenomas had a mean attenuation value of ≤ 10 HU on contrast-enhanced CT images, 52.7 % (97 out of 184) of them could be diagnosed by the presence of negative pixels using the CT histogram analysis method. In their series, none of the metastases had a mean attenuation value of ≤ 10 HU or contained negative pixels. Despite the absence of negative pixels in their metastases group they were not sure that the presence of any negative pixel could be regarded as a 100 % specific evidence for the diagnosis of an adrenal adenoma. Therefore they recommended using a 10 % negative pixel threshold as an appropriate criterion for diagnosis of adenomas due to the lowest percentage of negative pixels in their adenoma group which measured less than 10 HU on contrast-enhanced CT images that was detected as 9.8 %. In their study, using 5 % and 10 % negative pixel threshold values, they obtained sensitivities of 35.9 % and 27.7 % respectively, and even with these more stringent criteria that they used for the CT histogram analysis method, the results could be regarded as much better than the 10.9 % sensitivity value they obtained with the 10 HU mean attenuation threshold method. However, if anyone should use more than a 10 % negative pixel threshold value for the diagnosis of adenoma, this increase would result in a decrease of test sensitivity and may obviate the histogram analysis method to be used as a clinically useful adjunct to the mean attenuation method.

Jhaveri et al (11) pointed out that by using a CT histogram-derived threshold of more than 10 % negative pixel, adenomas can be diagnosed with a 100 % specificity on unenhanced CT. In spite of this perfect specificity value they achieved, the sensitivity was compromised and yielded a modest value of 46 %. Negative pixels were present in 25 out of 28 adenomas and the mean negative pixel percentage was found to be 9.8 % for adenomas. In their series, unlike Bae et al ' s, 9 out of 11 nonadenomas also demonstrated negative pixels and the mean negative pixel percentage was found as 5.7 % for the nonadenoma group. However by using a more than 10 % negative pixel threshold value, although 13 out of 28 adenomas were detected, none of the nonadenomas were consistent with this criterion. Based on this finding, they could not find a statistically significant relationship for diagnosing an adenoma by the simple presence of negative pixels in a mass and for this reason they did not recommend using the mere presence of negative pixels as a sufficient criterion for the diagnosis of an adenoma.

Remer et al (12) in the their retrospective study, included 187 patients with 204 adrenal masses to evaluate CT histogram analysis method in distinguishing adenomas from nonadenomas based on their pathology results. In this study, the interpreters found that 72 out of 76 and 63 out of 72 adenomas, respectively, with attenuation values of more than 10 HU contained negative pixels on unenhanced CT images. On contrast -enhanced CT images, none of the adenomas had a mean attenuation value of ≤ 10 HU, but 24 and 28, respectively, persisted to contain negative pixels. Negative pixels were detected on both unenhanced and contrast-enhanced CT images of the nonadenoma group including metastases, pheochromocytomas and adrenocortical carcinomas. However, none of the nonadenoma group showed an attenuation value of ≤ 10 HU on both unenhanced and contrast-enhanced CT images. Using a 10 % negative pixel threshold value to diagnose an adenoma, an approximately 88 % specificity and 71 % sensitivity was obtained on unenhanced CT images. But on contrast-enhanced CT images even a better specificity of 99 % was obtained, where sensitivity dropped to 12 %. This sensitivity level was similar to that obtained by Bae et al (5) on contrast-enhanced CT images. Due to this unacceptable low sensitivity value obtained, they concluded that despite the perfect specificity value achieved, CT histogram analysis using 10 % negative pixel threshold value on contrast-enhanced CT images has limited clinical usefulness for the diagnosis of an adenoma.

Boland et al (3) in their meta-analysis of 10 reported studies used unenhanced CT to characterize adrenal masses. They concluded that an increase in the 10 HU mean attenuation threshold value yielded more overlapping between adenomas and metastases. Consequently, although the diagnostic sensitivity of an adenoma increases, specificity drops. Similarly, as with Bae et al (5), the same trend can be observed in our study, too. When we used more than 10 HU threshold value for contrast-enhanced CT images, our sensitivity values substantially increased while specificity values decreased.

Jhaveri et al (13) recently published a study in which a 24 lipid-poor adenoma population was evaluated by CT histogram analysis method using more than 5 % negative pixel threshold value on unenhanced images. They obtained a sensitivity of about 91 % with a specificity of 100 % when compared with adrenal washout CT sensitivity and specificity of 100 % each. When they used a 10 % negative pixel threshold value, the sensitivity was still at a good level of 70 %, while maintaining a specificity of 100 % compared with adrenal washout CT at sensitivity and specificity of 100 %.

In a recently published study by Ho LM et al (14), the authors stated that by applying a 10 % negative pixel threshold, sensitivity increases in the diagnosis of adenoma from 68 % to 84 %, when the standard mean CT attenuation value of ≤ 10 HU was used, while maintaining a 100 % specificity. They concluded that a CT histogram analysis using a 10 % negative pixel threshold can be used to characterize some adenomas that would otherwise be considered as indeterminate by mean CT attenuation alone and consequently may help decrease referrals for additional imaging or biopsy of adrenal masses, particularly in patients with a known primary malignancy. They stated that the application of a threshold of 5 % negative pixels slightly increases sensitivity for the diagnosis of an adenoma compared to using a threshold of 10 % negative pixels ; however, the advantage of this higher sensitivity is compromised by decreased specificity. In an oncological patient population, decreasing specificity would lead to more metastases since they may be misclassified as benign adenomas which consequently could result in understaging of the primary tumor. They therefore recommended the application of a threshold of 10 % negative pixels for CT histogram analysis.

In our study, we obtained a 77.2 % sensitivity for ≤ 10 HU mean attenuation threshold value and a much better sensitivity of 90.9 % for 10 % negative pixel threshold value with CT histogram analysis method on unenhanced CT images. Both methods gave a 100 % specificity for the diagnosis of an adenoma. But at contrast-enhanced CT, our sensitivity substantially decreased to 12.1 % for ≤ 10 HU mean attenuation value. We obtained a sensitivity of 37.9 % for 5 % negative pixel threshold and a 28.8 % sensitivity for 10 % negative pixel threshold, respectively. For both methods, again a 100 % specificity was maintained on contrast-enhanced CT images. Our results suggest that a CT histogram analysis method using a 10 % negative pixel threshold performed on unenhanced CT images is superior to ≤ 10 HU mean attenuation threshold method and results in good sensitivity while maintaining perfect specificity for the diagnosis of an adenoma. But on contrast-enhanced images, in similarity with most of the studies we mentioned before, although a 100 % specificity was maintained, sensitivity values dramatically decreased to unacceptable levels for both 5 % and 10 % negative pixel threshold values, pointing to CT histogram analysis method as a less clinical useful adjunct on contrast-enhanced CT.

The sensitivity for diagnosing an adenoma using a CT histogram-derived threshold of more than 10 % negative pixel decreased as the unenhanced CT attenuation increased. The demonstration of a statistically significant relationship between increasing the percentage of negative pixels and decreasing mean CT attenuation supported this relationship. This relationship is consistent with the fact that adenomas having abundant lipid have lower CT attenuation and therefore are likely to have a higher percentage of negative pixels.

In our study, adrenal masses demonstrated an increase in mean attenuation and a decrease in the percentage of negative pixels on contrast-enhanced CT images compared to unenhanced CT images. This can be seen in many other studies and was attributed to the pseudoenhancement effect that has been described for renal cysts (15, 16). This phenomenon may cause a decrease in the percentage of negative pixels in adenomas on contrast-enhanced CT images as a result of artifactual enhancement of lipid tissue related to enhancing adjacent nonlipid tissue.

Clinical applications of CT histogram analysis and chemical shift MRI for the diagnosis of adrenal adenomas are based on the different lipid contents of benign and malignant adrenal masses. In fact, adenomas have higher lipid contents than metastases which account for their low attenuation on unenhanced CT and signal intensity loss on opposed-phased MR images. But whether a high correlation between CT histogram analysis and chemical shift MRI measurements exists is yet unclear, because a comparison of these techniques in the same cohort of patients has been previously published in only a few of the studies in the literature (11, 17).

In general radiology practice, qualitative visual assessment is a commonly used method to characterize adrenal adenomas without measuring signal intensity on chemical shift images. Mayo-Smith et al. (18) compared a qualitative assessment of adrenal masses with the adrenal-to-spleen chemical shift ratio and reported that there was no significant difference in terms of mass characterization. However, Israel et al. (17) found that there was a discrepancy in 15 out of 42 (36 %) adrenal masses between qualitative and quantitative analyses and stated that qualitative analysis should be regarded as less sensitive than quantitative analysis in adenoma diagnosis. The results of this study can be indicated that qualitative analysis should be regarded as less sensitive than quantitative analysis in terms of adrenal mass characterization on MRI and therefore it is a necessity to obtain quantitative measurements of adrenal masses. In our study, we did not use qualitative visual assessment for adrenal mass characterization on opposed-phase images.

In our study, using an adrenal-to-spleen chemical shift ratio of less than 0.71 and an adrenal signal intensity index of greater than 16.5 % formulas on chemical shift MRI, we were able to diagnose 65 out of 67 (97 %) adenomas. 2 out of 67 adenomas could not determined by MRI, but were also characterized as indeterminate by CT histogram analysis method due to containing less than 10 % negative pixels. But in 4 masses that were regarded as indeterminate by CT histogram, we were able to diagnose them as adenomas using chemical shift MRI formulas. Regarding metastases, none of them demonstrated a more than 10 % negative pixel by CT histogram analysis method. On the other hand, although 42 out of 42 metastases (100 %) exhibited an adrenal-to-spleen chemical shift ratio of more than 0.71, 39 out of 42 metastases (93 %) had an adrenal signal intensity index of less than 16.5 % leading to three false positive results and a subsequent decrease in specificity for adenoma diagnosis. Therefore we can state that although there was a high correlation between these two methods, chemical shift MRI using quantitative analysis was found to be more sensitive than CT histogram analysis method, because it enables us to discriminate more adenomas that would otherwise be regarded as indeterminate on CT. For metastases, CT histogram analysis and MRI using chemical shift ratio formula diagnosed all cases and was found superior to the signal intensity index formula.

Jhaveri et al. (11) compared CT histogram analysis method using 10 % negative pixel threshold on unenhanced CT and chemical shift MRI using a threshold of 20 % signal intensity drop in 39 adrenal masses that were indeterminate on CT. While CT histogram analysis using a more than 10 % negative pixel threshold yielded a 46 % sensitivity and 100 % specificity for adenoma diagnosis, MRI using a threshold of 20 % signal intensity drop increased sensitivity to a 71 % level, while maintaining 100 % specificity. Using MRI, the observers were able to characterize 7 more adrenal masses as adenomas whereas they were regarded as indeterminate by CT histogram analysis, similar to our study. They concluded that CT histogram analysis with a threshold of 10 % negative pixel increases sensitivity for adenoma diagnosis compared to mean CT attenuation alone. But chemical shift MRI with a threshold of 20 % signal intensity drop is more sensitive than CT histogram analysis for adenoma diagnosis.

In a similar study performed by Israel et al. (17), 42 adrenal masses were evaluated by both unenhanced CT and chemical shift MRI for further characterization. A lipid-rich adenoma was diagnosed if a mass showed equal or less than 10 HU mean attenuation value on unenhanced CT, had an adrenal-to-spleen chemical shift ratio of less than 0.71 and exhibited an adrenal signal intensity index of more than 16.5 %. 28 out of 42 (67 %) adrenal masses fulfilled all of the preceeding criteria and therefore were diagnosed as benign masses. Although 8 out of 42 (19 %) adrenal masses had a more than 10 HU mean attenuation value on unenhanced CT images, demonstrated an adrenal-to-spleen chemical shift ratio of less than 0.71 and a signal intensity index of more than 16.5 %, they were unchanged in size at follow-up imaging and were regarded as benign masses.Chemical shift MRI was able to characterize 8 out of 13 (62 %) adrenal adenomas that exhibited more than 10 HU mean attenuation value resulting in indeterminate masses on unenhanced CT images.

Outwater et al. (19) in their study investigated whether a correlation exists between mean attenuation value on unenhanced CT and chemical shift MRI using adrenal-to-spleen chemical shift ratio of 0.71 threshold in 49 adrenal masses. They reported that these measurements are highly correlated and support that both techniques rely on the lipid content within the adrenal lesions. But in this relatively small sample-sized study, they found no clear evidence as to which method used was more accurate to characterize adrenal masses.

In a study performed by Mayo-Smith et al. (18), a slightly higher adrenal-to-spleen chemical shift ratio of 0.75 was applied and all of the metastases were correctly identified. But with this threshold value, 5 out of 28 adenomas were misclassified. In this study similar to ours, both adrenal-to-spleen chemical shift ratio and adrenal signal intensity index formulas were used and it was mentioned that adrenal-to-spleen chemical shift ratio is a better quantitative test for discriminating adenomas from metastases. Conversely, Fujiyoshi et al. (20) reported that adrenal signal intensity index using a threshold value between 11.2 % - 16.5 %, resulted in 100 % accuracy and should be accepted as the best quantitative test for discriminating benign from malignant adrenal masses.They claimed that adrenal-to-spleen ratio, adrenal-to-muscle ratio and adrenal-to-liver ratio formulas demonstrated considerable overlap between benign and malignant adrenal tumors. Park et al. (21) compared delayed enhanced CT and chemical shift MRI for evaluating 43 lipid-poor adenomas. In this study, similar to the prior one, they revealed that adrenal signal intensity index exhibited a higher diagnostic accuracy than did adrenal-to-spleen chemical shift ratio.

In our study, as with the above, when we compared adrenal-to-spleen chemical shift ratio and adrenal signal intensity index formulas, we could not encounter any discrepancy between these two formulas in adenoma diagnosis. All of the adenomas, except for two cases, showed a less than 0.71 chemical shift ratio and had a more than 16.5 % signal intensity index. For these two adenomas, while a more than 0.71 chemical shift ratio was calculated, they also exhibited a less than 16.5 % signal intensity index. But regarding metastases, although all of them showed a more than 0.71 chemical shift ratio, 3 of them exhibited a signal intensity index of more than 16.5 % resulting in false positive adenoma cases. Hence, similar to Mayo Smith et al. (18), we can state that adrenal-to-spleen chemical shift ratio formula can be regarded as a better quantitative test for discriminating adenomas from metastases.

CT histogram analysis is influenced by variations in CT image quality and noise levels. CT image quality is affected by a number of other factors such as patient and technical properties which, as with other previous studies, were not standardized completely in this study.These factors include patient body habitus, breathing motion artifact, size and location of ROI, kilovolt peak and miliampere second values, slice collimation, section thickness, reconstruction kernel, IV contrast media injection rate, and scan delay. Other factors that could impact image noise include differences in CT scanner technology (Both dual and multi-detector row CT scanners were used in this study). Noisy pixels may simulate false-positive percentage negative pixels. The higher current reduces image noise and improves image quality, which is critical for thin-section extended-length studies, especially of large patients (22). This could reduce the number of spuriously negative pixels. However, thinner slice thickness may lead to noisier images.Therefore, thin slices or sharp kernels may be inappropriate for CT histogram analysis because of excessive image noise. Bae et al (5) recommended that CT images should be reconstructed with a smooth soft-tissue-kernel typically used for abdominal CT rather than a sharp lung or bone algorithm, which is usually noisier, prior to application of histogram analysis. Because image noise is inversely related to the square root of the tube current (23), CT images should be acquired with standard miliamper-second and peak kilovoltage used for the abdomen rather than with a low-dose technique (5, 23).

In spite of their several limitations, our studies carry the importance of being prospective in nature whereas many of the previous studies in the literature have been performed retrospectively and therefore carry a potential for subject-selection bias. Due to the prospective nature of the studies, we were able to standardize most of the imaging parameters such as slice thickness, collimation, bandwidth, coil type etc. An important limitation of our studies are that we used pathological data as a reference standard only in a small percentage of patients. This is partly due to daily practice where CT or MRI is used for characterizing adrenal adenomas and these patients seldom undergo biopsy or surgery for definitive diagnosis. Another limitation of both studies are the lack of long-term follow-up and although we used a minimum of 6 months follow-up time as a reference standard, there is a possibility that some adrenal metastases may have long doubling times leading to a confusion. In the literature although some authors have used a minimum 1 year follow-up (24, 25), many of the leading authors have agreed that 6 months follow-up time is sufficient as a reference standard for adenoma diagnosis (4, 18, 19, 26). Finally, in our studies we obtained high specificity values reaching out to 100 % level and this should be viewed with some scepticism.

11. Conclusion

In conclusion, our first study suggests that CT histogram analysis using a 10 % negative pixel threshold has a higher sensitivity than ≤ 10 HU mean attenuation threshold method to discriminate adenomas from nonadenomas on unenhanced CT while a 100 % specificity has been achieved for both methods. Therefore CT histogram analysis method has a promising potential in the diagnosis of adenoma and can replace the mean attenuation method. But with contrast-enhanced CT, although 100 % specificity is being maintained for both methods, sensitivities significantly decrease. Although better sensitivities are obtained with CT histogram analysis using 5 % and 10 % negative pixel threshold values compared to the mean attenuation method, this poor sensitivity levels would limit its clinical usefulness.

In our second study that comparing of CT histogram analysis using a 10 % negative pixel threshold on unenhanced CT with chemical shift MRI using adrenal-to-spleen chemical shift ratio and adrenal signal intensity index formulas demonstrate high correlation for adenoma diagnosis. Although CT histogram analysis and adrenal-to-spleen chemical shift ratio formula have perfect specificity values, adrenal signal intensity index formula has a relatively lower specificity. In the second study, we found that adrenal-to-spleen chemical shift ratio is superior to the other two methods in the diagnosis of adenoma. Hence we can state that chemical shift MRI using the quantitative method has a higher sensitivity than the histogram analysis method and may help further characterization of some adrenal masses which are regarded as indeterminate on CT histogram analysis.

12. References

[1] Korobkin M. 2000. CT characterization of adrenal masses : the time has come. Radiology 217 : 629-632.

[2] Lee MJ, Hahn PF, Papanicolaou N, Egglin TK, Saini S, Mueller PR, Simeone JF. 1991. Benign and malignant adrenal masses : CT distinction with attenuation coefficients, size and observer analysis. Radiology 179 : 415-418.

[3] Boland GW, Lee MJ, Gazelle GS, Halpern EF, Mc-Nicholas MM, Mueller PR. 1998. Characterization of adrenal masses using unenhanced CT : an analysis of the CT literature. AJR Am J Roentgenol 171 : 201-204.

[4] Pena CS, Boland GW, Hahn PF, Lee MJ, Mueller PR. 2000. Characterization of indeterminate (lipid poor) adrenal masses : use of washout characteristics at contrast enhanced CT. Radiology 217 : 798-802.

[5] Bae KT, Fuangtharnthip P, Prasad SR, Joe BN, Heiken JP. 2003. Adrenal masses : CT characterization with histogram analysis method. Radiology 228 : 735-742.

[6] Mayo-Smith WW, Boland GW, Noto RB, Lee M. 2001. State-of-the-art of adrenal imaging. RadioGraphics 21 : 995-1012.

[7] Slapa RZ, Jakubowski W, Januszewics A, Kasperlik-Zaluska AA, Dabrowska E, Fijuth J, Feltynowski T, Tarnawski R, Krolicki L. 2000. Discriminatory power of MRI for differentiation of adrenal non-adenomas vs. adenomas evaluated by means of ROC analysis : can biopsy be obviated ? Eur Radiol 10 : 95-104.

[8] Heinz Peer G, Honigschnabl S, Schneider B, Niederle B, Kaserer K, Lechner G. 1999. Characterization of adrenal masses using MR imaging with histopathologic correlation. AJR Am J Roentgenol 173 : 15-22.

[9] Korobkin M, Brodeur FJ, Yutzy GG, Francis IR, Quint LE, Dunnick NR, Kazerooni EA. 1996. Differentiation of adrenal adenomas from nonadenomas using CT attenuation values. AJR Am J Roentgenol 166 : 531-536.

[10] Al-Hawary MM, Francis IR, Korobkin M. 2005. Non-invasive evaluation of the incidentally detected indeterminate adrenal mass. Best Pract Res Clin Endocrinol Metab 19 : 277-292.

[11] Jhaveri KS, Wong F, Ghai S, Haider MA. 2006. Comparison of CT histogram analysis and chemical shift MRI in the characterization of indeterminate adrenal nodules. AJR Am J Roentgenol 187 : 1303-1308.

[12] Remer EM, Motta-Ramirez GA, Shepardson LB, Hamrahian AH, Herts BR. 2006. CT histogram analysis in pathologically proven adrenal masses. AJR Am J Roentgenol 187 : 191-196.

[13] Jhaveri KS, Lad SV, Haider MA. 2007. Computed tomographic histogram analysis in the diagnosis of lipid poor adenomas : comparison to adrenal washout computed tomography. J Comput Assist Tomogr 31 : 513-518.

[14] Ho LM, Paulson EK, Brady MJ, Wong TZ, Schindera ST. 2008. Lipid-poor adenomas on unenhanced CT : Does histogram analysis increase sensitivity compared with a mean attenuation threshold method ? AJR Am J Roentgenol 191 : 234-238.

[15] Coulam CH, Sheafor DH, Leder DA, Paulson EK, DeLong DM, Nelson RC. 2000. Evaluation of pseudoenhancement of renal cysts during contrast-enhanced CT. AJR Am J Roentgenol 174 : 493-498.

[16] Bae KT, Heiken JP, Siegel CL, Bennett HF. 2000. Renal cysts : is attenuation artifactually increased on contrast-enhanced CT images ? Radiology 216 : 792-796.

[17] Israel GM, Korobkin M, Wang C, Hecht EN, Krinsky GA. 2004. Comparison of unenhanced CT and chemical shift MRI in evaluating lipid-rich adrenal adenomas. AJR Am J Roentgenol 183 : 215-219.

[18] Mayo-Smith WM, Lee MJ, McNicholas MM, Hahn PF, Boland GW, Saini S. 1995. Characterization of adrenal masses (< 5 cm) by use of chemical shift MR imaging : observer performance versus quantitative measures. AJR Am J Roentgenol 165 : 91-95.

[19] Outwater EK, Siegelman ES, Huang AB, Birnbaum BA. 1996. Adrenal masses : correlation between CT attenuation value and chemical shift ratio at MR imaging with in-phase and opposed-phase sequences. Radiology 200 : 749-752.

[20] Fujiyoshi F, Nakajo M, Fukukura Y, Tsuchimochi S. 2003. Characterization of adrenal tumors by chemical shift fast low-angle shot MR imaging : comparison of four methods of quantitative evaluation. AJR Am J Roentgenol 180 : 1649-1657.

[21] Park BK, Kim CK, Kim B, Lee JH. 2007. Comparison of delayed enhanced CT and chemical shift MR for evaluating hyperattenuating incidental adrenal masses. Radiology 243 : 760-765.

[22] Rydberg J, Buckwalter KA, Caldemeyer KS, Phillips MD, Conces DJ Jr, Aisen AM, Persohn SA, Kopecky KK. 2000. Multisection CT : scanning techniques and clinical applications. RadioGraphics 20 : 1787-1806.

[23] Birnbaum BA, Hindman N, Lee J, Babb JS. 2007. Multidetector row CT attenuation measurements: assessment of intra- and interscanner variability with an anthromorphic body CT phantom. Radiology 242 : 109-119.

[24] Outwater EK, Siegelman ES, Radecki PD, Piccoli CW, Mitchell DG. 1995. Distinction between benign and malignant adrenal masses : value of T 1 weighted chemical-shift MR imaging. AJR Am J Roentgenol 165 : 579-583.

[25] Szolar DH, Kammerhuber FH. 1998. Adrenal adenomas and nonadenomas : assessment of washout at delayed contrast-enhanced CT. Radiology 207 : 369-375.

[26] Caoili EM, Korobkin M, Francis IR, Cohan RH, Platt JF, Dunnick NR, Raghupathi KI. 2002. Adrenal masses : characterization with combined unenhanced and delayed enhanced CT. Radiology 222 : 629-633.

5

CT-Guided Brachytherapy Planning

Cem Onal and Ezgi Oymak
Baskent University Faculty of Medicine/ Department of Radiation Oncology
Turkey

1. Introduction

Brachytherapy applications are not restricted to one method only; any method could be combined with another, as well as other radiotherapy techniques. In cervical cancer, intracavitary brachytherapy (ICBT) has been used for practical reasons. Lately though, combination of ICBT and and interstitial brachytherapy (ISBT) techniques are being evaluated in deference to feasibility, practicality and reproducibility. The possibilities are limited only to the physician's imagination.

Brachytherapy in cervical cancer is indicated in every stage. Currently, general approach is either to operate the patients who have tumors confined in the cervix or treat them with definitive radiotherapy, which consists of BT only or external beam radiotherapy (EBRT) plus BT. The rationale behind is to avoid unnecessary toxicity of surgery and radiotherapy combined in one patient.

2. Historical background

The word "brachytherapy" comes from Latin, meaning "short-distance therapy". That is exactly what brachytherapy is about. Soon after the discovery of radioactive seeds by Becquerel and Curies, radioactive radium seeds were planted inside the tumors. Radiating a target from within outshined delivering the same dose to a target externally in specific tumors. Tumor location, in other words, the accessibility of a tumor made the distinction. First experimentations were done on gynecologic, prostatic and breast tumors. It is not surprising to see brachytherapy approaches still focus on these tumors, as well as other tumor sites such as head and neck, esophagus and in limited cases in lung.

In gynecologic cancers, radiation doses delivered with brachytherapy has been used for more than 100 years. Possibly one of the first presented cases, Margaret Cleaves performed ICBT for cervical cancer in 1903 (Cleaves 1903). Since then, ICBT with or without external radiotherapy has played a major role in curative treatment of cervical cancer. Over the years, application methods as well as dose delivery methods have changed dramatically, reaching a less uncomfortable and much more effective treatment. Among gynecologic cancers, radiation therapy plays a role first and foremost in cervical cancer. Endometrial cancer and vulvovaginal cancers may also be treated with radiotherapy adjunct to surgery. In ovarian cancers, radiotherapy has limited use except for palliative setting.

3. Brachytherapy techniques

Brachytherapy methods can be listed as following:

- *Intracavitary brachytherapy (ICBT):* Suitable for tumors located in a body cavity, e.g. cervical cancer located at the end of vaginal cavity, or tumors located in the oral cavity.
- *Interstitial brachytherapy (ISBT):* Where radioactive sources are surgically implanted within the tumor or tumor bed; e.g. breast cancer, tumors floor of mouth or tongue, prostate cancer.
- *Intraluminal brachytherapy (ILBT):* In which tumors surrounding a luminal organ is accessed via the lumen, e.g. esophageal tumors, lung tumors, biliary tract tumors.
- *Mold brachytherapy (MBT):* Mold shaped out to fit the target surface is implanted with radioactive seeds, e.g. scalp tumors.

3.1 Dose rates

The dose rate of BT refers to the level or 'intensity' with which the radiation is delivered to the surrounding medium. The dose rate of BT is defined in Grays per hour (Gy/h). In clinical practice, commonly used BT dose rates are as follows:

- **Low-dose rate (LDR) brachytherapy**: Involves implanting radiation sources that emit radiation at a rate of less than 2 Gy per hour (Fu and Phillips 1990). LDR brachytherapy is commonly used for cancers of the oral cavity and oropharyngeal carcinomas (Bourgier et al. 2005; Mazeron et al. 2009), soft tissue sarcomas (Alektiar et al. 2011) and prostate cancer (Koukourakis et al. 2009).
- **Medium-dose rate (MDR) brachytherapy**: Characterized by a dose delivery rate ranging between 2 Gy to 12 Gy per hour (Guedea et al. 2010).
- **High-dose rate (HDR) brachytherapy:** The dose rate is more than 12 Gy per hour. The most common applications of HDR brachytherapy are gynecological cancers (Atahan et al. 2007; Atahan et al. 2008), esophageal carcinoma, lung and prostate cancers.
- **Pulsed-dose rate (PDR) brachytherapy:** Involves short pulses of radiation, typically once an hour, to simulate the overall rate and effectiveness of LDR treatment. Typical tumor sites treated by PDR brachytherapy are gynecological and head and neck cancers.

3.1.1 High-dose rate brachytherapy

Traditionally, cervical carcinoma has been treated with LDR brachytherapy. However HDR brachytherapy was developed to overcome potential disadvantages of LDR brachytherapy, such as unwanted radiation exposure to medical staff, prolonged treatment time, need for long time hospitalization, and possible applicator movement due to prolonged treatment time (Fu et al. 2000). Despite these potential advantages, the primary disadvantage of HDR brachytherapy is the late toxicity due to large doses per fraction, a problem that can be overcome through adequate fractionation schedules. Additionally, in HDR, late tissue complications might be minimized more effectively than in LDR, because greater normal tissue displacement is possible with either packing or some custom made retractors pushing bladder anteriorly and rectum posteriorly (Stitt et al. 1992; Thomadsen et al. 1992). Several studies have compared LDR brachytherapy to HDR brachytherapy in the management of cervical cancer.

Advantages of HDR vs. LDR in cancer of the cervix

- Eliminates undesired radiation exposure hazard to caregivers, visitors; and also diminishes radiation exposure during source preparation and transportation, which may reduce the risk of secondary cancer risk.

- Treatment times are shorter leading to:
  - Less discomfort to the patient
  - Ability to treat high risk patients who are unable to tolerate long period of isolation, such as patients with cardiopulmonary diseases, musculoskeletal diseases, etc.
  - Less risk of applicator movement during therapy.
  - Cost-effectiveness, since there is no need to hospitalization.
  - Larger number of patients treated in institutions that have a high volume of cervical cancer patients but insufficient inpatient facilities (for example, in some developing countries).
- Reduction in the need for heavy sedation or general anesthesia. Since the diameter of sources used in HDR brachtherapy is less than that of LDR brachytherapy, extra dilatation of cervix for insertion of larger sources into cervical os is eliminated.
- Treatment-dose-optimization. The variation of dwell time with the single stepping source allows an almost infinite variation of the effective source strength and source positions allowing greater control of the dose distribution and potentially less morbidity.
- Integration of EBRT and HDR, which can lead to a shorter overall duration of treatment and potentially better tumor control.

Many studies comparing HDR and LDR BT demonstrated comparable local control, survival, and morbidity (Akine et al. 1990; Fu and Phillips 1990; Orton 1991; Teshima et al. 1993; Patel et al. 1994; Petereit and Pearcey 1999), some studies even showed less rectal complications with the use of HDR (Fu and Phillips 1990; Patel et al. 1994). In order to standardize the treatment with HDR brachytherapy, The American Brachytherapy Society (ABS) formed a committee to issue guidelines specifically for the use of HDR brachytherapy for cervical carcinoma in 2000 (Nag et al. 2000).

The ABS recommends that brachytherapy must be delivered during EBRT time, based on the Patterns of Care studies that show that recurrences and complications are decreased when brachytherapy and EBRT were embedded (Coia et al. 1990; Montana et al. 1995). The relative doses given by EBRT vs. brachytherapy depend upon the initial volume of disease, the ability to displace the bladder and rectum, the degree of tumor regression during pelvic irradiation, and institutional preference. Another important recommendation of the ABS is to keep total treatment time less than 8 weeks, because prolongation of total treatment duration can adversely affect local control and survival (Girinsky et al. 1993; Petereit et al. 1995). The recommendation is therefore to interdigitate the implants during the EBRT (but EBRT is not given on the day of HDR). Typically, if the vaginal geometry is optimal, HDR brachytherapy is started after 2 weeks of EBRT. HDR is then continued once a week, with the ERT given the other 4 days of the week. If, due to large tumor volume, it is necessary to delay the start of HDR brachytherapy, it is advisable to perform two applications per week after the EBRT has been completed, so that the total treatment duration is kept within 8 weeks.

The ABS recognizes that the whole pelvic EBRT dose varies from one institution to another. Some institutions prefer to limit the whole pelvis dose for patients with early disease and to perform the first intracavitary insertion after 20 Gy, with further EBRT delivered with a central block in place. The ABS recommends careful attention to the complex matching between the intracavitary system and the edge of the midline block, which is critical to the success of this approach (Eifel et al. 1995). However, the individual fraction size should be kept to less than 7.5 Gy due to reports of higher toxicity with larger fraction sizes (Orton et al. 1991; Orton 1998).

There is no consensus regarding the use of midline blocks. The ABS recommends that, if used, simple rectangular blocks should routinely be between 4- and 5-cm wide at midplane when intracavitary brachytherapy applicators are used. Optimally, customized midline blocks based on radiographs taken with similar isocenters and reflecting the isodose distribution of the implant should be considered, if possible. When a midline block is inserted before 40 Gy, it should not extend to the top of the pelvic field because it will shield the common iliac and presacral nodes. When there is suspicion of uterosacral ligament involvement, it is safer to avoid early placement of a midline block, which could potentially shield disease posterior to the implant.

The ABS recommends use of multiple HDR insertions to allow progressive tumor volume reduction, allowing more effective disease coverage with the subsequent application. If there are any deficiencies in the initial insertions, adjusting applicator position and packing from fraction to fraction is recommended. Optimum applicator placement and attention to details are critical in both maximizing local control and minimizing complications. The ABS recommends considering placement with ultrasound and fluoroscopic guidance, particularly in patients with altered cervical anatomy because the narrow HDR tandem potentially presents a higher risk for uterine perforation.

It is important to choose an applicator that can optimally treat the disease and can be placed in an anatomically distorted vagina. When tandem and ovoids are used, the largest ovoid diameter that can be accommodated in the fornices without displacement should be inserted. The ring applicator is particularly useful when the vaginal fornices are asymmetric or absent and it is popular because it has a reproducible geometry and is easy to insert. It is important that the plastic caps of the ring applicator be in place with each insertion, because excessive vagina mucosal doses would be delivered without them. It is also important not to activate the entire ring circumference; usually the lateral 4–6 dwell positions are activated on each side of the ring, depending on the ring diameter.

4. Conventional brachytherapy planning

Before going into conformal BT, a short description of conventional BT planning will be given to enable a better comparison. As it is, conformal 3D BT is a result of the need for better treatment modalities.

In the second part of the 20th century, conventional BT planning played a prominent part up until the introduction of imaging techniques to BT in the 1990s. From 1950 to 1990, three major conventional BT planning systems were utilized.

The oldest one, the Paris system consisted of two cork colpostats in the form of a cylinder and an intrauterine tube. A dose of 7000-8000 mg-hrs of radium (Ra) was given in a period of five days. In this system, both the uterus and vagina were treated to similar doses, without any distinction between the tumor and adjacent normal tissues.

The following Stockholm system is where fractionated BT was first introduced. It consisted of 2-3 applications, each taking 20-30 hours. As an improvement after Paris system, uterus and vaginal doses were different, presenting a primitive conformality. In this system, intravaginal boxes and an intrauterine tube were used as applicators. A total dose of 6500-

7100 mg Ra was given, 4500 mg Ra of this by the vaginal box. Both Paris and Stockholm systems had a single line for radioactive sources, reaching to the most proximal end of the uterine cavity to ensure dose ranges in paracervical areas.

In later years, more intricate applicator systems were designed. One of the pioneers in the field, Fletcher designed an applicator system with an intrauterine tandem coupled with two colpostats, which was later improved by Suit and Delclos, respectively (Delclos et al. 1980). This applicator consisted of two ovoid colpostats placed bilaterally to a tandem that reaches to the whole length of the uterine cavity (Figure 1).

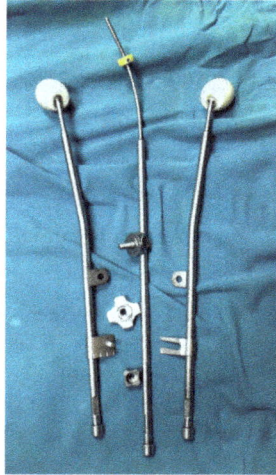

Fig. 1. Fletcher-Suit-Delclos applicator consisting of one intrauterine tandem flanked by two ovoids

Another common applicator in use was designed by Henschke, first introduced in 1960 (Henschke 1960). This applicator had the same intrauterine tandem, but instead of ovoid colpostats, a ring colpostat was used to hold the cervix in place (Figure 2).

A recent study comparing these two system showed that ring applicator was superior to tandem-ovoid applicator in dose distribution (Thirion et al. 2005). Here, an emphasis has to be made. The vital decision in the treatment of cervical cancer is whether brachytherapy is used, rather than how. Experience through skill and imagination is more critical than the choice of applicator (Nag et al. 1999). Hence, current guidelines are not recommending any type of applicator but one that the physician is familiar with.

When Manchester system was introduced in 1938 (Tod 1938) and later revised by Tod and Meredith in 1953 (Tod and Meredith 1953), it brought along a big improvement; a way to determine doses prescribed to points representing the targets. They defined anatomical points that would not change from patient to patient, also were independent on applicators of choice. They observed radiation necrosis in rectum and bladder due to high doses, consequently leading them to define a point corresponding to paracervical triangle, which is accepted as the main limiting factor in irradiation of the cervix. Point A, as they proposed, is 2 cm superior from the mucous membrane of the cervix and 2 cm lateral to the uterine canal. In later years, a second Point B was described, corresponding to parametrial wall, 3 cm lateral to Point A in the same horizontal plane (Figure 3).

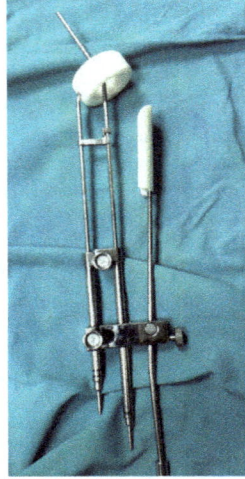

Fig. 2. Ring applicator consisting of one intrauterine tandem encircled by a shielded ring.

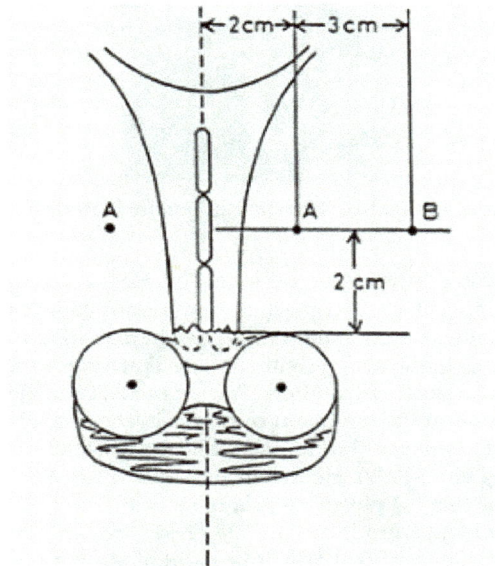

Fig. 3. Point A and B defined by International Commission on Radiation Units and Measurements (ICRU) 38 report published in 1985.

When dose distributions were inspected, it was noticed that Point A was located in a distance where the dose decreased steeply. This fired discussions regarding the reliability of Point A doses, when small changes in applicator placements could result in dire dose differences. In the International Commission on Radiation Units and Measurements (ICRU) 38 report published in 1985, recommendations were made to achieve a common ground in treating and reporting intracavitary brachytherapy for the cervical cancer. In addition to Point A and B, reference points corresponding to bladder wall, rectum and bony structures were described. The bladder reference point was located according to the Foley catheter inserted into the bladder. The posterior surface of the balloon of the catheter on the lateral radiograph was marked as the bladder reference point. Similarly, posterior vaginal wall was visualized on lateral radiographs; 5 mm posterior on a line drawn at the lower end of the intrauterine source was assigned as the rectal reference point (Figure 4 and Figure 5).

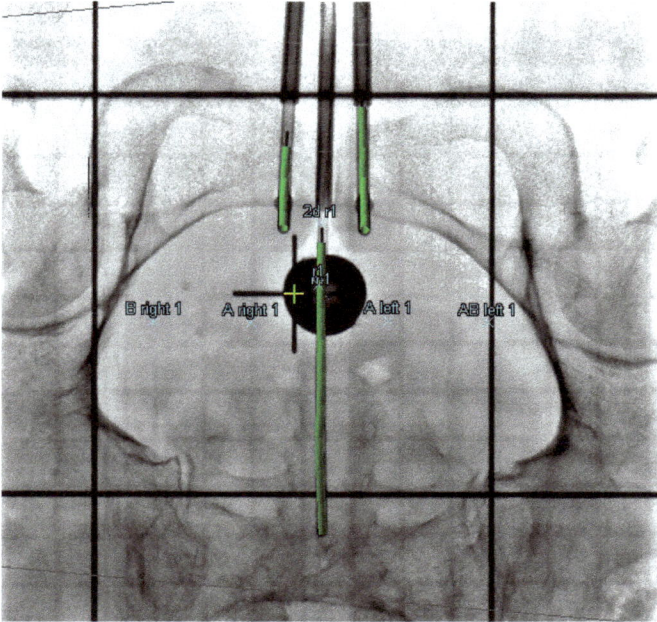

Fig. 4. Bilateral Points A, B, bladder reference point (m1), rectal reference point (r1) on antero-posterior radiograph. Rectal and bladder reference points are superimposed on this image.

The ABS published thoroughly detailed guidelines for intracavitary brachytherapy for carcinoma of the cervix (Nag et al. 2000; Nag et al. 2002). Again, the steep dose gradient where Point A is located was criticized and the many definitions of its location addressed (Nag et al. 2002). To overcome the diversity resulting from these differences, they suggested a detailed description of Point A, as well as other reference points for rectum, bladder and regional lymph nodes.

The main pitfall of the conventional brachytherapy planning stems from its basic idea to determine doses according to reference points which are thought to represent targets. The reference points in conventional BT does not change in accordance with tumor geometry, nor do the reference points for the organs at risk (OARs) in accordance to their respective positions or volumes. An ideal conventional BRT planning with strict respect to the guidelines ensure reproducible and comparable Point A doses between patients. However, that is not to say that each patient has similar dose coverage within their tumor, seeing they each are bound to have different tumor extensions. What is more, decrease in the tumor volume due to radiation effects presents different target volumes for each BT session. Timing of the BT present another struggle, drawing a line between facing the tumor at its initial size or the possibility of facing a completely recovered cervix at the end of EBRT. In that respect, Point A and B doses offer a false sense of security since both fail to show any undercoverage of the tumor.

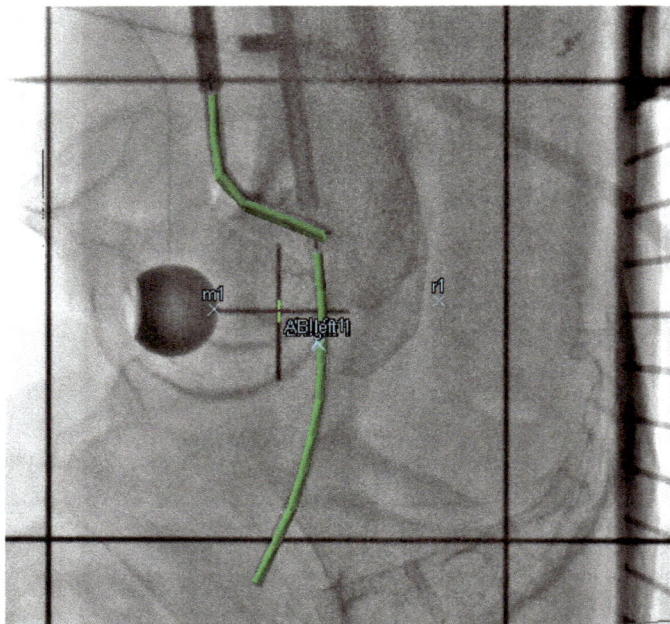

Fig. 5. Bilateral Points A, B, bladder reference point (m1), rectal reference point (r1) on lateral radiograph. Points A and B are superimposed on this image.

Same argument goes for OARs as well. Bladder reference point is reasonably better located, relying on the balloon of the intravesical catheter. This point coincides with the bladder wall, but in conventional BT planning systems, it is impossible to discern if this point is actually within the high dose zone on the bladder. In rectal reference point on the other hand, the point is located according to a visualized vaginal wall border. Except for the experienced eye, it is very hard to make this distinction. Therefore it is possible that the rectal reference point may be located somewhere between the posterior vagina and rectal lumen. Again, it is impossible to know whether this point coincides with the high dose zone within the rectum. In addition, considering both the bladder and the rectum are luminal voluminous organs, trusting a single point to represent the whole organ for every BT session is a big assumption to make.

5. 3D CT-based brachytherapy

Due to target volume irregularities and the close proximity of the target to surrounding organs, such as the rectum, bladder and bowel, it is technically difficult to deliver proper radiation doses to the target volume. It is therefore problematic to achieve a homogenous radiation dose distribution with conventional 2D plans. Furthermore, it is difficult to assess the organs at risk associated with each dose, especially for doses delivered to the rectum and bladder. The integration of computers and treatment planning systems, especially 3-dimensional (3D) computed tomography (CT) planning techniques, enables easier evaluation of the target volume coverage than previous techniques and allows accurate assessment of the dose delivered to OARs during treatment, which aids in the prediction of toxicity risk (Figure 6). In 3D conformal radiotherapy (CRT), dose-volume histograms (DVH) are delivered for assessment of target volume and OARs doses (Figure 7).

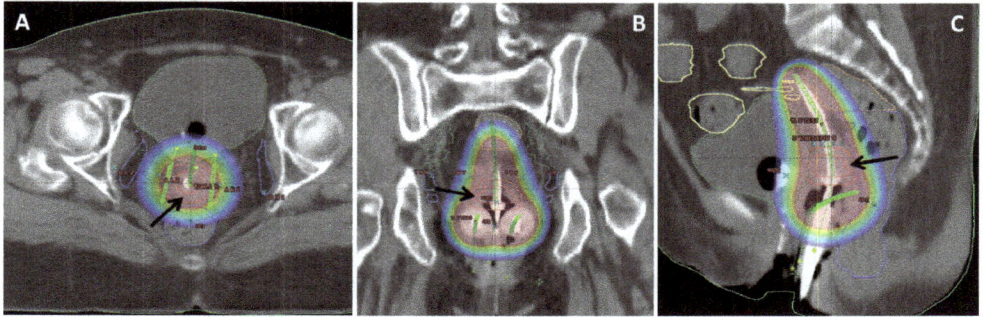

Fig. 6. Dose distribution of brachytherapy application in (A) axial, (B) coronal and (C) saggital images. The dose is prescribed to target volume (CTV) (arrow). The prescribed dose was demonstrated in red area.

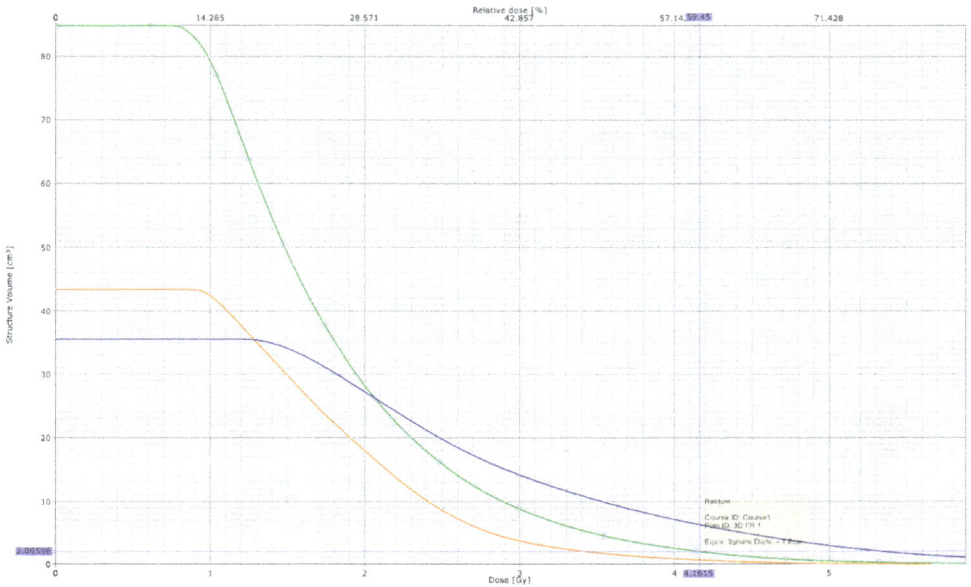

Fig. 7. Dose-volume histogram of a patient demonstrating doses of target volume (orange) and organs at risk (rectum, green; bladder, dark blue).

With the introduction of CT to radiotherapy planning, target delineation have come under spotlight. Instead of indirect ways to calculate doses received by the target, direct visualization of dose distributions within the target volume could be evaluated. What was more; organs at risk could now be delineated instead of assessment through reference points. It was no surprise this renovation happened in the field of brachytherapy. In 1987, Ling published the first CT guided ICBT for gynecological cancers (Ling et al. 1987). In 2004, guidelines were published by Image-Guided Brachytherapy Working Group (Nag et al. 2004). Many studies comparing image based planning techniques with conventional BT planning were published since then (Potter et al. 2000; Wachter-Gerstner et al. 2003; Shin et al. 2006; Onal et al. 2009). The common findings focus around accurate target delineation, better tumor coverage, accurate OARs dose determination and lower normal tissue doses (i.e. rectum, bladder and sigmoid colon). For compared local control and survival data, more studies with adequate follow-up are needed.

5.1 Target volumes

Whether 2D or 3D based, brachytherapy plays a major role in curative treatment of cervical cancer. As in other tumor sites, 3D image guidance in radiotherapy planning has introduced new concepts of gross target volume (GTV) and its derivatives clinical target volume (CTV) and planning target volume (PTV).

For conformal RT, as well as CT-guided BT, some volumes are defined according to ICRU.

- **Gross Tumor Volume (GTV):** Gross palpable or visible/demonstrable extent and location of malignant growth
- **Clinical Target Volume (CTV):** Tissue volume that contains a GTV and/or subclinical microscopic malignant disease, which has to be treated with RT. In fact, CTV is an anatomical-clinical concept, that has to be defined before a choice of treatment modality and technique is made
- **Planning Target Volume (PTV):** Defined to select appropriate beam sizes and beam arrangements, taking into consideration the net effect of all the possible geometrical variations and inaccuracies in order to ensure that the prescribed dose is actually absorbed in the CTV. Its size and shape depend on the CTV but also on the treatment technique used, to compensate for the effects of organ and patient movement, and inaccuracies in beam and patient setup
- **Treated Volume:** Volume enclosed by an isodose surface (e.g. 95% isodose), selected and specified by radiation oncologist as being appropriate to achieve the purpose of treatment. Ideally, Treated Volume would be identical to PTV, but may also be considerably larger than PTV
- **Irradiated Volume:** Tissue volume which receives a dose that is considered significant in relation to normal tissue tolerance. Dose should be expressed either in absolute values or relative to the specified dose to the PTV.

During CT-guided BRT, especially GTV delineation is essential; however either CTV or PTV is preferred for prescribing the radiation doses. Other volumes defined by ICRU are usually used for external beam RT rather than BT.

GTV is considered as one of the important prognostic factor for cervical cancer. However there are still some problems remaining in delineation of target volumes, especially GTV, CTV, PTV. For this reason, there are some guidelines and recommendations made for defining target volumes (Haie-Meder et al. 2005; Potter et al. 2005; Potter et al. 2006).

Accurate delineation of GTV, definition and delineation of CTV and PTV, as well as of critical organs has a direct impact on BT procedure, especially if it is possible to adapt the pear-shape isodose by optimisation allowing DVH analysis for a fixed dose and/or a fixed volume.

GEC-ESTRO decided in 2000 to support and promote 3D imaging based 3D treatment planning approach in cervix cancer BT. A Working Group (WG) was founded (Gynaecological (GYN) GEC-ESTRO WG), which was based on contribution of physicians and physicists from different centers actively involved in this field at that time. The task was to describe basic concepts and terms for this approach and to work out a terminology which would enable various groups working in this field to use a common language for appropriately communicating their results.

In order to take into account major concepts that are basically different and solve the problems in delineating the target volumes, but have both a significant clinical background, two CTVs are proposed by GEC-ESTRO WG:

*   A 'high risk' CTV (HR CTV): with a major risk of local recurrence because of residual macroscopic disease. The intent is to deliver a total dose as high as possible and appropriate to eradicate all residual macroscopic tumour.
*   An 'intermediate risk' CTV (IR CTV) with a major risk of local recurrence in areas that correspond to initial macroscopic extent of disease with at most residual microscopic disease at time of BT. The intent is to deliver a total radiation dose appropriate to cure significant microscopic disease in cervix cancer, which corresponds to a dose of at least 60 Gy.

In, 2004 The Image-Guided Brachytherapy Working Group, consisting of representatives from the Gynecology Oncology Group (GOG), Radiologic Physics Center (RPC), American Brachytherapy Society (ABS), American College of Radiology (ACR), American College of Radiology Imaging Network (ACRIN), American Association of Physicists in Medicine (AAPM), Radiation Therapy Oncology Group (RTOG), and American Society for Therapeutic Radiology and Oncology (ASTRO), proposed guidelines for image-based brachytherapy for cervical cancer (Nag et al. 2004). The Working Group proposes that the primary GTV be defined through imaging ($GTV_{(I)}$) plus any clinically visualized or palpable tumor extensions. This volume is meant to include the entire determinable tumor (the primary tumor in the cervix and its extensions to the parametria as determined by MRI plus the clinical examination). Because the actual target volume for ICBT remains uncertain, the GTV_{cx} is defined as the GTV plus the entire cervix. If the entire cervix is involved by tumor, the GTV and GTV_{cx} will be the same.

In 2003, the study group from Vienna University Hospital published their comparative evaluation of radiograph based BT plan versus CT and MR guided planning (Wachter-Gerstner et al. 2003). As one of the older schools practicing 3D image based brachytherapy, they also marked the differences between the three modalities. They introduced a parameter for conformity; a relation between the 95 % isodose volume and target volume. MRI based BT plans presented statistically significant conformity compared to radiograph based plans without any increase in the bladder and rectum doses. In the patients who had both CT and MRI at the beginning of BT, they found that target volumes delineated on CT images were 1.2 times larger than the volumes delineated on MRI images. Consequently, MRI plans enabled dose escalation compared to conventional plans by a factor of 1.38. In CT plans, this factor was 1.24. They were also one of the first groups that mentioned the need for interstitial brachytherapy, based on the fact that individualized dose distribution was limited by intracavitary BT only, particularly in patients with parametrial extension.

Shin et al. evaluated 30 brachytherapy plans in 2006 (Shin et al. 2006). To run a thorough comparison between conventional and CT based BT planning, they used the following entities: Coverage index (CI) is the fraction of target receiving a dose equal to or greater than the reference dose. External volume index (EI) is the ratio of the normal tissue volume outside the target receiving a dose equal to or greater than the reference dose. Conformal index (COIN), which was first introduced by van't Riet and Baltas (van't Riet et al. 1997; Baltas et al. 1998), is a formulation related to the ratio of CTV volume receiving the reference dose. In an ideal plan, it should be equal to 1 and best dose distributions are achieved when COIN is nearing to 1. In their report, they classified the patients into two groups; 20 patients were in Group 1 where the 100% reference dose (V_{ref}) to Point A fully encompassed the CTVs, and 10 patients were in Group 2, where the 100% reference dose to Point A failed to encompass the CTVs. They found that Group 2 CTVs were significantly larger than Group 1. Upon a closer look, all patients' pretreatment MRI findings and tumor diameter were similar; meaning Group 2 consisted of patients with poorer response to external radiotherapy. They found that V_{ref} for all patients and Group 1 was significantly reduced in CTV plans. CI of the CTV plan for all patients and Group 2 patients were better than conventional plan. EI was reduced in CTV plan for all patients and Group 1 patients. Similarly, COIN for all patients and Group 1 patients were greater in CTV plan, which corresponds, as expected, to higher conformity. As for OAR doses, their comparison yielded interesting results. They ascertained that conventional planning underestimates maximal bladder and rectum doses, both of which were significantly reduced in Group 1 patients with CTV plans. In their analysis, Group 2 patients (i.e. patients with larger CTVs) had significantly higher bladder and rectum volumes receiving 50%, 80% and 100% of the reference dose. They discussed the reason for this lack of decrease comes from the reference isodose line covering an irregularly shaped, large CTV, especially in lateral directions to meet parametrial extension. They emphasized that even if the conventional plan has lower mean OAR doses, it fails to cover the CTV to the full, thus resulting in cold spots particularly in parametria, consequently leading to local failure (Petereit and Pearcey 1999; Katz and Eifel 2000).

Closely following this report, Datta et al. published their comparative results (Datta et al. 2006). They pointed out that despite the common acceptance of ICRU 38 reference doses; these point doses were usually not reported (Potter et al. 2001). In their assessment they found that in larger tumors, particularly those with parametrial extension, conventional planning failed to fully cover the tumors. 100% coverage of the tumor ranged from 60.8% to 100%, with tumor volume at the beginning of the ICBT being inversely related. Again, they emphasized the underestimation of ICRU 38 maximal bladder and rectum point doses in light of literature even with large patient numbers (Katz and Eifel 2000).

In a similar study done by this group, Onal et al. evaluated 62 plans in 29 patients comparing conventional plans with CT based plans (Onal et al. 2009). The authors classified the patients into two groups on the basis of whether the 95% isodose line to Point A dose encompassed the CTV or not. The mean percentage of target coverage decreased with increasing tumor size and stage, especially in patients with vaginal or parametrial extensions. The mean percentage of GTV and CTV encompassed within Point A isodose level was 93.1% and 88.2%, respectively. According to guidelines, the minimum dose in the 2 and 5 cc volumes receiving the highest dose (D2cc and D5cc) for rectum and bladder were calculated. On the matter of whole organ volume versus organ wall contouring in assessing rectal and bladder doses, D2 provides a reliable value, since D2 for the whole organ volume is almost the same as the D2 for the organ wall, which represents the tissue exposed to the highest dose. The clinical importance of D5 in predicting fistula formation has been previously published (Cengiz et al. 2008). In this analysis, the mean D2 and D5 rectum doses were 1.66 and 1.42 times higher than the mean ICRU rectum dose. Likewise, the mean D2 and D5 bladder doses were 1.51 and 1.28 times higher than ICRU bladder dose, all statistically significant. In addition to rectum and bladder doses, sigmoid colon and small bowel have been shown to receive substantial dose (Kim et al. 2007). In their study, they demonstrated that the sigmoid colon received the highest mean D2 followed by small bowel and rectum. In the previous study, this group had revealed that the D2 for the small bowel was higher than D2 for sigmoid colon, and that both D2 and D5 doses for the sigmoid colon were significantly higher in larger tumors.

6. Conclusion

External RT together with ICBT are essential components in treatment of inoperable cervical cancer. With developing technology, especially integration of computer into treatment planning systems, either CT or MRI based treatment strategies both in external RT and BT achieves higher doses to target volumes and lower doses to surrounding organs, resulting in higher local control without increasing toxicities. For this reason, CT is essential for delivering better and homogenous dose distribution, which enables optimal treatment outcomes (Figure 8).

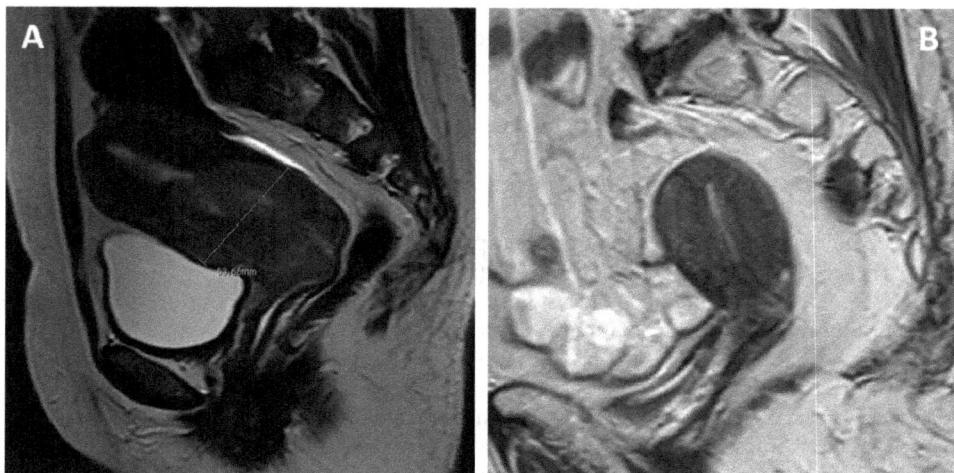

Fig. 8. (A) Magnetic resonance images of a corresponding patient demonstrating bulky tumor before treatment. Large cervical mass located in cervical os infiltrating the parametria and upper portion of the vagina. (B) Complete response after external RT and intracavitary brachytherapy.

7. References

"International Commission on Radiation Units. ICRU Report No. 38: Dose and volume specification for reporting intracavitary therapy in gynecology." *Bethesda, MD. International Commission on Radiation Units* 38: 1-23.

Akine, Y., N. Tokita, et al. (1990). "Dose equivalence for high-dose-rate to low-dose-rate intracavitary irradiation in the treatment of cancer of the uterine cervix." *Int J Radiat Oncol Biol Phys* 19(6): 1511-1514.

Alektiar, K. M., M. F. Brennan, et al. (2011). "Local control comparison of adjuvant brachytherapy to intensity-modulated radiotherapy in primary high-grade sarcoma of the extremity." *Cancer*.

Atahan, I. L., C. Onal, et al. (2007). "Long-term outcome and prognostic factors in patients with cervical carcinoma: a retrospective study." *Int J Gynecol Cancer* 17(4): 833-842.

Atahan, I. L., E. Ozyar, et al. (2008). "Vaginal high dose rate brachytherapy alone in patients with intermediate- to high-risk stage I endometrial carcinoma after radical surgery." *Int J Gynecol Cancer* 18(6): 1294-1299.

Baltas, D., C. Kolotas, et al. (1998). "A conformal index (COIN) to evaluate implant quality and dose specification in brachytherapy." *Int J Radiat Oncol Biol Phys* 40(2): 515-524.

Bourgier, C., B. Coche-Dequeant, et al. (2005). "Exclusive low-dose-rate brachytherapy in 279 patients with T2N0 mobile tongue carcinoma." *Int J Radiat Oncol Biol Phys* 63(2): 434-440.

Cengiz, M., S. Gurdalli, et al. (2008). "Effect of bladder distension on dose distribution of intracavitary brachytherapy for cervical cancer: three-dimensional computed tomography plan evaluation." *Int J Radiat Oncol Biol Phys* 70(2): 464-468.

Cleaves, M. (1903). "Radium therapy." *Med Rec* 64: 601.

Coia, L., M. Won, et al. (1990). "The Patterns of Care Outcome Study for cancer of the uterine cervix. Results of the Second National Practice Survey." *Cancer* 66(12): 2451-2456.

Datta, N. R., A. Srivastava, et al. (2006). "Comparative assessment of doses to tumor, rectum, and bladder as evaluated by orthogonal radiographs vs. computer enhanced computed tomography-based intracavitary brachytherapy in cervical cancer." *Brachytherapy* 5(4): 223-229.

Delclos, L., G. H. Fletcher, et al. (1980). "Minicolpostats, dome cylinders, other additions and improvements of the Fletcher-suit afterloadable system: indications and limitations of their use." *Int J Radiat Oncol Biol Phys* 6(9): 1195-1206.

Eifel, P. J., C. Levenback, et al. (1995). "Time course and incidence of late complications in patients treated with radiation therapy for FIGO stage IB carcinoma of the uterine cervix." *Int J Radiat Oncol Biol Phys* 32(5): 1289-1300.

Fu, K. K., T. F. Pajak, et al. (2000). "A Radiation Therapy Oncology Group (RTOG) phase III randomized study to compare hyperfractionation and two variants of accelerated fractionation to standard fractionation radiotherapy for head and neck squamous cell carcinomas: first report of RTOG 9003." *Int J Radiat Oncol Biol Phys* 48(1): 7-16.

Fu, K. K. and T. L. Phillips (1990). "High-dose-rate versus low-dose-rate intracavitary brachytherapy for carcinoma of the cervix." *Int J Radiat Oncol Biol Phys* 19(3): 791-796.

Girinsky, T., A. Rey, et al. (1993). "Overall treatment time in advanced cervical carcinomas: a critical parameter in treatment outcome." *Int J Radiat Oncol Biol Phys* 27(5): 1051-1056.

Guedea, F., J. Venselaar, et al. (2010). "Patterns of care for brachytherapy in Europe: updated results." *Radiother Oncol* 97(3): 514-520.

Haie-Meder, C., R. Potter, et al. (2005). "Recommendations from Gynaecological (GYN) GEC-ESTRO Working Group (I): concepts and terms in 3D image based 3D treatment planning in cervix cancer brachytherapy with emphasis on MRI assessment of GTV and CTV." *Radiother Oncol* 74(3): 235-245.

Henschke, U. K. (1960). ""Afterloading" applicator for radiation therapy of carcinoma of the uterus." *Radiology* 74: 834.

Katz, A. and P. J. Eifel (2000). "Quantification of intracavitary brachytherapy parameters and correlation with outcome in patients with carcinoma of the cervix." *Int J Radiat Oncol Biol Phys* 48(5): 1417-1425.

Kim, R. Y., S. Shen, et al. (2007). "Image-based three-dimensional treatment planning of intracavitary brachytherapy for cancer of the cervix: dose-volume histograms of the bladder, rectum, sigmoid colon, and small bowel." *Brachytherapy* 6(3): 187-194.

Koukourakis, G., N. Kelekis, et al. (2009). "Brachytherapy for prostate cancer: a systematic review." *Adv Urol*: 327945.

Ling, C. C., M. C. Schell, et al. (1987). "CT-assisted assessment of bladder and rectum dose in gynecological implants." *Int J Radiat Oncol Biol Phys* 13(10): 1577-1582.

Mazeron, J. J., J. M. Ardiet, et al. (2009). "GEC-ESTRO recommendations for brachytherapy for head and neck squamous cell carcinomas." *Radiother Oncol* 91(2): 150-156.

Montana, G. S., A. L. Hanlon, et al. (1995). "Carcinoma of the cervix: patterns of care studies: review of 1978, 1983, and 1988-1989 surveys." *Int J Radiat Oncol Biol Phys* 32(5): 1481-1486.

Nag, S., H. Cardenes, et al. (2004). "Proposed guidelines for image-based intracavitary brachytherapy for cervical carcinoma: report from Image-Guided Brachytherapy Working Group." *Int J Radiat Oncol Biol Phys* 60(4): 1160-1172.

Nag, S., C. Chao, et al. (2002). "The American Brachytherapy Society recommendations for low-dose-rate brachytherapy for carcinoma of the cervix." *Int J Radiat Oncol Biol Phys* 52(1): 33-48.

Nag, S., B. Erickson, et al. (2000). "The American Brachytherapy Society recommendations for high-dose-rate brachytherapy for carcinoma of the endometrium." *Int J Radiat Oncol Biol Phys* 48(3): 779-790.

Nag, S., B. Erickson, et al. (2000). "The American Brachytherapy Society recommendations for high-dose-rate brachytherapy for carcinoma of the cervix." *Int J Radiat Oncol Biol Phys* 48(1): 201-211.

Nag, S., C. Orton, et al. (1999). "The American brachytherapy society survey of brachytherapy practice for carcinoma of the cervix in the United States." *Gynecol Oncol* 73(1): 111-118.

Onal, C., G. Arslan, et al. (2009). "Comparison of conventional and CT-based planning for intracavitary brachytherapy for cervical cancer: target volume coverage and organs at risk doses." *J Exp Clin Cancer Res* 28: 95.

Orton, C. G. (1991). "Fractionated high dose rate versus low dose rate cervix cancer regimens." *Br J Radiol* 64(768): 1165-1166.

Orton, C. G. (1998). "High and low dose-rate brachytherapy for cervical carcinoma." *Acta Oncol* 37(2): 117-125.

Orton, C. G., M. Seyedsadr, et al. (1991). "Comparison of high and low dose rate remote afterloading for cervix cancer and the importance of fractionation." *Int J Radiat Oncol Biol Phys* 21(6): 1425-1434.

Patel, F. D., S. C. Sharma, et al. (1994). "Low dose rate vs. high dose rate brachytherapy in the treatment of carcinoma of the uterine cervix: a clinical trial." *Int J Radiat Oncol Biol Phys* 28(2): 335-341.

Petereit, D. G. and R. Pearcey (1999). "Literature analysis of high dose rate brachytherapy fractionation schedules in the treatment of cervical cancer: is there an optimal fractionation schedule?" *Int J Radiat Oncol Biol Phys* 43(2): 359-366.

Petereit, D. G., J. N. Sarkaria, et al. (1995). "The adverse effect of treatment prolongation in cervical carcinoma." *Int J Radiat Oncol Biol Phys* 32(5): 1301-1307.

Potter, R., J. Dimopoulos, et al. (2005). "Recommendations for image-based intracavitary brachytherapy of cervix cancer: the GYN GEC ESTRO Working Group point of view: in regard to Nag et al. (Int J Radiat Oncol Biol Phys 2004;60:1160-1172)." *Int J Radiat Oncol Biol Phys* 62(1): 293-295; author reply 295-296.

Potter, R., C. Haie-Meder, et al. (2006). "Recommendations from gynaecological (GYN) GEC ESTRO working group (II): concepts and terms in 3D image-based treatment planning in cervix cancer brachytherapy-3D dose volume parameters and aspects of 3D image-based anatomy, radiation physics, radiobiology." *Radiother Oncol* 78(1): 67-77.

Potter, R., T. H. Knocke, et al. (2000). "Definitive radiotherapy based on HDR brachytherapy with iridium 192 in uterine cervix carcinoma: report on the Vienna University Hospital findings (1993-1997) compared to the preceding period in the context of ICRU 38 recommendations." *Cancer Radiother* 4(2): 159-172.

Potter, R., E. Van Limbergen, et al. (2001). "Survey of the use of the ICRU 38 in recording and reporting cervical cancer brachytherapy." *Radiother Oncol* 58(1): 11-18.

Shin, K. H., T. H. Kim, et al. (2006). "CT-guided intracavitary radiotherapy for cervical cancer: Comparison of conventional point A plan with clinical target volume-based three-dimensional plan using dose-volume parameters." *Int J Radiat Oncol Biol Phys* 64(1): 197-204.

Stitt, J. A., J. F. Fowler, et al. (1992). "High dose rate intracavitary brachytherapy for carcinoma of the cervix: the Madison system: I. Clinical and radiobiological considerations." *Int J Radiat Oncol Biol Phys* 24(2): 335-348.

Teshima, T., T. Inoue, et al. (1993). "High-dose rate and low-dose rate intracavitary therapy for carcinoma of the uterine cervix. Final results of Osaka University Hospital." *Cancer* 72(8): 2409-2414.

Thirion, P., C. Kelly, et al. (2005). "A randomised comparison of two brachytherapy devices for the treatment of uterine cervical carcinoma." *Radiother Oncol* 74(3): 247-250.

Thomadsen, B. R., S. Shahabi, et al. (1992). "High dose rate intracavitary brachytherapy for carcinoma of the cervix: the Madison system: II. Procedural and physical considerations." *Int J Radiat Oncol Biol Phys* 24(2): 349-357.

Tod, M. and W. J. Meredith (1953). "Treatment of cancer of the cervix uteri, a revised Manchester method." *Br J Radiol* 26(305): 252-257.

Tod, M., Meredith, W. (1938). "A dosage system for use in the treatment of cancer of the uterine cervix." *Br J Radiol* 11: 809-824.

van't Riet, A., A. C. Mak, et al. (1997). "A conformation number to quantify the degree of conformality in brachytherapy and external beam irradiation: application to the prostate." *Int J Radiat Oncol Biol Phys* 37(3): 731-736.

Wachter-Gerstner, N., S. Wachter, et al. (2003). "The impact of sectional imaging on dose escalation in endocavitary HDR-brachytherapy of cervical cancer: results of a prospective comparative trial." *Radiother Oncol* 68(1): 51-59.

6

The Locally Adapted Scaling Vector Method: A New Tool for Quantifying Anisotropic Structures in Bone Images

Roberto Monetti et al.[*]

Max-Planck-Institut für extraterrestrische Physik, Garching
Germany

1. Introduction

Osteoporosis is a metabolic bone disorder in which bones become brittle and prone to fracture. According to the World Health Organization, it is characterized by the loss of bone mineral density and the deterioration of the bone micro-architecture (Prevention and Management of Osteoporosis, 2003). One of the most important factors in determining the risk of fracture is the bone strength. In clinical practice, the risk of fracture and the effects of drug therapy are assessed using only densitometric techniques as a quantitative measure (Kanis, 2002; Kanis, 2007).

Modern high-resolution imaging modalities like High-Resolution Computer Tomography (HRCT) and High-Resolution Magnetic Resonance Imaging (HRMRI) open up new possibilities to improve diagnostic techniques of osteoporosis since they are able to depict the architecture of trabecular bone. In particular, recent advances in MRI technology allow us to obtain images with in-plane spatial resolution as high as 50 µm in vitro and 150 µm in vivo, and a slice thickness of 128 µm in vitro and 280 µm in vivo (Link, et al., 1999; Carballido-Gamio et al., 2006; Wehrli, 2007; Krug et al., 2006). These figures should be compared with the actual thickness of the trabeculae, which ranges from 80 to 200 µm with an average size of approximately 120 µm. It has been shown that these imaging modalities enable the assessment of image data with respect to textural properties to detect structural differences (Boutry et al., 2003; Majumdar et al., 1996; Vieth et al., 2001).

HRCT is the preferred methodology to image bones. In contrast to MRI scans, CT scans can easily be calibrated using phantoms, thus rendering images with a standardize grey level distribution. In addition, CT images of the bone are free from the susceptibility artifacts and, in case of in vivo applications, have a less stringent requirement for patients to remain absolutely motionless during the scan as compared to MRI.

---

[*] Jan Bauer[2], Thomas Baum[2], Irina Sidorenko[1], Dirk Müller[2], Felix Eckstein[3], Thomas Link[4] and Christoph Räth[1]

[1]*Max-Plack-Institut für extraterrestrische Physik, Garching, Germany,* [2]*Institut für Röntgendiagnostik, Technische Universität München, München, Germany,* [3]*Institute of Anatomy and Musculoskeletal Research, Paracelsus Private Medical University, Salzburg, Austria,* [4]*Magnetic Resonance Science Center, Department of Radiology, UCSF, San Francisco, CA, USA*

Structure analysis techniques analogous to bone histomorphometry have been successfully applied in several in vivo studies of postmenopausal women to differentiate patients with and without osteoporotic fractures (Laib et al., 2002; Link et al., 2002; Majumdar et al, 1999; Phan et al., 2006; Link et al, 1998). However, these parameters, which are 2D linear measures, may show limitations when describing the complex 3D micro-architecture of human trabecular bone that contains non-linear correlations (Räth et al., 2003). It was shown in (Räth et al., 2003) that surrogate images generated from trabecular bone images which conserve the autocorrelation function display a different structure and can easily be distinguished using non-linear structure measures. On the other hand, texture measures extracted from HRMR and HRCT tomographic images of bone tissue using the Scaling Index Method (SIM) are well-suited for the description of the trabecular bone micro-architecture and its biomechanical properties (Baum et al., 2010; Müller et al., 2006). In contrast to the above mentioned 2D linear measures, bone structure parameters obtained using the SIM are 3D local texture measures which can account for the non-linear aspects of the trabecular network. The SIM is a tool inspired by the analysis of non-linear systems where it has been shown that global and local scaling properties of the phase space representation of a system provide useful information that characterize its underlying dynamics (Grassberger et al., 1998; Halsley et al., 1996; Paladini et al., 1987). This technique has also been successfully used in other fields of research, like astrophysics, biological applications and image processing (Räth et al., 2002; Räth et al., 2003; Jamitzky et al., 2000; Räth et al., 1997). Since the SIM considers different orientations on the image as equivalent, the derived structure parameters are isotropic. However, there are cases where the image structure reflects the anisotropy of the bone tissue. In fact, human proximal femur is a clear example where a large portion of bone tissue displays a mineralized trabecular network oriented along the major stress lines. The orientation of the trabecular structure is the result of the response of the mineral network growing mechanism to the external stimuli to maximize bone stability (Huiskes et al., 2000). Then, one expects that methods to predict bone mechanical properties based on image texture analysis will perform better when being able to quantify the intrinsic anisotropy of bone images.

Proximal femur fractures are the most severe complications of osteoporosis, with the highest morbidity and mortality (Center et al., 1999). Bone mineral density of the proximal femur measured using dual X-ray absorptiometry (DXA) is considered to be the standard technique for predicting fracture risk and the effects of drug therapy. DXA-based 2D-BMD is a bulk measure of mineralization that also accounts for the contribution of cortical bone, which is particularly important for the bone stability. Although BMD has already shown to have good correlation with bone strength, other properties of the bone like trabecular structure and connectivity may also contribute.

The aim of this chapter is to introduce a new methodology for the structure analysis of high-resolution tomographic images of human bone specimens able to account for orientations in the trabecular bone network. The so-called Locally Adapted Scaling Vector Method (LASVM) consists of two steps, namely the estimation of local main orientations and the subsequent application of an image structure analysis procedure that uses the previously obtained directional information. By means of the LASVM, we extract 3D non-linear texture measures, which locally take into account the anisotropic nature of the trabecular net. These measures are subsequently used to establish correlations with the biomechanical properties of bone specimens expressed via the fracture load. The purpose is to compare our results with those obtained using BMD, 2D morphometric parameters, and 3D isotropic texture measures derived from the (isotropic) SIM. In addition, we investigate if multifactorial models utilizing BMD and structural parameters can predict bone strength better than BMD alone.

2. Material and methods

2.1 Femur specimens

Femur specimens were harvested from 148 formalin-fixed human cadavers. The donors had dedicated their body for educational and research purposes to the Institute of Anatomy in Munich prior to death, in compliance with local institutional and legislative requirements. Aside from osteoporosis, all pathological bone changes like bone metastases, hematological, or metabolic bone disorders were exclusion criteria for the study. Therefore, biopsies were taken from the iliac crest of all donors and examined histologically. Furthermore, radiographs were obtained from all specimens. If fractures, osteolytic changes, or other focal abnormalities were detected in the images, the respective donor was excluded from the study. Femur specimens that fractured during preparation or had distal shaft fractures in the biomechanical testing were also excluded. Using these criteria, 94 donors were included in the study, 55 females and 39 males. The donors had a mean age ± standard deviation (SD) of 80±10 years (range 52–100 years). The body height (BH) and body weight (BW) of each donor were measured. Surrounding soft tissue was completely removed from the femora and femoral head and neck diameter were measured. The head diameter was defined as the largest diameter of the femoral head in a plane orthogonal to the femoral neck axis. The neck diameter was the smallest diameter of the neck in a plane orthogonal to the femoral neck axis. For the purpose of conservation, all specimens were stored in formalin solution during the study. The specimens were degassed at least 24 hours before imaging to prevent air artifacts.

2.2 CT Imaging

CT images of the proximal femora were acquired for the structure analysis of the trabecular bone by using a 16-row Multislice Spiral CT scanner (Sensation 16; Siemens Medical Solutions, Erlangen, Germany). The specimens were placed in plastic bags filled with 4% formalin–water solution. The plastic bags were sealed after air was removed by a vacuum pump. These bags were positioned in the scanner with mild internal rotation of the femur to simulate the conditions as in an in vivo examination of the pelvis and proximal femur. Three specimens were scanned twice with repositioning to determine reproducibility. The applied scan protocol had a collimation and a table feed of 0.75 mm and a reconstruction index of 0.5 mm. Further scanning parameters were 120 kVp, 100 mA, an image matrix of 512 x 512 pixels, and a field of view of 100 mm. From a high-resolution reconstruction algorithm (kernel U70u) resulted an in-plane spatial resolution of 0.29 x 0.29 mm^2, determined at δ=10% of the modulation transfer function. Voxel size was 0.19 x 0.19 x 0.5 mm^3. For calibration purposes, a reference phantom with a bone-like and a water-like phase (Osteo Phantom, Siemens Medical Solutions) was placed in the scanner below the specimens.

2.3 CT Image processing

Three volumes of interest (VOIs) were fitted automatically in the trabecular part of the femoral head, neck, and greater trochanter. The algorithm was described in detail by Huber (Huber et al., 2008) for trabecular BMD analysis. The outer surface of the cortical shell of the femur was segmented automatically by a threshold-based technique. The segmentation had to be corrected manually in 14 out of 94 cases due to thin cortical shell. Causes were focal bone loss due to advanced osteoporosis or adjacent anatomic structures, such as blood vessels, penetrating the cortex. After completed segmentation, an ellipsoid VOI was automatically fitted in the femoral head as well as a cylindric VOI in the femoral neck and an irregular VOI in the greater trochanter (Fig. 1). To obtain the head VOI, an ellipse was fitted to the superior bone surface points of the femoral head using a Gaussian– Newton least squares technique. The fitted ellipse was scaled down to 75% of its original size to account for cortical bone and shape irregularities of the femoral head and saved as head VOI. For the cylindrical neck VOI, an initial axis of the cylinder was established between the center of mass of the fitted ellipse and the intersection between the prolonged neck axis and the lateral bone surface. Based on this initial axis and the bone surface points of the neck, a first cube was fitted in the neck using a Gaussian–Newton least squares technique. The axis of the first cylinder was retained unchanged for the final cylinder. To account for cortical bone and shape irregularities, final cylinder length was defined as 65% of the radius of the first cylinder. The radius of the final cylinder was hereupon optimized by using the bone surface points of the neck. The final cylinder was saved as neck VOI. To define the trochanteric VOI, the cylinder axis was prolonged as far as the intersection with the lateral bone surface. Based on the relative position of the bone surface points to this intersection and the cylinder axis, surface regions corresponding to the trochanter, inferior part of the neck, and superior part of the shaft were determined. The surface region of the trochanter was used to fit a cone in the trochanter using a Gaussian–Newton least squares technique. The cone was discarded, but the relative position of the bone points to the fitted cone axis and the cylinder axis was assessed. According to their relative position, they were labeled as "trochanteric" or "nontrochanteric" bone points. The trochanteric bone points were saved as trochanteric VOI.

For all further image post-processing, images were interpolated to obtain isotropic datasets and reconstructed in a semi-coronal plane, oriented parallel to the axis of the femoral neck. For calibration purposes, a reference phantom (Osteo Phantom, Siemens) was placed below the specimens.

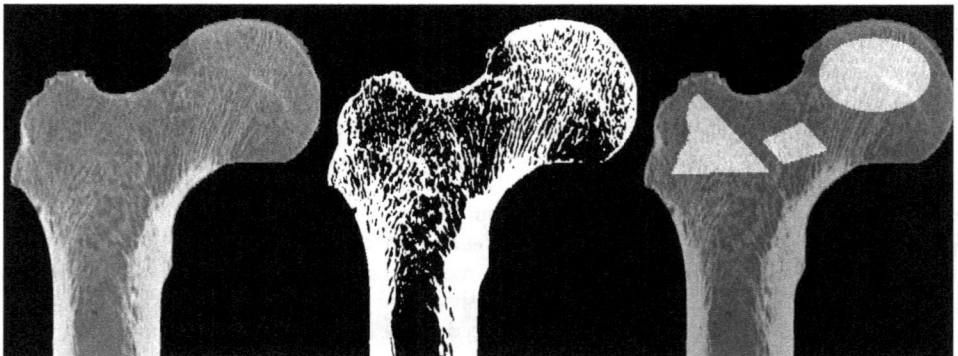

Fig. 1. Left: HRCT image of a human femur specimen with BMD = 0.69 g/cm^2 and FL = 3912 N (left). Middle: Binarized dataset according to the procedure explained in section 2.5. Right: Visualization of the fitted VOIs: head (ellipsoid), neck (cylinder), and trochanter (irregular) in the original CT data.

2.4 Biomechanical femoral bone strength

Absolute femoral bone strength was assessed with a biomechanical side-impact test measuring fracture load (FL), described in detail previously (Eckstein et al., 2004). In brief, a lateral fall on the greater trochanter was simulated. Femoral head and shaft were faced downward and could be moved independently from each other while the load was applied on the greater trochanter by using a universal testing machine (Zwick 1445; Zwick, Ulm, Germany) with a 10-kN force sensor and dedicated software. FL was defined as the peak of the load–deformation curve. Since FL depends on influencing variables such as bone size, relative femoral bone strength had to be appraised for better interpretation of the clinical utility. For appraisal of the relative bone strength, FL was adjusted femoral neck length (FNL). For this purpose, FL was divided by this parameter.

2.5 Morphometric parameters

In a first step, it was defined, which pixels should be interpreted as bone ("on"-pixels), and which as marrow ("off"-pixels). The binarization of the CT images was required to evaluate the 2D morphometric parameters. We applied an optimized global threshold to all images. To optimize this threshold, we evaluated thirty characteristic proximal femur images visually, and determined the best threshold to be 200 g/cm^3 hydroxyapatite. This hydroxyapatite threshold (Λ_{Ca}) was converted to Hounsfield units (HU) for every image using the following expression

$$\Lambda_{HU} = \frac{(B_{HU} - W_{HU})}{(B_{Ca} - W_{Ca})} \Lambda_{Ca} + W_{HU} , \qquad (1)$$

where Λ_{HU} is the grey level threshold in HU, Λ_{Ca} is the threshold evaluated in g/cm^3 of hydroxyapatite, B_{Ca} is the bone-like phase of the reference phantom in g/cm^3 of hydroxyapatite, B_{HU} is the bone-like phase of the reference phantom in HU, W_{Ca} is the water-like phase of the reference phantom in g/cm^3 of hydroxyapatite, and W_{HU} is the water-like phase of the reference phantom in HU. For further details see (Bauer et al., 2006).

After binarization, four morphometric parameters were calculated in analogy to standard histomorphometry using the mean intercept length method (Parfitt et al., 1987): bone fraction (BF) (resulting from bone volume divided by total volume), trabecular number (TbN), trabecular spacing (TbSp), and trabecular thickness (TbTh). It should be noted that the values of these parameters are considered as apparent values, since, given the limited spatial resolution, they cannot depict the true trabecular structure.

2.6 Local anisotropic structure analysis

A simple visual inspection of images of trabecular bone tissue reveals that the trabecular network and marrow bone areas are not evenly distributed. In addition, the trabecular structure of some human bones is essentially anisotropic, i.e. clear preferential directions of the mineral network are observed as a result of its growing mechanism. These image features suggest that a suitable method to assess the bone structure must be able to quantify local structure differences and account for the anisotropy of the mineral network. We propose a methodology which consists of two steps, namely the estimation of local main orientations and the subsequent application of a local image structure analysis procedure which uses the previously obtained directional information. This method, which is a variant of the Scaling Index Method (Böhm et al., 2003; Monetti et al., 2003; Müller et al., 2006), differs from previous approaches where only an average global directionality on images was considered (Monetti et al., 2004). Recently, the SIM has been applied to μ-CT images of trabecular bone (Monetti et al., 2007; Räth et al., 2008; Monetti et al., 2009) where it was demonstrated that the use of directional information allows identifying the most important load-bearing bone substructures.

As shown below, any suitable method to estimate directions in 2D or 3D can be coupled to this structure characterization procedure. Several methods have already been developed to measure the trabecular bone orientation like the tensor scale algorithm (Saha et al., 2004) or methods based on image skeletonization (Saha et al., 2000; Gomberg et al., 2000; Wehrli et al., 2001). Here, we will restrict ourselves to local directions on the image plane and estimate them using a local directional filter. For the sake of clarity, we first describe the image structure characterization procedure. Then, it becomes evident how the orientations can be coupled to it.

The SIM is a procedure to extract information from multidimensional, arbitrary point distributions by assessing local pointwise dimensions, i.e. the scaling indices, for each data point. Consider a 3D tomographic image where a gray value $g = G(x, y, z)$ is assigned to each pixel. Thus, each pixel contains space and gray value information that can be encompassed in a four dimensional vector $\vec{p} = [x, y, z, G(x, y, z)]$. Then, the 3D tomographic image $G(x, y, z)$ has been mapped onto a 4D point distribution which contains both the spatial and grey level information. For each point in the phase space, the number N of points located within an 4-dimensional sphere of radius L centered at $\vec{p}_i$ is counted,

$$N(\vec{p}_i, L) = \sum_j \Theta\left(L - \left\| \vec{p}_j - \vec{p}_i \right\|\right), \tag{2}$$

where $\Theta(x) = 1$ if $x \geq 0$ and $\Theta(x) = 0$ otherwise, is the Heaviside function. The distribution $N(\vec{p}_i, L)$ is evaluated within the so-called scaling range $L \in [L_1, L_2]$. In most of the cases, one finds that $N(\vec{p}_i, L)$ behaves approximately as a power-law when increasing L, i.e. $N(\vec{p}_i, L) \propto L^{\alpha_i}$. The scaling-index α_i can be estimated by the difference ratio

$$\alpha_i = \left[\log\left(N(\vec{p}_i, L_2)\right) - \log\left(N(\vec{p}_i, L_1)\right)\right] \Big/ \left[\log(L_2) - \log(L_1)\right], \tag{3}$$

where L_1 and L_2 are specified by the lower and upper limit of the scaling range. This scalar quantity contains information of the underlying local structure around $\vec{p}_i$. For instance, given a 3D point distribution, different structural elements like rods, plates, and a random background will lead to scaling index values $\alpha \approx 1$, $\alpha \approx 2$, $\alpha \approx 3$, respectively (Müller et al., 2006). The assessment of cancellous bone local structure type is an important issue already investigated using the so-called structure model index (SMI) (Hildebrand et al., 1997). This technique also allows the quantification of plate, rod objects or mixture of plates and rods by using an index value. The SMI was defined as a value between 0 and 3. For an ideal plate structure the structure model index value is 0 and it is 3 for an ideal rod structure. For a structure with both plates and rods of equal thickness, the value is between 0 and 3, depending on the volume ratio between rods and plates. The calculation of the SMI requires a binarization of the images. Typical applications of the SMI are connected to the use of μ-CT images. These studies (Hildebrand et al., 1999; Ding et al., 2000) address questions like age-related cancellous bone structure changes and demonstrate the cancellous bone structure variability for different skeletal sites.

Scaling indices can also be calculated using a different method. In general, instead of calculating $N(\vec{p}_i, L)$, it is possible to define a local weighted cumulative point distribution ρ as

$$\rho(\vec{p}_i, R) = \sum_j \exp\left(-\left(d(\vec{p}_i, \vec{p}_j)\Big/R\right)^q\right), \tag{4}$$

where R is the scale parameter and $d(\vec{p}_i, \vec{p}_j)$ a distance measure. The exponent q controls the weighting of points according to their distance to the point where the scaling index is calculated. For small values of q, points in a broad region around $\vec{p}_i$ significantly contribute to the weighted local density $\rho(\vec{p}_i, R)$. As q increases, the shaping function becomes more and more step-like counting all points with $d(\vec{p}_i, \vec{p}_j) < R$ and neglecting all points with $d(\vec{p}_i, \vec{p}_j) > R$. Here, we use $q=2$. The scaling index α_i is defined as the logarithmic derivative of ρ with respect to R, $\alpha = \dfrac{\partial \ln \rho}{\partial \ln R}$. Thus one obtains

$$\alpha_i = \frac{\sum_j 2\left(\dfrac{d(\vec{p}_i, \vec{p}_j)}{R}\right)^2 \exp\left(-\left(\dfrac{d(\vec{p}_i, \vec{p}_j)}{R}\right)^2\right)}{\sum_j \exp\left(-\left(\dfrac{d(\vec{p}_i, \vec{p}_j)}{R}\right)^2\right)}. \tag{5}$$

Using this procedure, scaling indices are expressed analytically and depend only on the parameter R. We call them weighted scaling indices.

Let us now focus on the distance measure $d(\vec{p}_i, \vec{p}_j)$. A generalized quadratic distance measure can be written as follows

$$d^2\left(\Delta\vec{p}_{ij}\right) = \Delta\vec{p}_{ij}{}^T A \Delta\vec{p}_{ij}, \tag{6}$$

where $A = U^T W U$ is a non-singular matrix, U is the rotation matrix and W is a diagonal matrix containing the eigenvalues of the matrix A. As in (Müller et al., 2006), the tomographic image $g = G(x, y, z)$ is mapped onto a 4D space as $\vec{p}(x, y, z, g) = (x, y, z, G(x, y, z))$. Thus, a 4D rotation matrix has to be used. The only meaningful rotations are rotations in the spatial 3D space. We consider rotations on the image plane, i.e. rotations around the z-axis. The reason for this choice is that we are using CT images of sagittal sections of the femur. We assumed no large directional changes outside the image plane ($z=$constant), since the mineralized trabeculae are mostly oriented along the major stress lines. The rotation matrix reduces to

$$U = \begin{pmatrix} \cos\theta & -\sin\theta & 0 & 0 \\ \sin\theta & \cos\theta & 0 & 0 \\ 0 & 0 & 1 & 0 \\ 0 & 0 & 0 & 1 \end{pmatrix}, \tag{7}$$

where θ is the rotation angle around the z-axis. The quadratic distance measure can be written as

$$d^2\left(\Delta\vec{p}_{ij}\right) = \lambda_x\left(\Delta x_{ij}\cos\theta + \Delta y_{ij}\sin\theta\right)^2 + \lambda_y\left(\Delta x_{ij}\sin\theta - \Delta y_{ij}\cos\theta\right)^2 + \lambda_z\left(\Delta z_{ij}\right)^2 + \lambda_g\left(\Delta g_{ij}\right)^2, \tag{8}$$

where the eigenvalues $\lambda_{k=\{x,y,z,g\}}$ are the weighting factors of the three orthogonal spatial directions and the grey-level axis, respectively. When all directions have the same weight, i.e. $\lambda_x = \lambda_y = \lambda_z = \lambda_g$, we obtain $A=I$, and d^2 becomes the (isotropic) Euclidean distance. We observe that the choice of different λ values allows us to assign different weights for the directions. It becomes clear from Eq. (8) that this variant of the SIM allows for the input of local orientations. For points where no clear directionality is observed it is always possible to set $\lambda_x = \lambda_y = \lambda_z$.

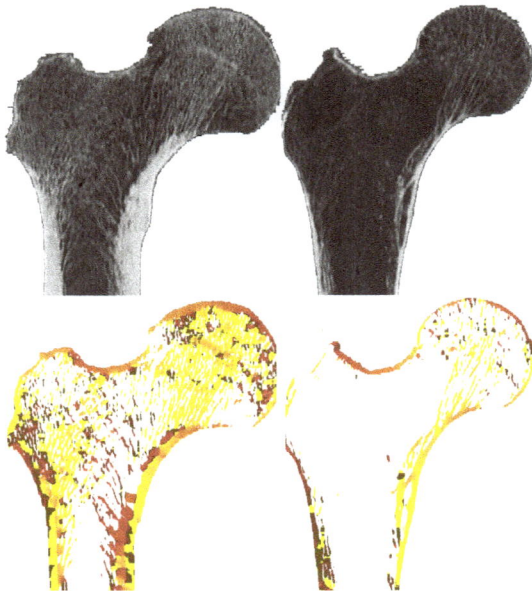

Fig. 2. First row: HRCT images of a healthy and an osteoporotic specimen. Second row: Color-represented orientation map. Trabeculae displaying the same directionality are coded with the same color. The orientations are calculated at every pixel for every bone slice.

Eq. (8) also indicates that the parameter λ_z can be used to account for the different in plane and normal to the plane resolutions and λ_g as a normalization factor for the grey level distribution. Because of the flexibility that this variant of the SIM offers, we call it the

"Locally Adapted Scaling Vector Method" (LASVM). It should be noted that the LASVM reduces to the original isotropic SIM when we set $\lambda_x = \lambda_y = \lambda_z$ for all points of the distribution. In the following, we will simply call scaling indices to the indices calculated using the "isotropic" SIM. Scaling indices obtained with LASVM are called "scaling vectors".

2.7 Calculation of the bone orientation map

To calculate local orientations of the trabecular network, we consider the CT images binarized according to the procedure given in section 2.5 (see Fig. 1 central panel). Then, the binarized images (2D CT slices) were skeletonized using the classical thinning algorithm. The predominant orientation Θ was calculated for every pixel having two neighbour pixels (defined as "rod-like" pixel), thus connection points or end points of the skeleton were excluded. To determine the final orientation map, every "bone" pixel of the binarized image was assigned the value of the orientation of the nearest rod-like pixel of the skeleton. The degree of anisotropy at every pixel was defined as $1/\sigma(\Theta)$, where $\sigma(\Theta)$ is the standard deviation of the orientations within a surrounding neighborhood of 7x7 pixels. Here, all orientations at "bone" pixels having a degree of anisotropy larger than 2 were considered. Image pixels that do not carry directional information were treated as isotropic, thus $\lambda_x = \lambda_y = \lambda_z$. Figure 2 shows typical examples of orientation maps for two femur specimens that have different bone mineral density. The colors indicate the angles evaluated using the procedure described above. It should be emphasized that the image structure characterization procedure is neither restricted to the use of orientations in 2D nor to the particular method to evaluate local directions. In fact, any suitable method to determine orientations can be coupled to the LASVM.

2.8 The structure measures

In order to quantify bone structural differences among specimens, the local information given by the scaling indices or scaling vectors is compiled in the so-called $P(\alpha) = \mathrm{Pr}(\alpha \in [\alpha, \alpha + d\alpha])$ probability density of scaling vectors or $P(\alpha)$ spectrum. As an example, we consider two dimensional binary toy images containing line-like elements and a noisy background (see Fig. 3). The purpose is to demonstrate how the sensitivity to the underlying anisotropy is enhanced, when using an anisotropic distance measure. Both images have exactly the same number of line-like elements and background points. The top-left image in Fig. 3 displays a pattern with no clear main directionality while the top right one shows a main direction given by an angle $\beta = 45°$ measured from the horizontal in the clockwise direction.

The bottom-left spectra shown in Fig. 3 were calculated applying the SIM to the upper images, i.e. using an isotropic distance measure. We observe that both spectra are quite similar, thus the clear anisotropy of the top right image is not accounted by the SIM. However, the bottom-right spectra (see Fig. 3) indicate that the use of an anisotropic distance measure enhances the contrast between the spectra and thus the sensitivity to the underlying anisotropy of the image.

Fig. 4 (upper row) shows $P(\alpha)$ spectra obtained using the (isotropic) SIM for the three segmented VOI's, i.e. femur head, neck and trochanter. We observe structural differences at the femur neck and trochanter, while the $P(\alpha)$ spectra from the femur head are quite similar.

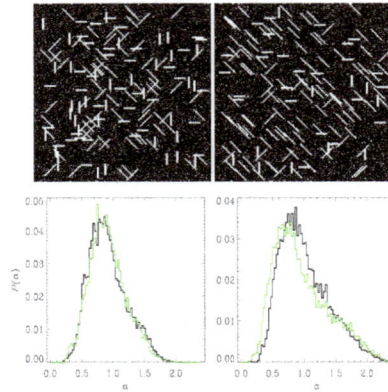

Fig. 3. Upper left: 2D toy image where a random background has been combined with randomly oriented lines. Upper right: 2D toy image where a random background has been combined with lines displaying a specific global orientation of $\beta = 45°$ with respect to the horizontal measured in the clockwise direction. The number of lines and background points is the same in both images. Lower left: $P(\alpha)$ spectra of the toy images obtained using the isotropic SIM. Lower right: $P(\alpha)$ spectra of the toy images obtained using the LASVM in 2D. Black curves are the spectra of the upper left image and green curves are the ones for the upper right image.

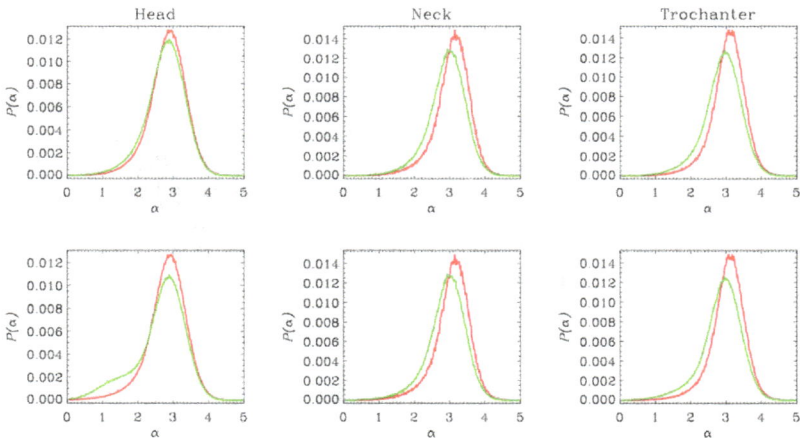

Fig. 4. $P(\alpha)$ spectra for the different VOI's of the proximal femur specimens. The green (red curve) spectrum corresponds to a specimen with BMD_DXA = 0.69 g/cm^2 and FL = 3910 N (BMD_DXA = 0.69 g/cm^2 and FL of 2450 N), respectively. From left to right, the plots show $P(\alpha)$ of the femur head, neck, and trochanter, respectively. Upper row: $P(\alpha)$ spectra obtained using an isotropic distance measure. Lower row: $P(\alpha)$ spectra for the same VOI's obtained using an anisotropic distance measure.

Figure 4 (lower row) shows the $P(\alpha)$ spectra calculated using the (anisotropic) LASVM. Now, the largest structural difference is observed in the femur head. These differences are the result of this novel structural characterization that takes into account the bone orientation map. Spectra corresponding to the femoral neck and trochanter are very similar to those calculated using the isotropic distance measure. This situation occurs in the absence of strongly oriented trabecula within the VOI, thus scaling vectors reduce to (isotropic) scaling indices. Then, we conclude that directionality assessment considerably enhances the contrast between $P(\alpha)$ spectra (see Fig 4, lower left) and improves the bone structure characterization procedure. This result is in agreement with that obtained from the analysis of the toy images.

Fig. 5 shows two HRCT image slices for specimens with equal BMD_DXA values but very different FL values. The color-coded femur sections are the corresponding α-images, i.e. the

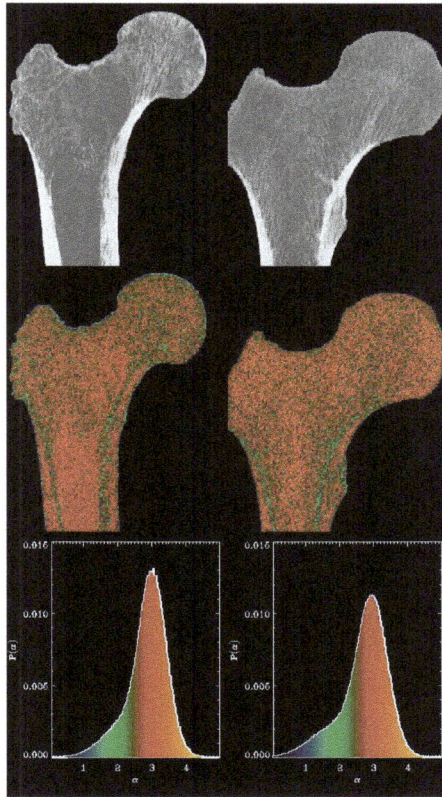

Fig. 5. First Row: HRCT images of two femur specimens with the same BMD_DXA = 0.83 and different FL = 2939 N (left) and FL = 6717 N. Second Row: Color-coded α-images of the specimens shown in the first row. Third Row: Color-coded $P(\alpha)$ spectra which helps identifying the local structures on the α-images. These results were obtained using scaling vectors.

images created using the values of the scaling vectors. Panels in the lower row of Fig. 5 show the color-coded $P(\alpha)$ spectra for the two femur specimens where the same color-coding as for the α-images was used. It is then clear that the trabecular bone structure mainly corresponds to the green-dark yellow region of the α-images, i.e. $1 < \alpha < 2.7$. We observe that the $P(\alpha)$ spectrum of the weaker femur specimen is shifted to higher α–values, thus reflecting a higher frequency of structureless (homogeneous) regions. However, the stronger femur specimen has a larger contribution of α–values corresponding to trabecular structure.

We perform a correlation analysis based on a filtering procedure applied to the $P(\alpha)$ spectrum, which considers one sliding window of variable width. Filtering procedures based on sliding windows have successfully been applied for the characterization of the bone micro-architecture in other studies (Böhm et al., 2003; Monetti et al., 2003). A characteristic quantity, called the α–fraction $\Delta_w P(\alpha)$, is extracted from the $P(\alpha)$ spectrum. Let α_i, and w be the position and width of the sliding window, respectively. We call α-fraction, the fraction of pixels with scaling vector values within the sliding window $[\alpha_i, \alpha_i + w]$. Thus, the α–fraction $\Delta_w P(\alpha)$ accounts for the structural content in window w. It should be noted that one has a simple scalar value $\Delta_w P(\alpha)$ for each individual specimen. The position and width of the window has been chosen to achieve optimal correlation between $\Delta_w P(\alpha)$ and FL. It should be noted that this kind of correlation analysis may lead to high correlation coefficients that must be disregarded. In order to avoid these outliers, one has to check if correlation coefficients are stable over a neighborhood of window positions and widths around the optimal value. Second, since our methodology allows us to retrieve the image pixels from the $P(\alpha)$ spectra, one has to check if the selected volume belongs to a particular bone substructure or corresponds to structureless marrow bone regions. It should be mentioned that our sample was not split into training and test samples due to its small size, which is otherwise the standard procedure to follow. All our results were obtained using $\lambda_g = (60/\sigma_g)^2$ and $R = 2.5$, where σ_g is the standard deviation of the grey level distribution in the VOI. We have chosen $\lambda_x = 50\lambda_y = 50\lambda_z$ to account for the local anisotropy of the trabecular structure. This defines an ellipse on the image plane of major axis approximately 14 pixels and a minor axis of 3. This eccentricity was suitable to account for anisotropy within a typical scale of the size of the apparent mean trabecular width. It should be noted that the value $\lambda_g = (60/\sigma_g)^2$ normalizes the standard deviation of the grey level distribution of the images to $\sigma_g = 60$. This is a suitable normalization choice that allows us to compare the spatial scales with the grey level scale and thus computing the distance in the above defined 4D space.

3. Results and discussion

Relationships among FL, $\Delta_w P(\alpha)$, BMD, and the 2D morphometric parameters were obtained using a linear regression analysis and a two-tailed t-test of significance as well. We have also studied the relationship between FL and the combination of a bone structure measure and BMD using a multivariate regression analysis. For the multiregression analysis, we have considered linear combinations of a structure measure and both the bone mineral density evaluated for the whole femur using DXA (BMD_DXA) and the bone mineral density evaluated for the individual VOI using QCT (BMD_QCT). In all cases, Spearman's correlation coefficients were calculated. We obtain a correlation $r=0.73$ for FL versus BMD_DXA of the whole femur. All other results are summarized in Tables 1 to 5. Table 1 shows the correlation coefficients of both the morphometric parameters and BMD_QCT versus FL for the different VOI. Tb.Sp is the morphometric parameter that correlates best with FL, when evaluated in the femur head ($r_H = 0.72$). All morphometric parameters evaluated in the femur head and neck lead to moderate correlations, while those calculated in the femur trochanter lead to lower correlation coefficients. Table 2 shows that for models combining the morphometric parameters and BMD_DXA, the prediction of femur mechanical properties is greatly improved. The best result is obtained for the femur head. However, Table 2 also indicates that BMD_QCT provides no additional information for the prediction of biomechanical strength, since some of the correlation coefficients become lower than those obtained using the morphometric parameters alone.

FL versus	BF	Tb.N	Tb.Sp	Tb.Th	BMD_QCT
r_H	0.64	0.31	-0.72	0.46	0.58
r_N	0.61	0.61	-0.51	0.58	0.58
r_{Tr}	0.49	0.52	-0.53	0.31	0.49

Table 1. Correlation coefficients calculated for the different VOI, i.e. femur head (r_H), neck (r_N), and trochanter (r_{Tr}), of the morphometric parameters versus the fracture load. The correlation coefficients of the bone mineral density evaluated using QCT versus FL are also shown.

FL versus	Tb.N	Tb.Sp	Tb.Th
r_H^D	0.78	0.76	0.76
r_N^D	0.76	0.76	0.76
r_{Tr}^D	0.76	0.76	0.76
r_H^Q	0.55	0.56	0.46
r_N^Q	0.54	0.55	0.55
r_{Tr}^Q	0.51	0.54	0.52

Table 2. Correlation coefficients indicated with a superscript "D" were calculated for the different VOI's using a linear multiregression model combining morphometric parameters and BMD_DXA. The coefficients indicated with a superscript "Q" were evaluated for the different VOI's using a linear multiregression model combining the morphometric parameters and the BMD_QCT of the respective VOI.

The results obtained using scaling indices are summarized in Tables 3-8. Table 3 shows that the α–fraction leads to low correlation coefficients versus FL for the three VOI's. For the femur head and femur neck, the bone structure that lead to the best correlations corresponds to trabecular structure. However, for the femoral trochanter, the α–fraction corresponds to marrow bone regions.

FL versus	r	Δ_w
$\Delta_w P_H(\alpha)$	0.42	$\alpha \in [2.09, 3.46]$
$\Delta_w P_N(\alpha)$	0.40	$\alpha \in [2.72, 2.86]$
$\Delta_w P_{Tr}(\alpha)$	0.13	$\alpha \in [4.43, 4.54]^*$

Table 3. Correlation coefficients for the α-fraction $\Delta_w P(\alpha)$ versus FL for the different VOI. The $P(\alpha)$ spectra were evaluated using an isotropic distance measure. The intervals show the region of the spectrum leading to the highest correlation coefficient. (*) Interval corresponding to marrow bone regions.

Table 4 shows results of a multiregression analysis combining the α–fraction and BMD_DXA for the three VOI's. We observe that the use of structural information lead to correlation coefficients higher than that obtained using BMD_DXA alone ($r=0.73$). However, only the α–fraction of the femoral head corresponds to the trabecular bone structure. Table 5 shows results of a multiregression analysis where the α–fraction has been combined with the BMD_QCT of the corresponding VOI's. We observe that correlations do not increase, thus the structural information is redundant in this case.

FL versus	r^D	Δ_w
$\Delta_w P_H(\alpha)$	0.79	$\alpha \in [2.03, 3.49]$
$\Delta_w P_N(\alpha)$	0.78	$\alpha \in [4.28, 4.42]^*$
$\Delta_w P_{Tr}(\alpha)$	0.78	$\alpha \in [3.68, 3.88]^*$

Table 4. Correlation coefficients calculated for the different VOI obtained using a linear multiregression model combining the α-fraction $\Delta_w P(\alpha)$ and BMD_DXA. The $P(\alpha)$ spectra were evaluated using an isotropic distance measure. (*) Interval corresponding to marrow bone region.

FL versus	r	Δ_w
$\Delta_w P_H(\alpha)$	0.52	$\alpha \in [2.12, 3.46]$
$\Delta_w P_N(\alpha)$	0.54	$\alpha \in [4.31, 4.51]^*$
$\Delta_w P_{Tr}(\alpha)$	0.56	$\alpha \in [3.62, 3.88]^*$

Table 5. Correlation coefficients calculated for the different VOI obtained using a linear multiregression model combining the α-fraction $\Delta_w P(\alpha)$ and BMD_QCT evaluated within the respective VOI. The $P(\alpha)$ spectra were evaluated using an isotropic distance measure. (*) Interval corresponding to marrow bone region.

Table 6 shows correlation results of FL versus the α-fraction extracted from $P(\alpha)$ spectra evaluated with the LASVM. We observe that the correlation coefficient for the femur head is significantly higher than that obtained using scaling indices ($r_H=0.42$). Even though moderate correlations are obtained at the femoral neck, the bone substructure leading to the highest correlation coefficient is the trabecular network. The femoral trochanter leads to a low correlation coefficient for an α–fraction corresponding to marrow bone regions. Note, however that this result is not significant. A multiregression analysis combining the α–fraction of the femoral head and BMD_DXA (see Table 7) leads to the highest correlation coefficient obtained in this analysis ($r_H{}^D$=0.80). Results for the multiregression model calculated for other VOI's are considered not significant.

FL versus	R	Δ_w
$\Delta_w P_H(\alpha)$	0.66	$\alpha \in [2.39, 3.21]$
$\Delta_w P_N(\alpha)$	0.37	$\alpha \in [2.72, 2.86]$
$\Delta_w P_{Tr}(\alpha)$	0.17	$\alpha \in [4.46, 4.54]$ *

Table 6. Correlation coefficients of the α-fraction $\Delta_w P(\alpha)$ versus FL for the different VOI. The $P(\alpha)$ spectra were evaluated using an anisotropic distance measure. The intervals show the region of the spectrum leading to the highest correlation coefficient. (*) Interval corresponding to marrow bone region.

FL versus	r^D	Δ_w
$\Delta_w P_H(\alpha)$	0.80	$\alpha \in [2.57, 3.07]$
$\Delta_w P_N(\alpha)$	0.78	$\alpha \in [4.28, 4.51]$ *
$\Delta_w P_{Tr}(\alpha)$	0.78	$\alpha \in [3.68, 3.94]$ *

Table 7. Correlation coefficients calculated for the different VOI obtained using a linear multiregression model combining the α-fraction $\Delta_w P(\alpha)$ and BMD_DXA. The $P(\alpha)$ spectra were evaluated using an anisotropic distance measure. (*) Interval corresponding to marrow bone region.

FL versus	r^Q	Δ_w
$\Delta_w P_H(\alpha)$	0.66	$\alpha \in [2.36, 3.25]$
$\Delta_w P_N(\alpha)$	0.54	$\alpha \in [4.31, 4.51]$ *
$\Delta_w P_{Tr}(\alpha)$	0.56	$\alpha \in [3.68, 3.88]$ *

Table 8. Correlation coefficients calculated for the different VOI obtained using a linear multiregression model combining the α-fraction $\Delta_w P(\alpha)$ and BMD_QCT evaluated within the respective VOI. The $P(\alpha)$ spectra were evaluated using an anisotropic distance measure. (*) Interval corresponding to marrow bone region.

Finally, Table 8 shows results of a multiregression analysis where the α–fraction has been combined with the BMD_QCT of the correspoding VOI's. We observe that the correlations do not increase, thus the information provided by the combined quantities is redundant.

In summary, the structure measure obtained using the LASVM leads to a correlation coefficient r=0.66 versus FL for the femoral head. This value is comparable to that given by BMD_DXA (r=0.73) and the best histomorphometric parameter Tb.Sp (r=0.72). It should be mentioned that our analysis was performed on VOI's which were defined automatically by means of geometrical considerations only. Since most of the fractures in the mechanical test occurred in the femoral neck, better correlations with *FL* might be obtained when using a larger VOI, including the whole femur neck and the distal part of the femur head. Considering that the α-fraction is a simple measure of structure, a better prediction of the biomechanical properties of the human femur is also expected when applying more refined quantities extracted from the bone structural characterization given by the LASVM.

A linear multiregression model combining the α-fraction calculated at the femoral head using the LASVM and BMD_DXA increases the correlation with the *FL* to $r=0.80$. This indicates that these two quantities are complementary and explain better the biomechanical strength of femur specimens. In contrast, a multiregression model combining the α-fraction and BMD_QCT does not explain better the biomechanical strength. BMD_DXA is a global measure of mineralization that contains a contribution of the cortical bone. However, BMD_QCT was evaluated in the VOI's, thus no contribution of the cortical shell was considered. This fact may explain the different performances of these two quantities when combined with bone structure measures in multiregression models.

A comparison between results obtained using scaling indices and scaling vectors indicates that structure measures that account for the anisotropic nature of the trabecular structure are best suited to describe the biomechanical properties of human femur in vitro.

4. Conclusions

We have introduced a new anisotropic methodology, the so-called Locally Adapted Scaling Vector Method, to characterize structures in HRCT images of human bone tissue. The LASVM is able to account for the intrinsic orientation of the trabecular net of the proximal femur. This study showed that a more accurate bone structure characterization is achieved when a detailed assessment of local orientations is performed. Because of this fact, results obtained using the new 3D non-linear local texture measure are superior to those obtained using a 3D non-linear local isotropic texture measure and comparable to those given by BMD. This suggests that anisotropic texture measures have a superior performance than isotropic ones in cases where the image structure orientation plays a relevant role. We also found that models combining bone structure measures with BMD can better predict the mechanical properties of femoral specimens. This finding is in agreement with other studies (Link et al., 2003; Monetti et al. 2004; Wigderowitz et al., 2000) where it is suggested that structure characterization and BMD measurements should regularly be applied since they are complementary techniques and provide a great deal of information on the biomechanical properties of bone specimens.

5. Acknowledgments

This study was supported by the Deutsche Forschungsgemainschaft (DFG) under the grant MU 2288/2-2. The authors are very thankful to Ernst Rummeny for stimulating discussions. We also thank Simone Kohlmann, Volker Kuhn, and Maiko Matsuura for performing the biomechanical tests, and Holger Böhm, Simone Kohlmann, and Cecilia Wunderer for scanning the specimens.

6. References

Bauer, JS.; Kohlmann, S.; Eckstein, F.; Müller, D.; Lochmüller, EM. & Link, TM. (2006). Structural analysis of trabecular bone of the proximal femur using multislice computed tomography: a comparison with dual X-ray absorptiometry for predicting biomechanical strength in vitro. *Calcif. Tissue Int.*, Vol. 78, No 2, pp.78–89

Baum, T.; Carballido-Gamio, J.; Huber, M.; Müller, D.; Monetti, R.; Räth, C.; Eckstein, F.; Lochmüller EM.; Majumdar, S.; Rummeny, E.; Link, T. & Bauer, JS. (2010). Automated 3D trabecular bone structure analysis of the proximal femur— prediction of biomechanical strength by CT and DXA. *Osteoporos. Int.*, Vol. 21, pp.1553-1564

Böhm, H.; Räth, C.; Monetti, R.; Müller, D.; Newitt, D.; Majumdar, S.; Rummeny, E.; Morfill, G. & Link, T. (2003). Local 3D Scaling Properties for the Analysis of Trabecular Bone extracted from High Resolution Magnetic Resonance Imaging of Human Trabecular Bone. *Investigative Radiology*, Vol. 38, pp.269-280

Boutry, N.; Cortet, B.; Dubois, P.; Marchandise, X. & Cotton, A. (2003). Trabecular bone structure of the calcaneous: preliminary in vivo MR imaging assessment in men with osteoporosis. *Radiology*, Vol. 227, pp. 708-717

Carballido-Gamio, J. & Majumdar S. (2006). Clinical utility of micro-architectural measurements of trabecular bone. *Curr. Osteoporos. Rep.*, Vol. 4, pp. 64-70

Center, J.R.; Nguyen, T.V.; Schneider, D.; Sambrook, P. & Eisman, J. (1999). Mortality after all major types of osteoporotic fracture in men and women: an observational study. *Lancet*, Vol. 353(9156), pp. 878-882

Ding, M. & Hvid, I. (2000). Quantification of age-related changes in the structure mdoel type and trabecular thickness of human tibial cancellous bone. *Bone,* Vol.26, No. 3, pp. 291-295

Eckstein, F.; Wunderer, C.; Böhm, H.; Kuhn, V.; Priemel, M.; Link, TM. & Lochmüller, EM. (2004). Reproducibility and side differences of mechanical tests for determining the structural strength of the proximal femur. *J. Bone Miner. Res.* Vol. 19, No 3, pp. 379– 385

Grassberger, P.; Badii, R. & Politi, A. (1988). Scaling laws for invariant measures on hyperbolic and nonhyberbolic atractors. *Journal of Statistical Physics*, Vol. 51, No. 1/2, pp. 135-178

Gomberg, B.R.; Saha, P.K.; Song, H.K.; Hwang, S.N. & Wehrli, F. (2000). Application of topological analysis to magnetic resonance images of human trabecular bone. *IEEE Trans. Med. Imaging*, Vol. 19, pp. 166-174

Halsley, T.; Jensen, M.; et al. (1986). Fractal measures and their singularities: the characterization of strange sets. *Phys. Rev. A*, Vol. 33, pp.1141-1151

Hildebrand, T. & Rüegsegger, P. (1997a). A new method for the model-independent assessment of thickness in three-dimensional images. *J Microsc*, Vol. 185, Pt 1, pp. 67-75

Hildebrand, T. & Rüegsegger, P. (1997b). Quantification of bone microarchitecture with the Structure Model Index. *CMBBE*, Vol.1, pp.15-23

Hildebrand, T.;Laib, A.; Müller, R.; Dequeker, J. & Rüegsegger, P. (1999). Direct three-dimensional morphometric analysis of human cancellous bone: microstructural data from spine, femur iliac crest, and calcaneus. *J Bone Miner Res,* Vol. 14, No. 7, pp. 1167-1174

Huber, M.; Carballido-Gamio, J.; Bauer, JS; Baum, T.; Eckstein, F.; Lochmüller, EM; Majumdar, S. & Link, TM. (2008). Proximal femur specimens: automated 3D trabecular bone mineral density analysis at multidetector CT-correlation with biomechanical strength measurement. *Radiology*, Vol. 247, No. 2, pp. 472-481

Huiskes, R.; Ruimerman, R.; van Lenthe, G. & Janssen, J. (2000). Effects of mechanical forces on maintenance, adaptation of form in trabecular bone. *Nature*, Vol. 405, pp. 704-706

Jamitzky, F.; Stark, RW; Bunk, W.; Thalhammer, S.; Rath, C.; Aschenbrenner, T.; Morfill, G. & Heckel, W. (2000) Scaling-index method as an image processing tool in scanning-probe microscopy. *Ultramicroscopy*, Vol. 86, pp.241-246

Kanis, J.A. (2002). Diagnosis of osteoporosis and assessment of fracture risk. *Lancet*, Vol. 359, pp. 1929-1936

Kanis, J.A., on behalf of the World Health Organisation Scientific Group (2007). Assessment of osteoporosis at the primary health care level. *WHO Collaborating Centre for Metabolic Bone Diseases*, University of Sheffield

Krug, R.; Banerjee, S.; Han, E.; Newitt, D.; Link, T. & Majumdar, S. (2005). Feasibility of in vivo structural analysis of high-resolution magnetic resonance images of the proximal femur. *Osteoporos. Int.*, Vol. 16, pp. 1307-1314

Prevention and Management of Osteoporosis. (2003). *World Health OrganizationTechnical Report Series*, Vol. 921, pp. 1-164

Laib, A.; Newitt, D.; Lu, Y. & Majumdar, S. (2002). New model independent measures of trabecular bone structure applied to in vivo high-resolution MR images. *Osteoporos. Int.*, Vol. 13, pp. 130-136

Link, T.; Majumdar, S.; Grampp, S.; Gugliemi, G.; van Kuijk, C.; Imhof, H.; Glueer, C. & Adams, J. (1998). A comparative study of trabecular bone properties in the spine and femur using high resolution MRI and CT," *J. Bone Miner. Res.*, Vol. 13, pp. 122-132

Link, T.; Majumdar, S.; Lin, J.; Newitt, D.; Augat, P.; Ouyang, X.; Mathur, A. & Genant, H. (1999). Imaging of trabecular bone structure in osteoporosis. *Europ. Radiol.*, Vol. 9, pp. 1781-1788

Link, T.; Vieth, V.; Matheis, J.; Newitt, D.; Lu, Y.; Rummeny, E. & Maj, S. (2002). Bone structure of the distal radius and the calcaneous versus BMD of the spine and proximal femur in the prediction of osteoporotic spine fractures. *Eur. Radiol.*, Vol. 12, pp. 401-408

Majumdar, S.; Newitt, D.; Mathur, A.; Osman, D.; Gies, A.; Chiu, E.; Lotz, J.; Kinney, J. & Genant, H. (1996). Magnetic resonance imaging of trabecular bone structure in the distal radius: relationship with X-Ray tomographic microscopy and biomechanics. *Osteoporos. Int.*, Vol. 6, pp. 376-385

Majumdar, S.; Link, T.; Augat, P.; Lin, J.; Newitt, D.; Lane, N. & Genant, H. (1999). Trabecular bone architecture in the distal radius using MR imaging in subjects with fractures of the proximal femur. *Osteoporos. Int.*, Vol. 10, pp. 231-239

Monetti, R.A.; Böhm, H.; Müller, D.; Newitt, D.; Majumdar, S.; Rummeny, E.; Link, T.M. & Räth, C. (2003). Scaling Index Method: a novel nonlinear technique for the analysis of high-resolution MRI of human bones. *Proceedings of Medical Imaging Conference of SPIE,* Vol. 5032, pp. 1777-1786

Monetti, R.A.; Böhm, H.; Müller, D.; Rummeny, E.; Link, T. & Räth, C. (2004). Assessing the biomechanical strength of trabecular bone in vitro using 3D anisotropic non- linear texture measures: The Scaling Vector Method. *Proceedings of Medical Imaging Conference of SPIE,* Vol. 5370, pp. 215-224

Monetti, R.A.; Bauer, J.; Müller, D.; Rummeny, E.; Matsuura, M.; Eckstein, F.; Link, T. & Raeth, C. (2007). Application of the Scaling Index Method to μ-CT images of human trabecular bone for the characterization of biomechanical strength. *Proceedings of Medical Imaging Conference of SPIE,* Vol. 6512, pp. 65124H

Monetti, R.A.; Bauer, J.; Sidorenko, I.; Müller, D.; Rummeny, E.; Matsuura, M.; Eckstein, F.; Lochmüller, E.M.; Zysset, P. & Räth, C. (2009). Assessment of the human trabecular bone structure using Minkowski Functionals. *Proceedings of Medical Imaging Conference of SPIE,* Vol. 7262, pp. 72620N

Müller, D.; Link, T.M.; Monetti, R.; Bauer, J.; Böhm, H.; Seifert-Klauss, V.; Rummeny, E.J.; Morfill, G.E. & Räth, C. (2006). The 3D-based scaling index algorithm: a new structure measure to analyze trabecular bone architecture in hifh-resolution MR images in vivo. *Osteoporos. Int.,* Vol. 17, pp. 1783-1493

Osteoporosis: Clinical Guidelines for Prevention and Treatment. (1999). *Royal College of Physicians.* Lavenham Press, Sudbury, Suffolk

Parfitt, M.; Drezner, M.; et al. (1987). Bone Histomorphometry: Standardization of nomenclature, symbols and units. Report of the ASBMR histomorphometry nomenclature committee. *J. Bone Miner. Res.,* Vol. 2, pp.595-610

Paladini, G. & Vulpiani, A. (1987). Anomalous scaling laws in multiftactal objects. *Phys Reports,* Vol. 156, No. 4, pp. 147-225

Phan, C.M.; Matsuura, M.; Bauer, J.; Dunn, T.; Newitt, D.; Lochmueller, E.; Eckstein, F.; Majumdar, S. & Link, T. (2006). Trabecular bone structure of the calcaneous: comparison of MR imaging at 3.0 and 1.5 T with micro-CT as the standard of reference. *Radiology,* Vol. 239, pp. 488-496

Räth, C. & Morfill, G. (1997). Texture detection and texture duscrimination with anisotropic scaling indices. *J. Opt. Soc. Am. A,* Vol. 14, No. 12, pp. 3208-3215

Räth, C.; Bunk, W.; Huber, M.B.; Morfill, G.E.; Retzlaff, J. & Schücker, P. (2002). Analysing large-scale structure –I. Weighted scaling indices and constrained randomization. *Mon. Not. R. Astron. Soc.,* Vol. 337, pp. 413-421

Räth, C.; Monetti, R.; Böhm, H.; Müller, D.; Rummeny, E. & Link, T. (2003). Analysing and selecting measures for quantifying trabecular bone structures using surrogates. *Proceedings of Medical Imaging Conference of SPIE,* Vol. 5032, pp. 1748-1756

Räth, C. & Schücker, P. (2003). Analysing large scale structure - II. Testing for primordial non-Gaussianity in CMB maps using surrogates. *Mon. Not. R. Astron. Soc,* Vol. 344, pp.115-128

Räth, C.; Monetti, R.; Bauer, J.; Sidorenko, I.; Müller, D.; Matsuura, M.; Lochmüller, E.-M.; Zysset, P. & Eckstein, F. (2008). Strength through structure: visualization and local assessment of the trabecular bone structure. *New Journal of Physics,* Vol. 10, pp. 125010-125027

Saha, P. & Wehrli F. (2004). A robust method for measuring trabecular bone orientation anisotropy at in vivo resolution using tensor scale. *Patt. Recog.*, Vol. 37, pp. 1935-1944

Vieth, V.; Link, T.; et al. (2001). Does the trabecular structure depicted by high-resolution MRI of the calcaneous reflect the true bone structure? *Invest. Radiol.*, Vol. 36, pp. 210-217

Wehrli, F.W. (2007). Structural and functional assessment of trabecular and cortical bone by micro-magnetic resonance imaging. *J. Magn. Reson. Imaging*, Vol. 25, pp. 390-409

Wigderowitz, C.A.; Paterson, C.R.; Dashti, H.; McGurty, D. & Rowley, D. (2000). Prediction of bone strength from Cancellous structure of the distal radius: Can we improve on DXA? *Osteoporos. Int.*, Vol. 11, pp. 840-846

Part 2

General Science Application

7

Gas Trapping During Foamed Flow in Porous Media

Quoc P. Nguyen
The University of Texas at Austin
USA

1. Introduction

Two pore-scale constituents of foam mobility are effective yield stress and viscosity. These rheological quantities have been related directly to foam texture, flow rate, and morphology of the porous medium. It would be ideal to observe these relationships in natural rocks to capture more realistic foam behavior in the field. Since a technique for directly visualizing foam texture in natural porous media is not available, the interpretation of foam mobility on the basis of texture is impossible. Generally, all that is available is the measured pressure drop. Consider two typical foam processes commonly studied in the laboratory: liquid displacement by foam (LDF), and foam displacement by liquid (FDL). These processes represent many of the field applications of foam for gas/liquid mobility control.

Experimental study of local foam mobility does not seem to have been reported in literature. The few existing investigations on in-situ foam-induced fluid partitioning have provided only partial insight into the conditions for foam generation. Apaydin and Kovscek [2000] verified their "bubble population balance" model by fitting the experimental one-dimensional pressure drop and fluid saturation profiles during the transient foam displacement in sandpacks. The local liquid saturation profiles were determined using an X-ray Computed Tomography (X-ray CT) technique. Wassmuth et al. [2001] conducted several foam-flood experiments, where distribution of local fluid saturations was visualized using a Magnetic Resonance Imaging (MRI) technique. The authors have not reported the corresponding pressure drop data, thus limiting the interpretation.

Although most of the reported experimental studies [Zerhboub et al., 1994; Parlar et al., 1995; Siddiqui et al., 1997; Behenna, 1995; Thompson and Gdanski, 1993] on the FDL process have been focused on the acid diversion process, their outcomes are expected be relevant for water shut-off by foam. The insight gained into the FDL process is mainly due to Rossen and co-workers [1994, 2001], who conducted systematic studies using two-stage experiments of foam placement followed by liquid injection. Rossen et al. [1994, 2001] found that the pressure gradient declines in two steps. The pressure gradient first falls rapidly, but levels off to a value that remains relatively high. This is followed by a rather gradual decrease that leads to a quasi-steady state of liquid flow in the presence of significant trapped foam. The authors explained their results using a picture of foam flow in porous media in which the foam is separated in two parts. A (small) fraction of the foam is mobile following a mechanism of lamellae displacement. The remaining part exists in the form of trapped bubbles. When liquid is injected into the porous medium containing foam, the mobile bubbles are driven out which causes the pressure to drop steeply. The gas contained in the trapped bubbles then slowly expands and dissolves in the liquid and leads to the final gradual decline of the pressure gradient. The quasi-steady-state fraction of trapped gas was estimated using the pressure drop profile and the Darcy law for the liquid phase. The amount of stationary foam relates closely to the kinetics of foam generation by virtue of lamella mobilization and division. On the other hand, for foam displacement by liquid (FDL), the characteristic flow regime is liquid fingering, which reflects a wide spectrum of local foam mobility. This leads to a hypothesis that if the quasi-stationary foam domain observed during the FDL is approximately the same as that during the steady state foam flow, one can predict the structure of the liquid finger for known distribution of local foam mobility, and vice versa. However, the blocking/diverting capacity of foam depends on not only the trapped gas fraction, but also on the pattern of foam displacement by liquid. As we shall show later, these factors are not always correlated. The in-situ fluid partitioning profile is thus needed to strengthen the interpretation of the experiments. Note that most of the above studies on the LDF or FDL process used bead- and sandpacks, missing the important effect of natural rock layering.

This work is concerned with the macroscopic mechanisms of foam propagation, trapping and resistance to liquid flow, with a focus on the less-explored issues addressed above. For this purpose, a systematic investigation on both LDF and FDL processes was conducted through –CT-visualized, two-stage foam core-flood experiments: foam flood followed with liquid injection using the X-ray CT imaging technique and different types of sandstones. A new method for determining the distribution of local foam mobility during the macroscopically steady-state flow in sandstone cores was developed based on the X-Ray CT imaging technique and Xenon gas (Xe) as a visual tracer. Due to the enhanced X-ray absorption of the tracer, one can track the mobile foam and thus estimate the saturation of trapped foam. Beyond this, the results also provide insight into the convection-diffusion problems in porous media.

2. Experimental description

2.1 Principle and apparatus
a.   Principle
A CT scan is a special type of X-ray that can reconstruct the cross-sectional internal structure of an object from multiple projections of the object. The latter represents the attenuation of X-rays through the object. Consider a parallel beam of X-ray photons with sufficiently small width propagating through a slab of a porous rock, which confines mobile and stationary nitrogen foams at the quasi-steady state. The slab is divided into regular voxels whose size is sufficiently small that they can represent the differential properties of the slab. The incident beam attenuates due to photons either being absorbed by the atoms of the materials (core-holder materials, rock, surfactant solution, and gas) or being scattered away from their original directions of travel. For a range of photon energies most commonly encountered in practice (from 20 to 150 keV), the mechanisms responsible for these two contributions to the attenuation are the photoelectric and the Compton effect. The former, (much more energy dependent than the latter), becomes dominant at energies below about 100 KeV. For convenience, these effects are customarily evaluated together through a single constant, $\hat{\mu}$, representing the attenuation coefficient of the material. Although it is customary to say that a CT scanner calculates the linear attenuation coefficient of the materials (at some effective

energy), the numbers actually put out by the computer attached to the scanner are integers, called the CT values. These values are measured in Hounsfield units, denoted by HU. The relationship between the linear attenuation coefficient and the corresponding Hounsfield unit HU is

$$HU_m(t,s,E_r) = \left(\frac{\hat{\mu}_m(t,s,E_r)}{\hat{\mu}_w(E_r)} - 1 \right) \times 1000 \tag{1}$$

where $\hat{\mu}_w$ (E_r) is the attenuation coefficient of water. The value HU_m = 0 corresponds to water; and the value HU_m = -1000 corresponds to $\hat{\mu}_m$ (t,s,E_r) = 0, which is assumed to be the attenuation coefficient of air ($\hat{\mu}_a$). Since the latter is difficult to obtain in practice, it is more convenient to use the following normalized form of HU_m (equivalent to liquid saturation S_w), assuming linearity between the measured HU_m and the actual value of the attenuation coefficient $\hat{\mu}_m$.

$$S_w = \frac{HU_m - HU_{mw}}{HU_{mw} - HU_{ma}} \times 1000 \tag{2}$$

where HU_{mw} and HU_{ma} are the measured Hounsfield units for water and air, respectively. Note that for those materials having atomic numbers higher than water, such as natural rocks, their CT values are far above zero. Assuming the linearity between HU and bulk density for this range of CT value, the contribution of rock to the total measured attenuation can be eliminated by the linear image subtraction algorithm [McCullough, 1975; Kak and Roberts, 1986]

b. **X-ray CT scanner**

The X-ray CT system used is of the fourth-generation SAMATOM AR produced by Siemens. For the whole object examinations, the X-ray source-detector system rotates continuously, utilizing the traversing slice method. The main technical data of this scanner is presented in Table 1.

Specification	Quantity
Max tube voltage	134 kV
Filtering	6.5 mm AL equivalent
Tube current range	50, 70, 100 mA
Projections per second	333
Number of channels	704, 1024
Scan time (seconds)	1.3, 1.9, 2, 3, 5 s
Scan field	28/45, 45
Table speed	0.5 - 100 mm/s ± 15%
Arbitrary tabletop movement	± 0.5 mm

Table 1. Main technical data of the X-ray CT system

The imaging system uses the Somaris software to reconstruct CT images from the measurement data received. However, we only use this system for monitoring real time propagation of the components during core floods and for obtaining online statistical data of the X-ray adsorption of the fluid system at steady states. A standalone image processing software developed by the author reads the absorption data of CT slices stored in a binary form into 512x512 image matrices. The CT values of the matrix components are then converted into the saturation scale according to Eq. (2). Different built-in coloring schemes are also available for mapping the image matrices.

c.   Foam Core flood Setup

The schematic of the foam core flood setup is presented in Fig. 1. It consists of a core holder in line with, on one end, a double effect piston displacement pump (Pharmacia Biotech P-500) in parallel with a gas mass flow controller (SIERRA) and, on the other end, a backpressure regulator set at 1.0 bar and a collector for the produced fluids. The gas mass-flow controller is used to ensure the supply of nitrogen gas (N_2) at a constant rate. The pump is used to inject the surfactant solution also at a constant rate. Four pressure ports along the core enable the monitoring of the local absolute pressures using transducers (ENRESS-HAUSER) and a personal computer equipped with a Kettley data acquisition system. All experiments are conducted in a thermostat room at 20 ± 1 C.

d.   Core holder

The core holder is placed horizontally on the platform of the CT scanner apparatus and kept in place using a polymethyl methacrylate (PMMA) stand. The coreholder is made of polyether etherketone (PEEK), which combines good mechanical properties with a low X-ray attenuation. PEEK is also believed to transmit X-rays within a narrow energy window (refiltering the polyenergetic source X-rays), which appreciably minimizes the beam-hardening artifact due to the polychromaticity (sometimes called the interpetrous lucency artifact [Brooks et al., 1998]). This effect gives the appearance of dark streaks and flares in the vicinity of the boundary between the coreholder and the core (note that streaks can also be caused by aliasing [Millner et al., 1978]). The geometry and structure of the coreholder are also designed to minimize beam hardening and scattering artifacts in longitudinal imaging where the detected energy spectrum may vary with the projection direction. To eliminate the boundary flow effect at the inner surface of the coreholder, the core (diameter = 44 ± 1 mm and length = 180 ± 1 mm) is encapsulated in a thin layer of low X-ray attenuation Araldite (CW 2215) superglue, with CIBA HY 5160, Araldite CW 2215 as the hardener. During core mounting, the high viscosity of the superglue mixture ensures a very low penetration (less than 1.0 mm) of the core. The four pressure taps divides the core into three sections of 60, 40, and 80 mm: the sections are noted 1, 2, and 3, respectively.

2.2 X-ray CT-imaging settings

The fixed imaging settings for all foam core flood experiments are presented in Table 2. The X-ray tube of the CT-Scanner is operated at either 130 kV or 110 kV. The corresponding effective energies, at which a given material will exhibit the same attenuation coefficient as measured by the scanner, are typically about 50 to 60% of these values (see Refs. Millner et al., 1978; Alvarez and Macovski, 1976 for a practical procedure for determining the effective energy of a CT scanner). The use of low X-ray energy gives rise to the undesirable X-ray scattering effect. Moreover, because rock is high radio-dense, it is advisable to operate at the lowest energy and the highest ray density.

All CT images contain noise, that is pixel-to-pixel variations in the pixel value in the image of an object of uniform linear attenuation coefficient. It typically ranges from 3 to 20 HU. In the case of quasi-steady state foams in sandstones, the noise appears when subtracting two subsequent images of a fixed CT slice. Note that the quasi-steady state denotes the time-averaged foam behavior at pore scale. The noise therefore may include local fluctuations, which cause detectable changes of the voxel compositions in time. It is also important to mention that the noise is proportional to the reciprocals of the squared X-ray tube current (mA), the scan time and the thickness of the CT slice. However, the longest scan time and the thickest CT slice are not always preferable, particularly in the imaging of dynamic processes such as transient foam and liquid displacements. A voxel is the three dimensional pixel, including the slice width. The average linear attenuation coefficient of the voxel thus reflects both resolution and partial volume effects.

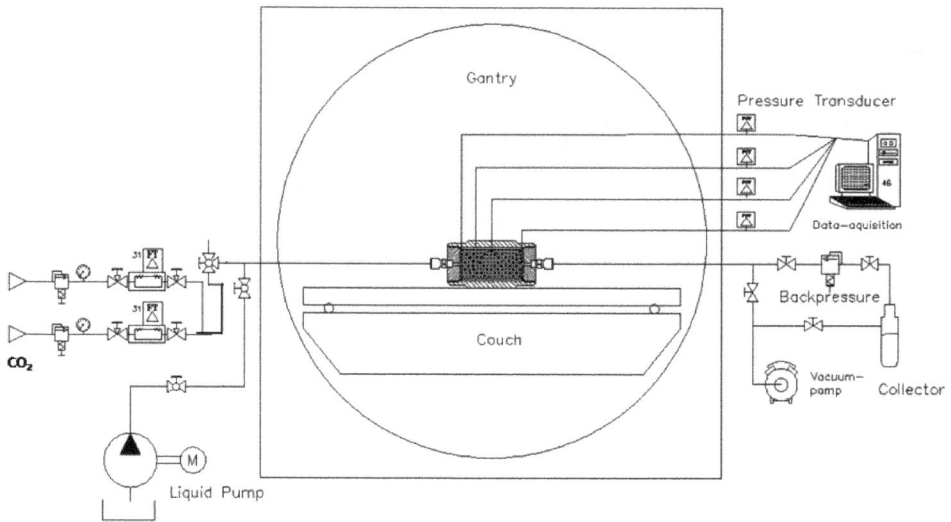

Fig. 1. The experimental setup used to investigate foam flow in porous media. Nitrogen (N_2) or Carbon Dioxide (CO_2) supplied via two dedicated mass flow controllers. CO_2 is used only for core saturation. Liquids (water or surfactant solution) are supplied using a precision piston displacement pump. Fluids are collected using a graded tube and gas counter. The core is placed with its axis in the flaming plane of the gantry of the X-ray tomograph, for the real-time visualization of rock features and in-situ foam induced fluid partitioning.

Specification	Quantity
Tube Voltage	110 kV
Tube curent	100 mA
Slice thickness	3 mm
Scan time	3 s
Field of View	160 mm
Image reconstruction kernel	Standard
Scan mode	Sequence
Couch feeding	6 mm span

Table 2. Imaging settings

2.3 Materials

Sandstone cores. Bentheim sandstone is used to carry out the experiments. This sandstone is macroscopically homogeneous according to its X-ray absorption data (for porosity and bulk density) and bulk X-ray diffraction data (for composition). The main physical properties of the Bentheim cores are presented in Table 3.

Permeability (mD)	Porosity (%)	Density (g/ml)	Main composition
1010	22.1	2.34	Quartz

Table 3. Properties of Bentheim sandstone

Gases. The analytical grade Nitrogen (N_2) and Xenon (Xe) are purchased from Scott High Pressure Technology. The qualities of these gases are presented in Table 4. We use these pure gases to make calibration gas mixtures of N_2 and Xe. For the foam core-flood experiments, a mixture of N_2 and Xe is used, and this mixture is also purchased from the Scott High Pressure Technology.

Quality	Xenon gas (%)	Nitrogen gas (%)
Xe	99.995	0.00
N_2	0.001	99.09
Ar	0.002	0.18
O_2	0.001	0.70
CO_2	0.000	0.04

Table 4. Qualities of bulk and tracer gas

2.4 Procedures

a.   Core saturation

Since the X-ray absorption depends on the compositions of the attenuating system, the chemical properties of the Bentheim sandstone cores should be stabilized before carrying out the experiment. For this purpose, the Soxhlet method is used to extract native contaminants such as oil (using toluene) and other minerals (using a mixture of chloroform and methanol in distilled water). The core is then dried in a vacuum oven at 90 C. The initial saturation process starts with the injection of 200 pore volumes of brine (0.5 M $NaCl$) under vacuum (note that one pore volume is defined as the total volume of pore space of the core), and is followed with 200 pore volumes of surfactant solution at 1 bar backpressure to satisfy surfactant adsorption and ion exchange.

b.   Fluid core-flood

Foam injection. The nitrogen gas and surfactant solution are co-injected directly into the saturated core at fixed rates. To investigate the fluid-rate effect on the displacement pattern in the Bentheim cores, three experiments with different total flow rates are conducted. An overview of fluid rates used is presented in Table 5.

The foam displacement process is visualized by constructing a series of 8 parallel images slicing vertically the core parallel to its axis. The central image is on the plane of the core axis (axis plane), whereas the other ones are placed two by two, symmetrically with respect to the axis plane. The spacing between two adjacent images (i.e., the couch feeding) is 4 mm.

Each five-image series is scanned in sequence from a couch position (CP) set to zero for the central image.

Foam types	Gas rate* (cm3/min)	Liquid rate (cm3/min)	Foam quality (%)
Foam-A	5.0	0.5	90.90
Foam-B	10.0	0.5	95.24

*Standard conditions

Table 5. Fluid rates used in the LDF experiments

Liquid injection following steady-state foam. Liquid is injected at a fixed rate after foam reaches full development. The first experiment is conducted with Foam-A, using a liquid rate of 2 cm^3/min. The effect of foam strength is investigated with Foam-B at the same post-foam liquid injection rate.

c.   Determination of trapped gas based on a visual tracer method

The general principle of determining local foam mobility, using the X-ray CT technique and a tracer gas, is similar to that of visualizing gas-liquid displacement, as described in Section 2.1. However, some important differences are worth discussing. The mobility field of steady-state foam (native foam) in a porous medium can be identified through the visualized percolation of a tracer-foam, which is identical to the injected native foam, except for a small fraction of the tracer added to the bulk gas. To enhance the resolution of the mobility field, the tracer foam must have a significantly higher X-ray attenuation than the native foam. Having an atomic number of 54, Xenon gas possesses an attenuation coefficient much higher than nitrogen gas (atomic number of 7), thus is an ideal tracer.

It is important to note that the presence of the tracer should not cause a significant disturbance to the local equilibrium of the native foam, which is determined by two state-parameters of individual voxels: (1) phase saturation, and (2) average pressure. The former parameter is practically difficult to monitor during the transient displacement of the tracer foam since a detectable change in the X-ray attenuation reflects changes in both tracer concentration and phase saturation. The latter parameter is indirectly determined from the pressure drops measured over a large number of voxels along the main flow direction, which thus may not indicate precisely the fluctuation of the local pressure gradient due to foam trapping and remobilizing. However, intermittent foam trapping is an inherent feature of any quasi-steady state foam flow. Therefore, the fraction of the tracer foam, X_f, percolating through a single voxel containing the native foam can be determined through Eq. (3).

$$X_f(t,s,E_r) = \frac{HU_m - HU_{nf}}{HU_{tf} - HU_{nf}} \times 1000 \qquad (3)$$

where HU_{nf} and HU_{tf} are the CT values of the native and tracer foams, respectively. Eq. (3) can be used to quantify exactly the fraction of mobile foam in the voxel, assuming a sharp compositional interface between the tracer foam and the native foam. However, the diffusion of Xenon across this interface and/or the instability of the foam films smear out the local tracer concentration profile (the mixing effect), thus leading to a poor interpretation of the reconstructed compositional image. Fortunately, these effects can be minimized with highly stable foams, and by ensuring the dominance of convective over diffusive tracer transfers.

It is important to emphasize that foam trapping is a dynamic process. Gas trapping and remobilizing takes place at the pore scale, even in a macroscopic steady state foam process. This means that the propagation of the tracer foam observed in a CT slice reflects a local distribution of foam mobility. In this mobility field, trapped foam is defined as the lowest mobility (i.e. zero mobility and mobility of the same order of magnitude as the tracer diffusion rate in foam). Trapped foam also includes trapped and remobilized foam if this foam does not show a considerable net transport of the tracer in the main flow direction.

Selection of tracer concentration. The volume fraction of the tracer gas used should produce sufficient contrast between the native steady state and the injected tracer foams. It is thus necessary to quantify the sensitivity of the image resolution to the tracer concentration. For this purpose, the average CT values due to different tracer concentrations must be determined in both types of sandstones used. The procedure for the calibration measurement is as follows. First, the sandstone core must be cleaned and dried, as described in the core saturation procedure below. Three vertical longitudinal CT slices capturing most features of the entire core are selected for the sequence scanning: one slice on the plane of the core axis (central image) and the other two placed symmetrically with respect to the central image. The distance between two adjacent slices is 10 mm. An image series of the core without tracer gas is used as the reference for the image subtraction (see the core preparation procedure below). The imaging setting is presented in Table 2. Next, Xenon and nitrogen premixed to a chosen volumetric ratio are injected into the core where the system pressure is maintained at 1 bar (equal to the fixed core backpressure during foam flooding). The injection rate of the tracer mixture is 5 cm^3/min (standard conditions), fixed in all the calibration measurements. Note that the measured CT values of the individual voxels are in principle influenced by the voxel pressures because of the proportional relationship between the Hounsfield units and the tracer density. However, the injection gas rate used is chosen so that the ensuing pressure drop over the entire core is negligible with respect to the backpressure. This allows assuming a uniform density of gas throughout the core. The sequence scanning continues until the CT value of each image in series (obtained by averaging the CT values of its voxels) stays constant, signaling a full saturation of the tracer gas. The excess CT value due to the Xenon concentration is determined by subtracting the full-tracer-saturation images from the corresponding reference ones.

Tracer transport in dry cores. Without foam, the convection-dispersion of the tracer gas is mainly influenced by the topological disorder of the pore networks. However, with foam it is further modified by the local foam mobility and the effective tracer diffusivity due to liquid films. Therefore, the effect of pore-network heterogeneity on the tracer transport can be better distinguished in the absence of foam (dry cores). For this purpose, we conduct a tracer injection experiment on the Bentheim core. The procedure starts with the injection of 100 pore-volumes of nitrogen into the dry core at 1 bar backpressure. The injection rate is maintained at 3 cm^3/min (standard conditions). The tracer gas mixture with the tracer concentration being used for determining trapped foam is then injected at the same rate. Note that the use of a higher injection rate helps the convective from diffusive dispersion of the tracer. Moreover, it also causes a fast breakthrough of the tracer, thus limiting the number of image series needed to capture important features of the advancing compositional front.

Core recovery. To obtain the reproducibility of the data, the sandstone core of each type is recovered for use in a new experiment as follows. First, it is flushed with 200 pore volumes of distilled water in the presence of 40% ethanol. Taken out of the holder, it then undergoes a 24-hour-cleaning process to remove the remaining surfactant, using the Soxhlet extraction apparatus as described in Section 3.4 A. The cleaning solvent is a mixture of chloroform and methanol in distilled water. Finally, the core is dried in the vacuum oven at 100 C before going through the saturation process.

Tracer-Foam flood. Nitrogen foam is injected into the saturated core until reaching a steady state as indicated by (a) the sectional pressure drop profiles, and (b) the average CT values of the fluid system. The latter is determined from a set of seven parallel image planes with the same arrangement as that for the measurement of tracer transfer in the dry core above. The injection nitrogen is then switched to the tracer gas mixture, and the sequence scanning takes place every three minutes to produce successive image series of the transient tracer displacement. A full saturation of the tracer over the entire core is signaled by constant CT values of the images.

3. Results and discussion

3.1 Liquid displacement by foam (LDF)

Fig. 2 shows the CT images of the fluids during the liquid displacement by Foam-A (Q_g = 5 cm³/min, Q_w = 0.5 cm³/min) in a Bentheim core. Unless otherwise stated the images presented in this section are the central images (corresponding to CP = 0), which capture most of the features of the transient displacement. Note that the real elapsed time is presented in a dimensionless form (called dimensionless time, DT), defined as: tQ/PV, where t is the real time, Q is the total injection volumetric flow rate, and PV is the pore volume of the core.

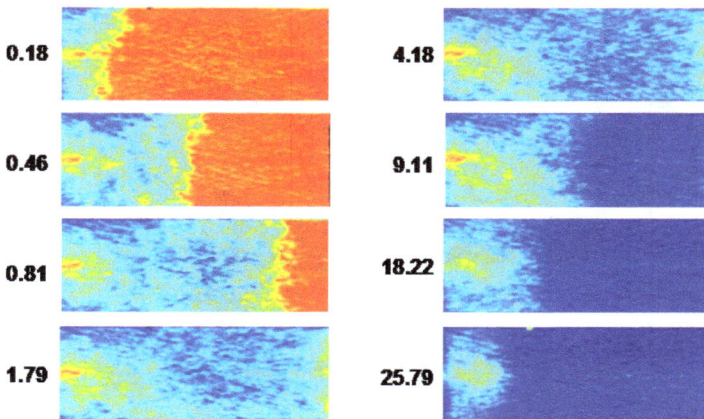

Fig. 2. The displacement by Foam-A (green/blue) in a Bentheim sandstone core, initially saturated with surfactant solution (red/yellow). Nitrogen and surfactant solution are directly co-injected at 5 (standard) cm³/min and 0.5 cm³/min, respectively. The images correspond to the centered longitudinal CT slice (CP = 0). First, a sharp foam front traverses throughout out the core after about 0.8 DT. After foam breakthrough, a second front develops and moves backwards to the inlet. Steady state is reached at about 25 DT.

Two foam displacement stages can be distinguished in the figure. The *first* stage runs from the beginning of the injection up to the breakthrough of foam at 1.79 DT. At first sight, the foam displaces the surfactant solution in a characteristic piston-like manner. However, a closer examination of the images reveals that we should consider three regions along the flow direction: (1) an upstream region characterized by a low liquid saturation, (2) a downstream region where liquid saturation is uniform and (3) a frontal region where a mixture of foam and free liquid gives rise to a fine fingering pattern. The *second* stage (indicated by the darkening of the blue region) starts after foam breakthrough and reaches maturity at 25.79 DT, corresponding to the establishment of the steady state flow regime. This stage is characterized by a strong secondary liquid desaturation (SLD), which initiates in the central portion of the core and propagates towards the inlet and the outlet. The well-known "capillary end" effect causing a relatively high liquid saturation near the core outlet is completely suppressed as the SLD drives through this region. However, this does not happen in the near-inlet region where the SLD could not exhaust a significant liquid-filled fraction.

To quantify the evolution of fluid saturations over the entire core, the CT data of five longitudinal image planes in each sequence scan are averaged in the transverse direction, resulting in one-dimensional liquid saturation profiles, as shown in Fig. 3. This figure shows more distinctly the two stages observed with the images in Fig. 2. Indeed, all profiles up to 0.81 DT, excepting the one at 0.11 DT, exhibit roughly the same trend: (1) a low (less than 55%) upstream liquid saturation, (2) a high (100%) downstream liquid saturation, and (3) a transition zone where the liquid saturation increases smooth, and rapidly towards the downstream.

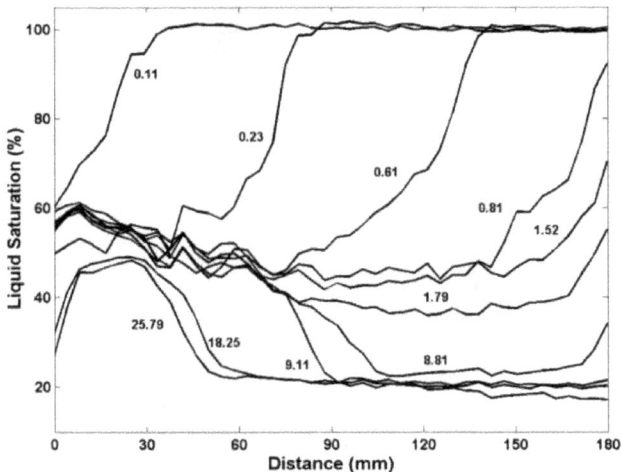

Fig. 3. Liquid saturation profiles (saturation versus distance from the inlet) at different times during the liquid displacement by Foam-A (Q_g = 5, Q_w = 0.5 cm³/min).

The profile at 0.11 DT exhibits only a transition zone and the downstream saturation. Within the upstream region, the liquid saturation gradually declines from the inlet. For example, at

0.61 DT the saturation decreases by almost 10% from the inlet to the position 75 mm. Note that high capillary forces still retain a higher liquid saturation near the outlet at this time, which soon disappears as the second front propagates towards the inlet. However, the front does not approach the inlet at the steady state, leaving about 48% unswept liquid over 30 mm from the inlet.

Fig. 4 shows the pressure drops versus the dimensionless time for three different core sections (overall pressure drop over the core at the foam breakthrough is about 120 mbar). In the first and second sections, the pressure drops remain almost constant up to about 17 and 12 DT respectively, at which time the pressure in the third section reaches a steady value, corresponding to the time at which secondary liquid desaturation ceases in the third section. Then, the pressure drop in Section 2 increases. Similarly, the pressure drop in section 1 starts to increase as the pressure drop and the liquid saturation in Section 2 reach plateau values. The process of foam generation associated with liquid desaturation is self-amplifying as the former requires the local viscous pressure gradients to be sufficiently high, while, on the other hand, further foam generation leads to high local pressure gradients. Moreover, since gas expansion increases with the pressure drop induced by the steady state foam before liquid injection, it may contribute to foam/free liquid mobilization, and thus foam generation, especially far from the injection point.

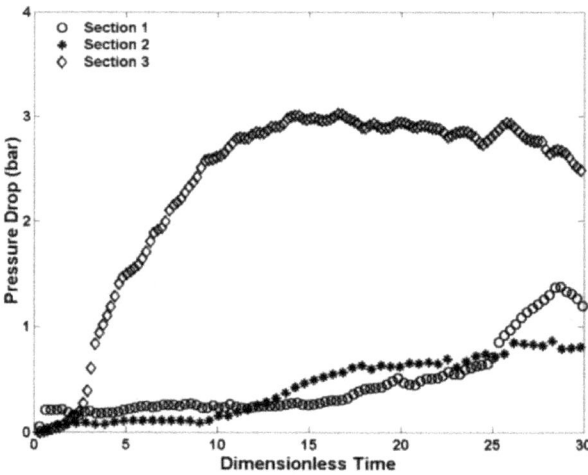

Fig. 4. Pressure drop histories of three successive sections during the liquid displacement by Foam-A (Q_g = 5, Q_w = 0.5 cm³/min). No steady state is shown

However, liquid desaturation ceases as the capillary number reaches a critical value N_c^* (or the limiting capillary pressure P_c^*) defining the local equilibrium between foam generation and destruction. The capillary number, i.e. the ratio of viscous to capillary forces, has been commonly used to determine the relative importance of these forces on the mobilization of fluid in porous media. The capillary number can be expressed as

$$N_c \equiv |\nabla P| \frac{K}{\sigma_{gw}} \tag{4}$$

where ∇P is the local viscous pressure gradient. Note that several expressions have been used in the literature to express the ratio of viscous and capillary forces [Gauglitz et al., 2002; Tanzil et al., 2002; Fulcher et al., 1985], but they have the same generic meaning as Eq. (2). The concept of critical capillary number explains the above observation that the quasi-steady state is obtained, for instance in Section 3, regardless of the substantial foam development in the preceding section. The liquid saturation corresponding to N_c^* is not necessarily the irreducible saturation (that is mainly determined by rock properties). Hence, if the system reaches an irreducible saturation state, foam may develop (indicated by increasing pressure drop) without necessarily a change of the liquid saturation as observed in some previous studies [Kovscek and Radke, 1994; Osterloh and Jante, 1992]. We believe that in this particular regime, mobilization and division of stationary foam will play an important role in foam generation.

3.2 Effect of fluid rate on LDF

For given properties of a porous medium, one way to increase the capillary number consists of increasing the interstitial fluid velocities. Although the latter is mainly determined by the local foam mobility, we assume that it increases with the superficial (injection) fluid velocities. For the sake of comparison, first consider the case where Q_w is the same as used for the previous Foam-A, and Q_g is increased by a factor of two (= 10 cm³/min, Foam-B in Table 5). The displacement of liquid is shown in Fig. 5. The first discernible difference from Foam-A is the gravity effect on the traveling foam front, as foam first breaks through in the upper part of the core (see image at 0.70).

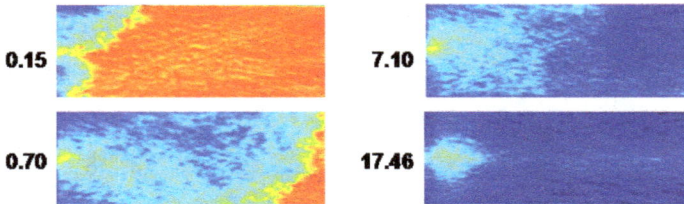

Fig. 5. The displacement by Foam-B (green/blue) in a Bentheim sandstone core, initially saturated with surfactant solution (red/yellow). Nitrogen and surfactant solution are directly co-injected at 10 (standard) cm³/min and 0.5 cm³/min, respectively. The images correspond to the centered longitudinal CT slice (CP = 0).

The gravity override is normally suppressed when foam in the frontal region develops strongly enough to raise the relative importance of viscous to bouyancy forces. However, this is not observed with Foam-B, possibly due to the fact that the high gas rate in Foam-B might be unfavorable for foam generation, particularly in Section 1. Additionally, gas saturation in this section for Foam-B is somewhat higher than that for Foam-A, resulting in a relatively higher bouyancy force.

The gravity effect leads to an earlier emergence of the SLD as compared with Foam-A. This is illustrated with the liquid saturation profiles shown in Fig. 6. Similar to Foam-A, the evolution of liquid saturation is composed of two distinct stages, except that, in the first stage, the elevated gas rate results in a rather uniform liquid saturation within the upstream region, and reduces somewhat the "entrance" effect. The sharp decrease in liquid saturation visible in the first few millimeters near the inlet is consistent with the desaturation in the corners as observed in the images (see Fig. 5). Additionally, the second liquid-saturation front propagates towards the inlet distinctly faster than that of Foam-A (comparing the profiles at 9.11 and 38 DT in Figs. 3 and 6, respectively), and approaches closer to the inlet. Foam still does not propagate as strongly in the near-inlet region as it does further downstream, even though injection gas rate is higher by a factor of 2. This suggests that foam generation is less dependent on the gas rate. In fact, comparing the pressure drop profiles of Foam-A and B shown in Figs. 5 and 7, respectively, the pressure drop over the first section at 30 DT is roughly 1.20 bar for Foam-A, which is slightly higher than that for Foam-B (about 0.90 bar).

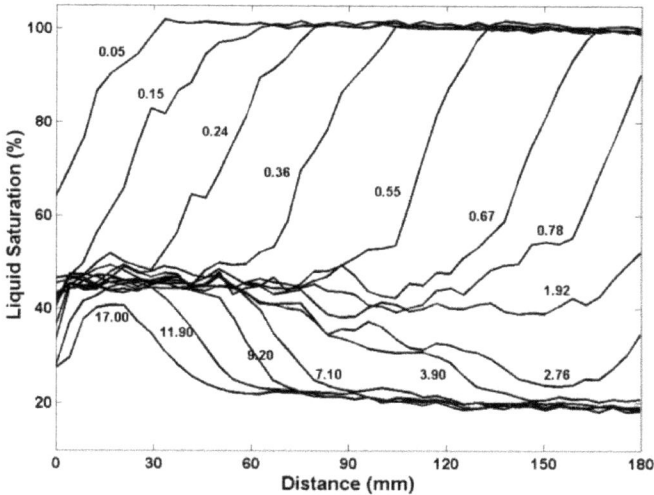

Fig. 6. Liquid saturation profiles (saturation versus distance from the inlet) at different times during the liquid displacement by Foam-B (Q_g = 10, Q_w = 0.5 cm³/min).

3.3 Foam displacement by liquid (FDL)

Fig. 8 shows a set of images (CP = 0, +8, +16) of the fluid partitioning during the injection of the surfactant solution (at 2 cm3/min) in the Bentheim core. At 3 DT, the images show that the liquid flows according to a characteristic finger pattern. This flow structure may be ascribed to the non-uniform foam mobilization by the injected liquid. The size and shape of the finger seem to be controlled by two effects. The first is the compressibility of foam and the second is the "wetting film" flow through the space occupied by the stationary foam (i.e. liquid flows preferentially in the wetting film). In particular, the downward bending of the liquid finger, in the midst of the trapped and expanding foams, is due to the gravity effect. Liquid saturation is approximately 82.0% within the finger, while in the surrounding foam region it remains at about 22.3%. The former indicates about 30% of gas probably trapped within the network of percolating liquid. Considering images taken at successive times (e.g. CP = +8, at 1.75, 3.0, and 6.0 DT), it can be seen that the liquid content of the finger increases in time, corresponding to the diminishing of the isolated gas blobs, as the correlation length

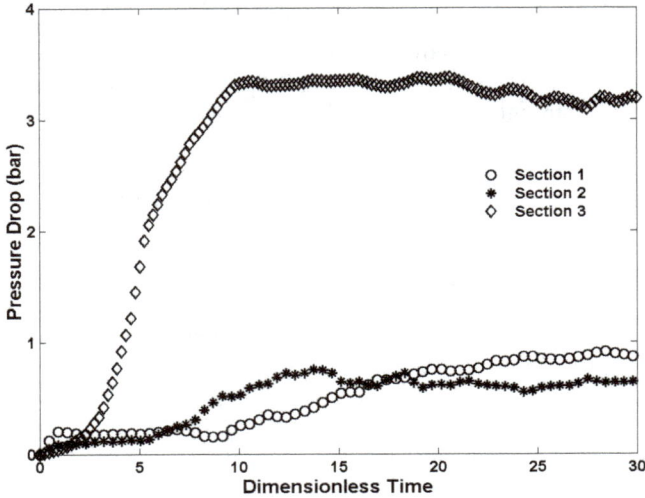

Fig. 7. Pressure drop histories of three successive sections during the liquid displacement by Foam-B (Q_g = 10, Q_w = 0.5 cm³/min). Steady state is shown.

of the liquid network is refined. Moreover, the finger grows from the beginning of the injection of liquid until it breaks through. It is thicker near the inlet, but becomes thinner as the distance from the inlet increases. The lateral development of the finger near the inlet can be explained by the fact that foam developed much more strongly towards the outlet during the foam injection (see Fig. 2), and that the invasion energy of liquid is dissipated due to the viscous flow. In addition, the inherent gas expansion tends to reduce foam density more near the inlet than in the downstream region (because of no foam injection and one-dimensional flow). As a result, the probability of a foam-filled pore being invaded by liquid is higher towards the inlet.

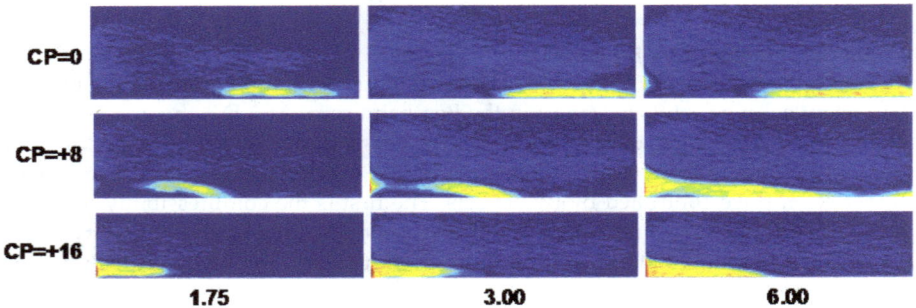

Fig. 8. Macroscopic pattern of fluid partitioning during the FDL process. Liquid fingering emerges after the injection of surfactant solution, following the steady state Foam-A in the Bentheim core (see Fig. 2). The liquid finger has an asymmetrical structure spanning over three image planes (CP= 0, +8, +16).

The pressure drops corresponding to the above images are shown in Fig. 9. The pressure drops over Sections 1 and 2 are added because the former is extremely low. In both core sections (1+2 and 3), the pressure drop evolves in three regimes. In the first regime (from 0 to about 1.2 DT), the pressure drop first increases and then falls sharply. Reporting similar pressure drop profiles, Cheng and co-workers [2001] attributed the brief increase in the pressure drop to the fact that the liquid rate is higher than the actual foam rate in the core, (near the inlet). To be more precise, in the range of flow rates used, this can actually be due to the compression of the small volume before the inlet core surface, where the gas and the surfactant solution were mixed during foam injection. In the second regime (1.2 to 5.5 DT), the pressure drop declines gradually, consistent with the "wetting film" flow and the development of the finger, as discussed above. Gas expansion also contributes considerably to the pressure decline. Finally, in the third regime, which runs from 5.5 to over 40 DT (only data up to 7 DT are shown in Fig. 9), a quasi-steady state flow has been is established. Foam remains trapped in the porous medium, since no gas production was observed during this time. The liquid finger also reaches an apparent stability in this regime.

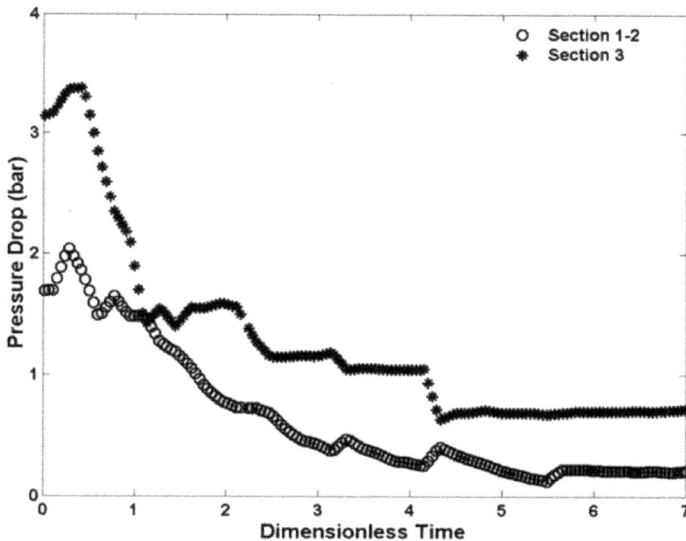

Fig. 9. Pressure drop histories of Section 1 Plus 2 and Section 3 during the injection of surfactant solution at 2 cm3/min, following the steady state Foam-A in the Bentheim core (Fig. 2).

3.4 Effect of the initial steady-state-foam strength on FDL

Fig. 10 shows the development of the liquid finger at 1.22 and 3.00 DT, during the injection of surfactant solution (at 2 cm³/min) following Foam-B (see Fig. 5 for the foam injection stage). Note that - for the sake of comparison on the same time scale, the definition of the dimensionless time is the same, except that the total injection flow rate Q is fixed at 1 cm³/min (even for the actual injection rate of 2 cm³/min).

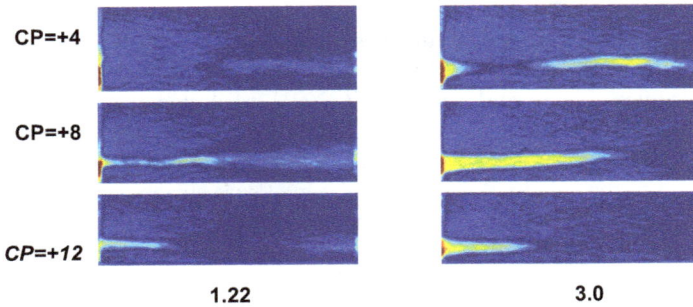

Fig. 10. Macroscopic pattern of fluid partitioning during the FDL process. Liquid fingering emerges after the injection of surfactant solution, following the steady state Foam-B in the Bentheim core (see Fig. 5). The liquid finger has an asymmetrical structure spanning over three image planes (CP= +4, +8, +12).

Unlike Foam-A (see Fig. 8), Foam-B reduces greatly the tortuosity of liquid percolation as the finger is confined only within the CT slices from CP = 4 to +12, (instead of 0 to +16 for Foam-A). Additionally, the finger lies away from the boundary of the core and gradually grows upwards along the core axis, indicating the decreasing gravity effect. This is because Foam-B is somewhat stronger than Foam-A, as indicated by the corresponding pressure drops during the foam injection in Figs. 4 and 7.

The image CP = +8 at 1.22 DT exhibits a distinct contrast in density of the percolating liquid network: high (low) in the first (second) half-length of the core (image CP = +8). More importantly, within the low liquid-density region, the finger grows into the image plane CP = +4 at the expense of the part in image CP = +8 at 3.00 DT. This provides an insight into the percolation pattern of liquid controlled by foam mobilization and gas expansion. Qualitatively, after driving "easy-to-mobilize" foam out of a certain pore fraction, the percolating liquid may then encounter "difficult-to-mobilize" foam, which leads to a buildup of the local liquid pressure. Once (a portion of) this foam is mobilized, the liquid pressure decreases as a result, causing a temporary increase in the local pressure gradients around the liquid-invaded region. The latter promotes the gas expansion, especially when the pressure energy of the foam domain is sufficiently high. This mechanism is most likely responsible for the simultaneous growth and decay of the liquid finger. It also implies that when the gas expansion becomes insignificant, the finger simply grows by virtue of foam mobilization, thus reaching a stable structure as observed in the images at 3.00 DT. The average liquid saturations within the stable finger and over the entire core at this time (roughly 77.1 and 26.7%, respectively) are a bit lower than in Foam-A (roughly 82.0 and 29.8%, respectively), consistent with a relatively stronger Foam-B.

3.5 Effect of liquid rate on FDL
One might expect that a decrease in liquid rate could results in a "weaker" liquid fingering, or on the other hand a clarifying of the picture of the "wetting film" flow regime. Let us clarify this with the result of Foam-B displacement at a lower liquid rate (1cm³/min), as shown in Fig. 11. The images in this figure show a mature liquid finger at 4.25 DT, which

initiates in both CT slices CP = - 8 and - 12 and then grows mainly into the latter slice before coming back in the former slice.

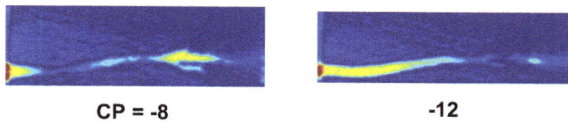

CP = -8   **-12**

Fig. 11. Macroscopic pattern of fluid partitioning during the FDL process. Liquid fingering emerges after the injection of surfactant solution at 1 cm3/min, following the steady state Foam-B in the Bentheim core (see Fig. 5). Images are taken at 4.25 DT.

Compared with the case of 2-cm³/min-liquid rate in Fig. 10, the first important difference is that the finger is now situated in the opposite side of the central image plane, as indicated by the native CP values. The only difference between these two experiments is the liquid injection rate. This implies that the position of the finger is not just determined by the properties of the medium, but also by the flow properties. In particular, lowering the liquid rate leads to a "delay" between the liquid invasion and gas expansion processes, and, as discussed previously, the latter strongly influences the evolution of the percolating liquid network. In fact, the finger obtains a smaller size as the liquid rate is decreased (comparing the finger structures in Figs. 10 and 11). Remarkably, its high-liquid-density-region does not approach the outlet as observed with the previous foams, suggesting the emergence of the "wetting film" flow regime in the subsequent region. In this regime, the initial liquid saturation is of the order of liquid saturation induced by the previous foam flow, and does not change significantly during the liquid percolation. As a result, the displacement of foam by liquid is constrained by the effective foam yield stress. Although the Bentheim core is macroscopically homogeneous, the finger "tip" is still branching. Therefore, the apparent discontinuity of the liquid saturation across the branching finger "tip" may stand as proof of a transition from "pore-scale, piston-like displacement" to "wetting film" flow regime. Furthermore, one can expect that an increase in the liquid rate may counteract the gravity force throughout the foam bank. This can be seen through comparing the mature finger structures in Figs. 10 and 11.

3.6 Calibration of contrast enhancement using Xenon for gas trapping measurement

Fig. 12 shows CT enhancement as a linear function of the Xenon concentration in the Bentheim core. The discrete data points designate the steady state CT values of the flowing tracer gas averaged over three CT slices. The pressure drop across the core is 0.8 ± 0.2 mbar, which is much smaller than the backpressure (1 bar). Note that for the tracer concentrations used we found the steady-state CT values to be insensitive to the variation of the injection rate over a rather wide range from 2 to 15 cm³/min (standard conditions). The slope of the fitting line in Fig. 12 gives a contrast enhancement of 0.68 HU per added percentage of the Xenon gas. This value reflects the bulk density and the composition of the Bentheim sandstone used. As shown later, the overall pressure drop induced by steady state foams is roughly 8 for the Bentheim core. Therefore, for a given Xenon concentration, the CT contrasts of the Xenon gas shown in Fig. 12 will be slightly enhanced as the tracer density increases with the system pressure.

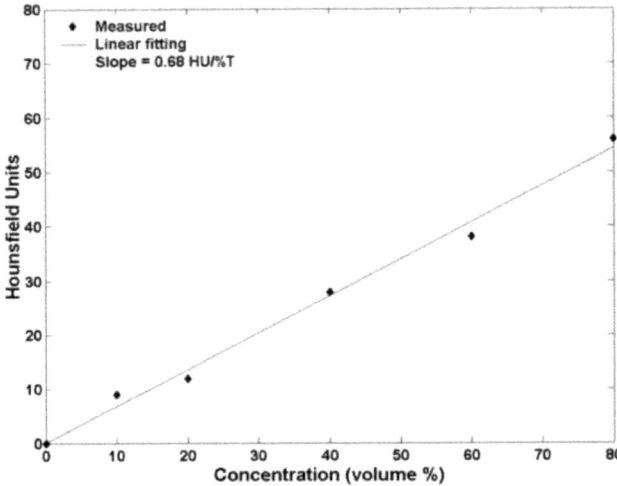

Fig. 12. The incremental CT value (HU) as a linear function of Xenon concentration for Bentheim core. The discrete data indicate the CT value of the tracer mixture flowing steadily in the cores at 1 bar backpressure, determined from averaging CT values over 3 image planes CP=-10, 0, and +10. The slopes of the linear fitting lines show increments of 0.68 due to one additional volume percentage of the tracer in the Bentheim core.

However, the use of very high tracer concentration is not recommended since it might lead to a substantial difference in the rheological properties between the native and tracer foams. We thus chose to use a mixture of 25% Xe in all trapped gas measurements. In tests of Xenon up to 40% for 90%-quality foam for both types of sandstones, we have found an insignificant change in the steady state overall pressure drops, suggesting a minimum disturbance of the tracer foam to the local fluid mobilities. It is worth mentioning that, by scaling the tracer foam saturation according to Eq. (3), the effect of the voxel-to-voxel variations in pressure due to foam is localized and averaged out. Additionally, the noise found in the CT images of steady state nitrogen foams normally ranges from zero to 12 HU. Since the image pixel's size is normally fixed for a fixed CT field of view, larger CT slice-width can be used to increase the total mass of the tracer per voxel, thus improving the signal-to-noise ratio, especially for a relatively high average fraction of quasi-stationary foam per voxel.

3.7 Tracer transport in dry Bentheim core

Fig. 13 shows the percolation of the tracer (green/red) in the Bentheim core after 501 and 1134 second injections of the tracer mixture. Only images CP = 0 and +12 are shown since they capture most of the features of the transient displacement of nitrogen by the tracer. The steady state pressure drop over the core is 0.5 ± 0.2 mbar, resulting in quasi-isobaric CT values of the voxels. The four-second delay between two adjacent images does not seem to cause a discernable shift of the advancing apparent tracer fronts over the image planes. The lateral distribution of the tracer concentration is rather uniform, confirming the macroscopic homogeneity of the Bentheim sandstone core. The longitudinal dispersion of the tracer is remarkably demonstrated by a 'hairy' pattern of the tracer concentration distribution in the main flow direction.

Consider a typical core section denoted by the white rectangle in the images CP = 0 in Fig. 13. Although the tracer first broke through this section after 501 seconds, its concentration continues increasing afterwards, indicating a wide distribution of the pore-scale travel times of the tracer molecules. Particularly, in the image CP = 0 at 1134 seconds, the tracer concentration around the core axis near the inlet is lower than in the surrounding radial region, even though the images in Fig. 13 show that there is uniform distribution of the tracer in the volume before the core inlet.

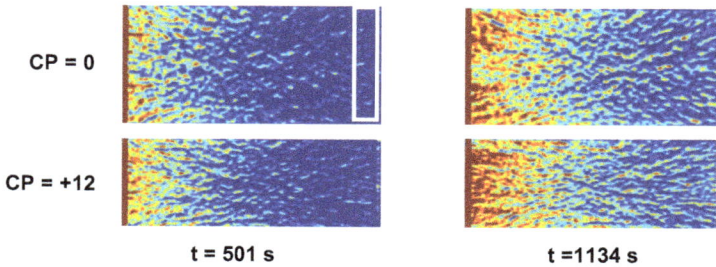

Fig. 13. Propagation of the tracer gas mixture with 25 vol.% Xe in the Bentheim core, following steady state nitrogen flow at 1 bar backpressure. The injection rate of 3 cm³/min (standard conditions) is applied equally for both Nitrogen and tracer mixture. The white rectangles show the non-uniform advancement of the tracer saturations in flow direction due to the significant tracer dispersion. Distribution of tracer concentration is rather uniform in the transverse direction.

Since the longitudinal dispersion of the tracer is relatively dominant for this Bentheim core, the magnitude of tracer dispersivity can be evaluated through one-dimensional tracer saturation profiles (S_T) at different points in time, plotted versus positions along the core as shown in Fig. 14. The saturation value at each position is determined by averaging the voxel tracer saturations over the corresponding cross sections of the seven CT slices. Examine first the 91s-profile in Fig. 14. The tracer percolates almost one-third of the total core length, while it displaces roughly just 35% of the native nitrogen gas near the inlet region. Comparing with the images in Fig. 13, this is due to the significant dispersion effect. This effect is observed more obviously in the subsequent profiles. The typical 501s-profile exhibits three distinct saturation regions: (1) the near inlet region with $S_T \approx 100\%$, (2) the transition region with an abrupt fall of S_T from 100 to roughly 50%, and (3) the relatively largest region with a further gradual decrease of S_T to slightly above 22%. Obviously, the tracer transport is mainly governed by convection in the first region, whereas the last region is characterized by convection and dispersion.

3.8 Foam tracer transport in a horizontal Bentheim core

Fig. 15 shows the displacement of the steady state mobile nitrogen Foam-A by Tracer-Foam-A. Both foams have the same quality of 90.90% with the liquid and (standard) gas rates of 0.5 and 5 cm³/min, respectively. The pressure gradient of 0.54 ± 0.03 bar/cm in Foam-A remained almost constant during the tracer foam injection. The five image planes in Fig. 15 show a three-dimensional structure of the relatively high mobility foam region. The images on the plane CP = 0 resemble its neighboring planes CP = ± 6 (not shown). Consider the first

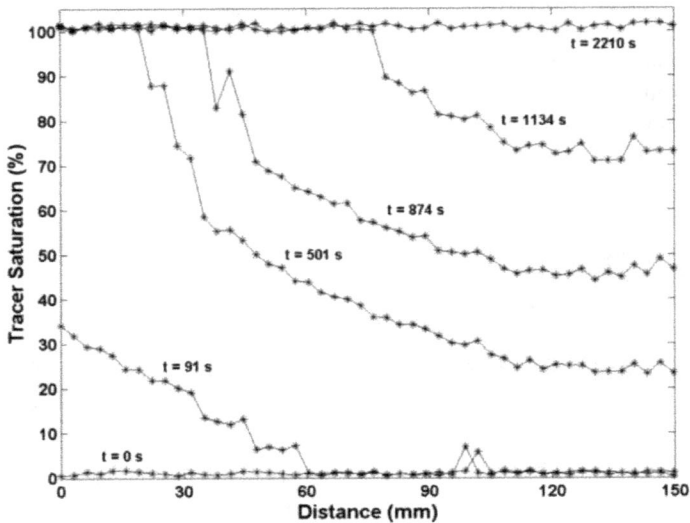

Fig. 14. One-dimensional tracer concentration profile plotted versus distance from the inlet, during the injection of the tracer mixture in the Bentheim core (see Fig. 13). The tracer saturation at each position along the core is determined from averaging the corresponding tracer saturations of individual voxels in the transverse direction over the three CT slices CP =-12, 0, and +12.

Image series in Fig. 15 taken after 990 seconds injection of Tracer-Foam A. The tracer penetrates, about 10 mm deep into the core, uniformly over the cross-sectional area. Further downstream, it propagates preferentially in the upper half of the cylindrical core, and apparently has broken through at the outlet by this time. The most mobile foam forms a cap at the top of the core growing laterally from the upper circumference of the core. A further development of this cap shown in the subsequent 1590-seconds-image series suggests an increase in the spreading of the tracer saturation with the gradually growing cap size. The tracer-saturation spreading reflects the degree of the dispersion effect on the tracer transfer within the cap, while the gradual growth of the cap indicates the diffusion rate of the tracer from the high mobility foam into the surrounding liquid and the quasi-stationary foam. It has been established that the foam films impose significant resistance to the tracer diffusion process. Therefore, for a sufficiently high interstitial velocity of foam, we expect the macroscopic structure of the high mobility foam region to become stably distinct soon after breakthrough of the tracer. This is confirmed in Fig. 15 where the tracer exhibits its stable profile at 2116 seconds. The cap size is well established while the spreading of tracer saturation within the cap is still evolving. Particularly, examining the three images CP = 0 reveals that the tracer near the inlet region around the core center percolates much slower than at the top of the cap. This suggests that the cap contains almost mobile foam. A large remaining fraction of foam is thus either stationary or has a very low mobility relative to that of foam in the cap.

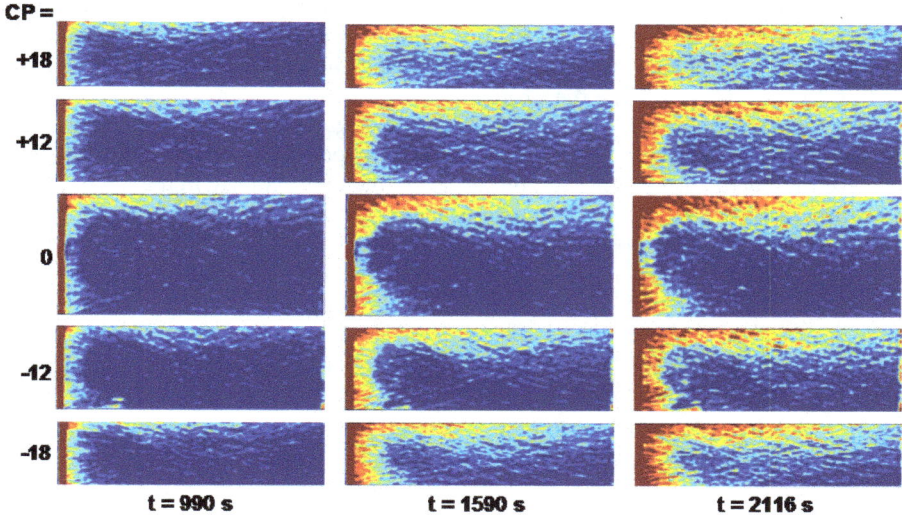

Fig. 15. Displacement of steady state nitrogen Foam-A by the tracer foam in the horizontal Bentheim core. Both foams have the same quality of 90.9% with (standard) gas and liquid rate rates of 5 and 0.5 cm³/min. Tracer concentrations (red/green) reflect the mobile foam, forming a cap-shaped structure in the upper half part of the core. The tracer foam saturation is highly dispersed within the cap. The remaining region (blue) exhibits the quasi-stationary foam.

Fig. 16a presents the corresponding one-dimensional tracer saturation (S_f) profiles, determined by the same averaging method as used for the dry case above. The profile at 990 seconds shows two distinct saturation regions. In the first region (region 1), from the inlet to around 30 mm downstream, the tracer saturation (S_f^1) falls from 40% to slightly above 10%. In the remainder of the core (region 2), tracer saturation (S_f^2) is quite uniform around 10% up to 110 mm, and then decreases gradually to about 8% near the core outlet. Subsequently, the slope of the tracer saturation profile in the main flow direction remains almost the same, but the rate of increase of saturation at a fixed position slows down after about 1500 seconds. This is demonstrated in Fig. 16b, where tracer saturation averaged over the cross-section at the middle position of the core is plotted versus time. The rate of change of saturation in at this position is significantly reduced after roughly 2116 seconds. The images in Fig. 15 show that the significant increase of S_f up to 1590 seconds reflects the fraction of highly mobile native foams displaced by the tracer foam in the cap. The short invasion of the tracer foam in the lower part of the core can result from the intermittent trapping and remobilizing of foam near the inlet region associated with the tracer diffusion. This particular transport phenomenon, that is analogous to the convection-diffusion of the tracer in the fraction of very low mobility foams within the cap, explains the uniform gradual increase of S_f as observed after 1590 seconds. Since the one-dimensional distribution of trapped foam fractions S_t equals to $(100 - S_f)$, the selection of any S_f profile far before 1590 seconds can lead to the overestimating of trapped foam due to a fraction of low mobility native foams, which have not yet been displaced by the tracer foam. The profiles far after this time, on the other hand, can underestimate trapped foam due to the tracer diffusion. Therefore, a good estimate of trapped foam (or quasi-stationary foam) can be obtained at the time where the rate of increase of saturations along the core slows down. In this sense, according to Fig. 16b we chose the profile at 2116 seconds, and found the average quasi-stationary foam fractions of 58 ($\overline{S}_t^1$) and 77% ($\overline{S}_t^2$) in regions 1 and 2, respectively. Note that $\overline{S}_t^1$ and $\overline{S}_t^2$ are used instead of an average of trapped foam $\overline{S}_t$ over the entire core only to emphasize the fluctuation of gas trapping near the inlet, particularly in the lower part of the core as discussed above. The best estimate of the trapped gas fraction under the given flow conditions is $\overline{S}_t^2$ =77%.

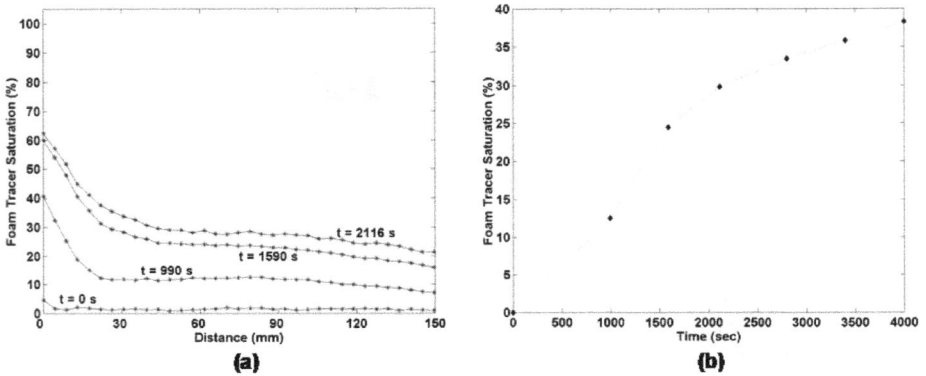

Fig. 16. Cross-section averaged tracer saturation during the displacement of the nitrogen Foam-A in the Bentheim core: (a) One-dimensional foam-tracer saturation profile plotted versus distance from the inlet, (b) The tracer saturation at the middle position of the core (75 mm from the inlet) plotted versus time. This figure shows that the rate of increase of tracer saturation is significantly reduced after 2116 seconds, indicating most of highly mobile native foam being displaced by the tracer foam.

3.9 Effect of gas rate on foam tracer transport in a horizontal Bentheim core

Consider Foam-B with 95.24% quality, having the injection (standard) gas rate twice that in Foam-A and the same liquid rate. The displacement of the steady state Foam-B by Tracer-Foam-B is shown in Fig. 17 at three different points in time. The structure of the high mobility foam cap is similar to that observed with Foam-A (Fig. 15), except that part of it in the image CP = 0 tends to grow away from the upper core circumference. This trend becomes more obvious after 976 seconds, as shown by the last two images series in Fig. 17. Particularly, a small finite cluster of the high tracer saturation propagates slowly in the lower half of the core in images CP = -6. It is possible that it originates from a small percolating cluster of mobile foam near the inlet, which is then somehow trapped. The diffusion process can thus be responsible for the subsequent growth of this cluster. More remarkably, the boundary between the high mobility foam cap and the surrounding region is much sharper than in Tracer Foam-A (see Fig. 15), and does not change significantly in structure and size even after the tracer breakthrough. Furthermore, the high tracer saturation within the cap propagates steadily and faster according to the recorded elapsed times in Fig. 15 and 17. More than likely this results from the increase in the injection gas rate, and the ensuing modification of foam rheology through rate-dependent mobility [Kovscek and Radke, 1994; Alvarez, 1996; Osterloh and Jante, 1992]. In our experiments above, doubling gas rate resulted in the steady state pressure gradient of 0.72 ± 0.03 bar/cm, slightly higher than that in Foam-A (0.54 ± 0.03 bar/cm), suggesting a shear thinning-like foam behavior. This will increase the relative dominance of the convection over diffusion of the tracer, which helps estimate more precisely the actual trapped foam fraction.

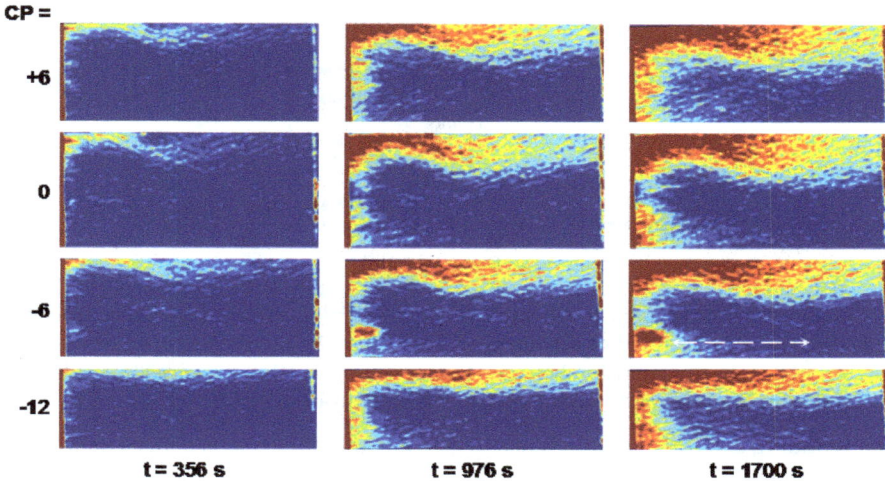

Fig. 17. Displacement of steady state nitrogen Foam-B by the tracer foam. Both foams have the same quality of 95.24% with (standard) gas and liquid rate rates of 10 and 0.5 cm³/min. The highly mobile foam (red/green) concentrates in the half upper part of the core. A small cluster of tracer foam in the lower part of the core near the inlet reflects most likely the fluctuation of gas trapping. The remaining region (blue) exhibits the quasi-stationary foam.

Consistently, the rate of increase of tracer saturations in Foam-B along the core is higher than for Foam-A as shown in Fig. 18, while the shapes of tracer saturation profiles due to both foams are very much similar. A closer examination of the saturation differences between two adjacent profiles reveals that the maximum difference apparently advances downstream in time. This most likely corresponds to the advancement of high tracer saturations in the high mobility foam cap as observed in Fig. 17 (red color). In particular, the profiles at 1700 and 2300 seconds are very close up to around 80 mm from the inlet, and then diverge gradually towards the outlet. The former indicates a rather complete displacement of most of mobile native foams in this region at about 1700 seconds, while the latter reflects the continuous displacement of the low mobility native foams up to 2300 seconds. Note that Fig. 18 does not show the profiles after this time since the subsequent tracer saturations along core changed uniformly and very slowly. Therefore, for the reasons previously mentioned in the section 31.3 A (on Foam-A), we used this profile to determine the average fractions of quasi-stationary foam for regions 1 and 2, which gives $\overline{S}_t^1 = 45$ and $\overline{S}_t^2 = 65\%$.

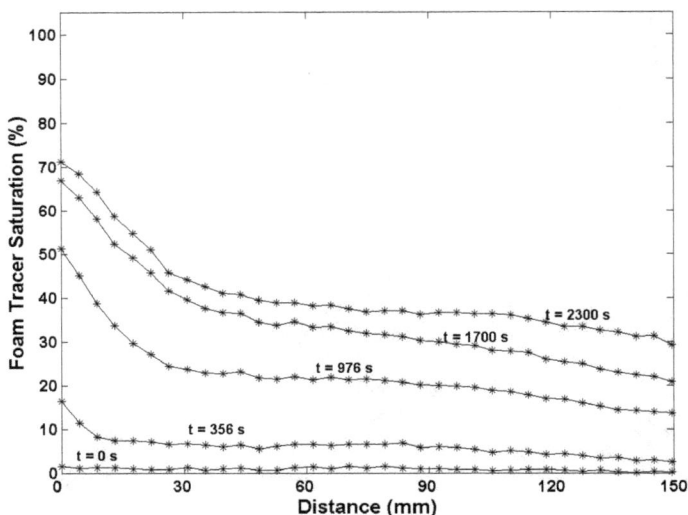

Fig. 18. One-dimensional foam-tracer saturation profile plotted versus distance from the inlet, during the displacement of the nitrogen Foam-B in the Bentheim core (see Fig. 17). The maximum difference in saturation between two adjacent profiles advances towards the outlet, indicating the propagation of the high tracer saturation front.

Notwithstanding a substantial difference in gas rate, the three foams above exhibit a similar macroscopic pattern of quasi-stationary foam. Due to the high foam qualities used, we surmise that the limiting capillary pressure (P_c^*) governs the "shear thinning" rheology of foam as observed in these cases [Khatib et al., 1988; Rossen and Zhou, 1995]. In this regime, foam texture self-regulates to maintain P_c^*. For instance, foam coalescence increases in response to the elevated gas rate. The experimental results suggested a decrease of P_c^* with increasing gas rate. We attribute this to the fact that the instability of foam at high gas rate affects primarily the mobility of flowing foams through the mechanical disturbance and high gradients of dynamic film surface tension at the pore scale. Moreover, if P_c^* is still somewhat smaller than the average critical disjoining pressure of (mobile/stationary) foam films, the trapped gas is strongly influenced by the mobilization capillary number, defined as the ratio of the viscous to foam mobilization pressure gradients

$$N_c = \frac{\left|\nabla P_v(n_f, X_t, v_f)\right|}{\left|\nabla P_m(n_t, K)\right|} \tag{5}$$

where ∇P_v is the viscous gradient as a function of flowing-foam density n_f, fraction of trapped gas X_t, and the mean interstitial velocity of foam flow v_f. ∇P_m is the mobilization pressure gradient determined by the trapped gas density n_t and permeability K [Friedmann et al., 1991; Rossen, 1990]. Since n_f may also be dependent on v_f, ∇P_v might not considerably change with the variation of gas rate at P_c^*, in agreement with Khatib et al. [1988], who reported experimentally a quasi-linear relationship between the gas fractional flow and the relative gas mobility in foam. As a result, the trapped gas fraction would be less sensitive to the gas rate for high quality foams at P_c^*, as found above.

3.10 Foam tracer transport in vertical Bentheim core

For horizontal flow, the highly mobile foam concentrates mainly in the upper part of the core, regardless of the gas rate, while the liquid rate apparently plays an important role in the mobilization of foam in the lower part. We surmise that gravity causes foam to be dryer towards the top of the core. As a result, foam in the upper region becomes less stable at the elevated gas rate, and thus the limiting capillary pressure governs its rheological behavior. On the contrary, increased liquid rate can increase in the liquid fraction of foam in the lower part of the core (particularly near the inlet region), resulting in low quality foam. To obtain a better understanding of the gravity effect, we next consider the distribution of foam mobilities in vertical flow.

Fig. 19 shows the displacement of Foam-A by Tracer-Foam-A in the central image plane at three different points in time. The high mobility foam cap observed with the horizontal flow (Fig. 15) is drastically modified as the foam flows vertically upwards.

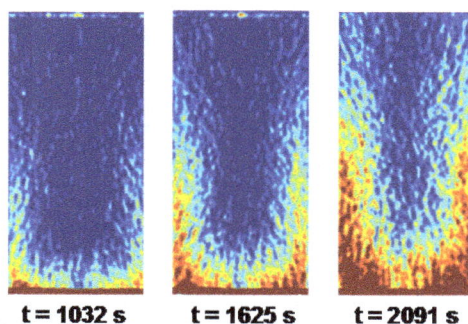

t = 1032 s   t = 1625 s   t = 2091 s

Fig. 19. Displacement of steady state nitrogen Foam-A (90.90 % quality) by the tracer foam in the vertical Bentheim core. The high foam mobility region has a 'cup'-shaped structure (outer annulus foam), leading to a higher total fraction of mobile foam, compared to the cap structure in the horizontal core (see Fig. 15).

The cap expands around the core center to form a symmetric annular shape, whose thickness slightly increases towards the inlet. Comparison with the images CP = 0 in Fig. 15 reveals that the tracer saturation is less variable for the vertical flow, suggesting a more uniform distribution of foam mobilities in the annular region (called outer-annulus foam). This is shown in the corresponding one-dimensional tracer saturation profiles shown in Fig. 20.

Consider the profiles at around 1000 seconds after injection of the tracer mixture for both core arrangements (Fig. 16a and 20), the tracer saturation for the vertical flow is about 5% higher in region 1, and decreases rapidly in region 2 to below 5% near the outlet, with a smoother transition between these regions. The profile at 1625 and 2091 seconds in Fig. 20 demonstrate the uniform slowdown of the rate of increase of tracer saturation, signaling most of the high mobility foams were displaced throughout the core. Note that the annular structure of the flowing foam region is expected to give a higher overall mobile foam fraction than in the cap. However, this was not observed near the outlet region for the vertical flow where the mobile foam fraction was found to be lower. This conflicting result is most likely ascribed to a higher convective dispersion in the horizontal cap, which drove a relatively larger fraction of the high mobility foams to the outlet for a given elapsed time. Thus, it is appropriate to use the average quasi-stationary foam fractions for regions 1 and 2. For the profile at 2091 seconds in Fig. 45, $\bar{S}_t^1 = 45$ % and $\bar{S}_t^2 = 70$ %. These values are consistently lower than those for the horizontal foam flow determined at almost the same elapsed time.

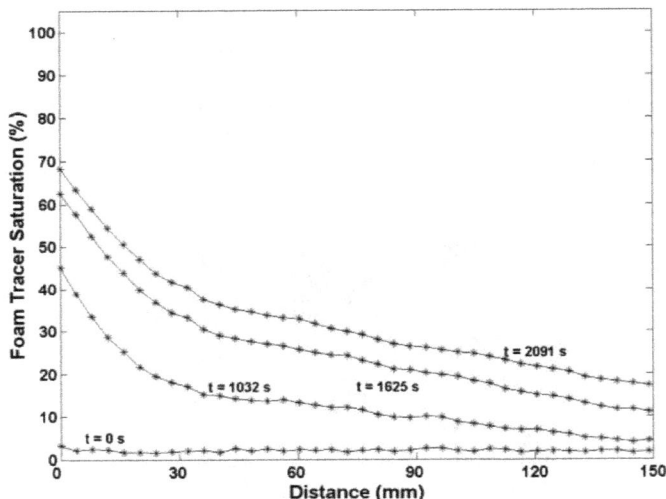

Fig. 20. One-dimensional foam-tracer saturation profile plotted versus distance from the inlet, during the displacement of the nitrogen Foam-A in the vertical Bentheim core (Fig 19).

4. Main conclusions

- The macroscopic conditions for foam propagation and the characteristic regimes of liquid flow in a quasi-stagnant foam matrix are crucial issues in the upscaled description of foam behavior in the majority of foam applications. These issues have been systematically investigated through the LDL and FDL processes, where the in-situ fluid mobility and partitioning are determined by the pressure drop measurement and the X-ray CT aided visualization. The theoretical and experimental framework elucidates several aspects that seem to be missing in the literature.

- For liquid displacement by foam, the pressure drop corresponds well with fluid saturation throughout a two-stage displacement. While the first stage has been commonly observed in previous work, the second stage seems to be a new phenomenon, which is characterized by a secondary liquid desaturation (SLD) initiating around the middle region of the core and propagating towards the inlet and outlet. Where and when the second saturation front emerges is important in designing a field foam process. For instance, for foam-improved sweep efficiency or gas blockage in underground gas storage, the development of foam far way from injection wells is desired, whereas a strong foam development near the well-bore is essential for the success of foam induced acid diversion.

- Except the "entrance" effect, the two-stage liquid desaturation is not affected by the fluid rates. Unlike the "capillary-end" effect that is suppressed as the SLD emerges, the "entrance" effect is much more sensitive to the increase in the liquid rate than the gas rate. This is attributed to two factors: (1) foam generation by snap-off is dependent more on the liquid rate, and (2) the elevated gas rate results in a lower value of the limiting capillary pressure, as a refection of the well known detrimental effect of high gas rate on foam stability.

- For foam displacement by liquid, the conventional imbibition process changes substantially in the presence of foam. According to our theory, for an insignificant gas expansion and dissolution effect, the percolation of the liquid phase is determined not only by the injection rate, but also by the magnitude and uniformity of foam yield stresses, and the gravity effect. As a result, on the pore scale the "piston-like displacement" and/or the "wetting film" flow regimes are expected to characterize the imbibition process. This is consistent with most of the experimental results, which show both fingering- and dispersed-flow regimes on the macroscopic scale.

- The structure of the liquid finger associated with the trapped gas fraction is strongly influenced by the initial steady-state foam strength. Particularly, the finger becomes less tortuous and orientates upwards against gravity as the foam strength increases. As a result, the trapped gas fraction over the entire core at the quasi-steady state increases significantly (e.g. from 70.2 to 78.1% for surfactant-solution injection). Moreover, the fingering region encapsulates a significant gas fraction, which also increases with the foam strength (e.g. from 18.0 to 31.2% for surfactant-solution injection). Therefore, strong foam tends to hinder the "fingering-flow" regime, consistent with our simple theoretical analysis.

- The liquid rate has different effects on the fingering pattern. On one hand, the finger dimensions decrease with the liquid rate, but on the other hand, the gravity effect is aggravated.

- The inherent gas expansion obviously reduces the foam-mobilization pressure, and thus favors the 'fingering-flow" regime. This helps explain partially why the finger grows more laterally towards the inlet. An important practical implication of the gas expansion is that in a stratified formation, the gas expansion is normally faster in high permeability layers, potentially reducing the diversion capacity of foam in these layers. On the other hand, the gas expansion can also be resisted if it triggers foam generation. The latter is particularly true if the injected liquid is the surfactant solution.

- The experimental results have demonstrated that the X-ray CT aided tracer technique developed is a powerful tool for investigating foam-trapping phenomenon in porous media, as well as characterizing the micro-heterogeneity of the pore networks through different patterns of tracer convection-dispersion. The use of tracer concentration of 25 vol.% at 1 bar backpressure provides sufficient contrast between the tracer gas mixture (tracer foam) and the native gas (foam). A higher tracer concentration might be required for a lower system pressure, and vice versa.

- Since diffusion rate of the tracer in stationary foam is small, but not zero, a reliable interpretation of the in-situ tracer concentration profile can be obtained if convection dominates over diffusion. The dominant convection may increase the convective dispersion of the tracer, which modifies the actual distribution of the stationary and flowing components for a relatively short observation time. Therefore, the system length should be limited to ensure the consistency of the measured tracer concentration profile with the actual distribution of local fluid mobilities. If the system dimensions are large, the use of the regional concentration profiles is advisable.

- For the Bentheim sandstone core, the transient displacement of the tracer gas without foam demonstrates typical one-dimensional single-phase flow in a homogeneous medium. Foams strongly modify this flow pattern due to persistent and/or temporary foam trapping. For the horizontal core Foam-A with 90.9% quality shows its mobile fraction concentrated only in the upper half part of the core, with a small fluctuation of stationary foam very near the inlet in the lower part. An increase in foam quality up to 95.24% (by increasing the standard gas rate from 5 to 10 cm³/min at a fixed liquid rate of 0.5 cm³/min) primarily enhanced the mobility of the flowing foam and the fluctuation of stationary foam near the inlet region without a significant change of the macroscopic structure ($\bar{S}_t^2$ = 77% for Foam-A with 90.90% quality, 65% for Foam-B with 95.24% quality).

- The same trends for the mobility distribution to the variation of gas and liquid rates were also observed when the foams flowed vertically upwards. However, in this flow direction, for a given foam quality, the mobilities of flowing foams were reduced and rather uniformly distributed compared with the horizontal case. This resulted from the restructuring of the macroscopic pattern of foam mobility distribution in which the mobile foam formed an annular region, whose center was filled with quasi-stationary foam.

- The macroscopic quasi-stationary gas domain during the foam stage is distinctly different from that during the post-foam liquid injection. This is attributed to: (a) change in local equilibrium between foam generation and destruction, (b) gas expansion and dissolution, and (c) gravity effect.

5. Acknowledgment

I would like to thank Prof. Peter K. Currie and Prof. Pacelli Zitha for their valuable scientific discussions. I would also like to thank Shell for supporting this work.

6. References

Alvarez, R.E and Macovski, A.: "Energy-Selective Reconstructions in X-ray Computed Tomography," Phys. Med. Biol. (1976), 21, 733.

Alvarez, J.M.: "Foam-Flow Behaviour in Porous Media: Effects of Flow Regime and Porous-Medium Heterogeneity," PhD Dissertation (December) 1996, the university of Texas at Austin.

Apaydin, O.G. and Kovscek, A.R., "Transient Foam Flow in Homogeneous Porous Media: Surfactant Concentration and Capillary End Effects," SPE paper 59286 presented at the SPE/DOE Improved Oil Recovery Symposium, Tulsa, OK, 2000.

Behenna, F. R: "Acid Diversion from an Undamaged to a Damaged Core Using Multiple Foam Slugs," paper SPE 30121 presented at the SPE European Formation Damage Conference, The Hague, 1995.

Brooks, R.A., Weiss, G.H., and Talbert, A.J., J. Comput. Assist. Tomog. 1978, 2, 577.

Burganos, V.N., J. Chem. Phys. 1998, 109, 16, 6772.

Cheng, L, Kam, S.I., Delshad, M., and Rossen, W.R.: "Simulation of Dynamic Foam-Acid Diversion Process," paper SPE 68916 presented at the European Formation Damage Conference, The Hague, 2001.

Friedmann, F., Chen W.H., and Gauglitz, P.A.: "Experimental and Simulation Study of High-Temperature Foam Displacement in porous Media," SPE Reservoir Engineering 1991, 37.

Fulcher, Jr. R.A., Ertekin, T., and Stahl, C.D.: "Effect of Capillary Number and Its Constituents on Two-Phase Relative Permeability Curves," JPT 1985, 249.

Gauglitz, P.A., Friedmann, F., Kam, S. I., and Rossen, W. R.: "Foam Generation in Porous Media," paper SPE 75177 presented at the SPE/DOE Symposium on Improved Oil Recovery, Tulsa, OK, 2002.

Kak, A.C. and Roberts, B., in Handbook of Pattern Recognition and Image Processing, Young, T.Y. and Fu, K.S. (Eds.), New York Academic Press 1986.

Khatib, Z.I., Hirasaki, G.J., and Falls, A.H.: "Effects of Capillary Pressure on Coalescence and Phase Mobilities in Foam Flowing through Porous Media," SPE Reservoir Engineering 1988, 3, 919.

Kovscek, A.R., and Radke, C. J.: "Fundamentals of Foam Transport in Porous Media," in Foams: Fundamentals and Applications in the Petroleum Industry, ACS Advances in Chemistry series 242, Washington, DC (1994), 110.

Kibodeaux, K.R., Zeilinger, S.C., and Rossen, W.R.: "Sensitivity Study of Foam Diversion Process for Matrix Acidizing," paper SPE 28550 presented at the SPE Annual Technical Conference and Exhibition, New Orleans, LA, 1994.

McCullough, E.C., "Photon Attenuation in Computed Tomography" Med. Phys. 1975, 2, 307.

Millner, M., Payne, W.H., Waggener, R.G., McDavid, W.D., Dennis, M.J. and Sank, V.J., Med. Phys. 1978, 5, 543.

Osterloh, W.T. and Jante, M.J.: "Effects of Gas and Liquid Velocity on Steady-State Foam Flow," paper SPE 24179 presented at the SPE/DOE Symposium on Improved Oil Recovery, Tulsa, OK, 1992.

Parlar, M., Parris, M.D., Jasinski, R.J., Robert, J.A.: "An Experimental Study of Foam Flow Through Berea Sandstone with Applications to Foam Diversion in Matrix Acidizing," paper SPE 29678 presented at the SPE Western Regional Meeting, Bakerfield, CA, 1995.

Rossen, W.R. and Zhou, Z.H.: "Modeling Foam Mobility at the Limiting Capillary Pressure," SPE Advanced Technologies Series 1995, 3, 1.

Siddiqui, S., Talabani, S., Yang, J., Saleh, S., Islam, M.R.: "An Experimental Investigation of the Diversion Characteristics of Foam in Berea Sandstone Cores of Contrasting Permeability," paper SPE 37463 presented at the Production Operations Symposium, OK, 1997.

Tanzil, D., Hirasaki, G.J., and Miller, C.A.: "Conditions for Foam Generation in Homogeneous Porous Media," paper SPE 75176 presented at the SPE/DOE Symposium on Improved Oil Recovery, Tulsa, OK, 2002.

Thompson, K.E. and Gdanski, R.D.: "Laboratory Study Provides Guidelines for Diverting Acid with Foam," SPE Production & Facilities 1993.

Wassmuth, F.R., Green, K.A, and Randall, L.: "Details of In-situ Foam Propagation Exposed with Magnetic Resonance Imaging," SPE Reservoir Evaluation & Engineering 2001, 135.

Zerhboub, M., Ben-Naceur, K., Touboul, E, and Thomas, R.: "Matrix Acidizing: A Novel Approach to Foam Diversion," SPE Production & Facilities 1994.

8

3D-μCT Cephalometric Measurements in Mice

F. de Carlos[1,2], A. Alvarez-Suárez[2,3], S. Costilla[4],
I. Noval[5], J. A. Vega[6] and J. Cobo[1,2]
[1]Departamentos de Cirugía y Especialidades Médico-Quirúrgicas (Section of Odontology)
[2]Instituto Asturiano de Odontología, Oviedo
[3]Construcción e Ingeniería de la Fabricación (Section of Mechanic Engineering)
[4]Medicina (Section of Radiology)
[5]Servicio de Radiología, Hospital Universitario Central de Asturias, Oviedo
[6]Morfología y Biología Celular (Section of Anatomy and Human Embryology)
Universidad de Oviedo
Spain

1. Introduction

The skull of all vertebrates is a structure made up of the neurocranium, which surrounds and protects the encephalon, and the viscerocranium, which protects the initial segment of the digestive and respiratory systems. The separate bones that form the skull are articulated among them forming sutures and synchondroses in the adjacent margins of the membrane bones of the calvaria and of the bones of the skull base, respectively (see for a detailed review and references Wilkie and Morriss-Kay, 2001; Morriss-Kay and Wilkie, 2005).

Advances in molecular genetics over the past two decades have revealed some of the key genes for skull vault development (Verdyck et al., 2006). Then, the genetic engineering has been used to construct mice that lack these genes resulting in abnormal craniofacial development, equivalent to those of some human conditions. Therefore, the murine model has been chosen as a surrogate for studying the biologic behavior of human cranial bones and joints-sutures. For example, we have recently analyzed the cranial, mandible and tooth defects of a mouse strain which mimics a human progeroid syndrome (De Carlos et al., 2008). These mouse models are basics for understanding the developmental mechanisms leading to skull malformations, and may eventually help in the development of new therapeutic strategies.

The image technique modalities used to quantitatively asses the changes in size and shape in the skull in these animal varies from simple radiology to three-dimensional (3D) micro-computed tomography (μCT; Figure 1; see for a review Tobita et al., 2010). Nevertheless, 3D-μCT is becoming more and more a common technique for the anatomical analyses of these mice models (Paulus et al., 2001; Song et al., 2001; Recinos et al., 2004; Schambach et al., 2010), especially in the field of the skeletal development and growth (Guldberg et al., 2004). For example, 3D μCT quantitative evaluations have been made in mouse to study different functional skull changes (Enomoto et al., 2010; Saito et al., 2011a,b), or several kinds of developmental or genetic skull malformations (Perlyn et al., 2006; De Carlos et al., 2008;

Coleman et al., 2010; Purushothaman et al., 2011), or the distribution of some genetic characters in different strains of mice (Nishimura et al., 2003).

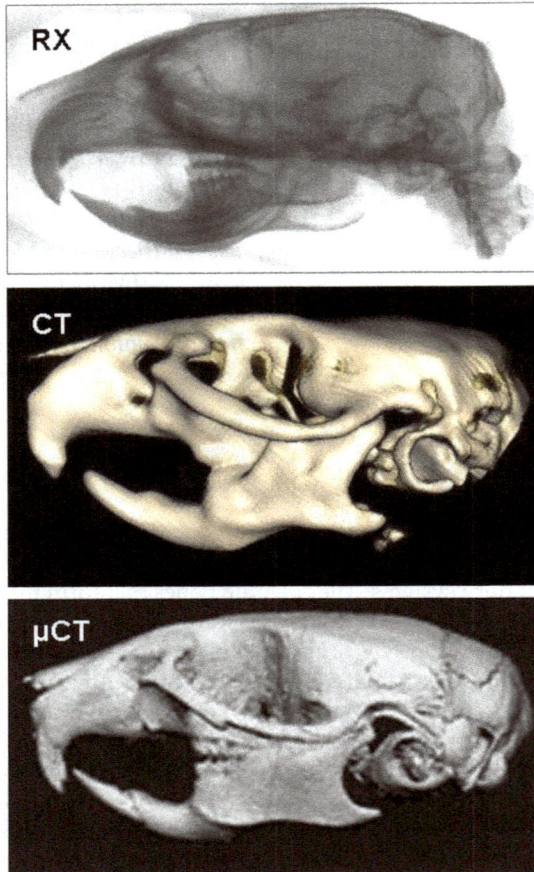

Fig. 1. Lateral view, left, of a mice skull using simple radiology (RX), conventional computed tomography (CT), and micro-computed tomography (µCT). Only simple radiology and µCT show detailed morphology of the skull and therefore consent an accurate localization of landmark points for cephalometry.

Cephalometric radiography analyses have been developed for the evaluation of specific skull of rodents, but no comprehensive standardized cephalometric methods have been generated for mice. Moreover, most of the 3D-µCT studies were used to show differences between wild-type and mutated mice evaluating a few number of lineal or volumetric parameters. These measurements are sufficient to quantitatively evidence the main skull changes induced by an experimental manipulation but are insufficient to accurately evaluate the length, height and width of the different segments of the cranium and the mandible. Thus, we consider that the skull measurements in mice must be more detailed in order to acquiesce to all the skull defects induced by an experimental condition or a mutation.

In this chapter we first establish landmarks which can be easily identified in 3D-µCT images from mice skull. Thereafter, in order to define the skull phenotype we propose a cephalometric study based on the osseous landmarks currently used in human orthodontics and orthopedics. Also we compare the results of cephalometric measurements obtained using simple radiology and those obtained using 3D-µCT. Finally, we underline the advantages and disadvantages of 3D-µCT for evaluating the morphology of mice skull. The 3D-µCT database of the skull size and shape in different mouse strains are necessary to provide references for future studies involving large-scare mutant screening.

2. Localization of cephalometric landmarks in mice skull using µCT

To perform 3D-µCT cephalometric analysis the first step is the identification and localization of cranial and mandible reference landmarks directly on the bone surfaces. Accurate location of landmarks and user skill are important factors to achieve reliable data. Here we have identified a series of landmarks than can be extrapolated to those used in human cephalometric, and therefore consent a detailed measurement of the mice skull. Some authors (Nishimura et al., 2003), however, limit cephalometric analysis to a small number of reliable and informative landmarks.

To perform cephalometric study we purpose, the the following landmarks were identified (Figure 2):

Norma dorsalis o superior (Fig. 2A): 1: internasal point; 2: occipital point; 3: nasal points; 4: orbital point (right and left infraorbital foramina); 5: zygomatic points; 6: jugal process of squamosal bone.

Norma basalis (Fig. 2B): 7: interdental point; 8: posterior nasal spine.

Norma posterior (Fig. 2C): 2: occipital point; 5: zygomatic points; 6: jugal process of squamosal bone.

Norma anterior (Fig. 2D): 4: orbital point (right and left infraorbital foramina); 5: zygomatic points.

Norma lateralis (dextra; Fig. 2E): 9: naso-maxillary point; 10: superior incisor-alveolar point; 11: prostion; 12: superior incisor point; 13: parietal point; 14: tympanic point.

The use of 3D-µCT imaging allows for the demonstration of structures and landmarks that are impossible to identify by conventional radiographic methods. It also allows for the selection of images at any desired angulation, and the calculation of 3D distance between any two points. Of particular interest are measurements that cannot be easily obtained by plain radiographs, such transverse distances between the same points on the two sides of the maxilla or mandible.

3. A proposal for the cephalometric analysis by µCT in mice

The dimensional analysis of the skull using 3D-µCT is based on measurements between reference landmarks, whereas topological analyses provide 3D geometrical reference frames using the reference landmarks. The shape measurements can be defined by ratios of inter-landmark distances or angles, or by principal components from outline data or landmark configurations.

For a correct cephalometric study we purpose ten measurements for the cranium, and seven for the mandible. All these measurements are distances between recognizable landmarks on digitalized images of the *normae dorsalis, basalis* and *lateralis* of the skull. The measurements

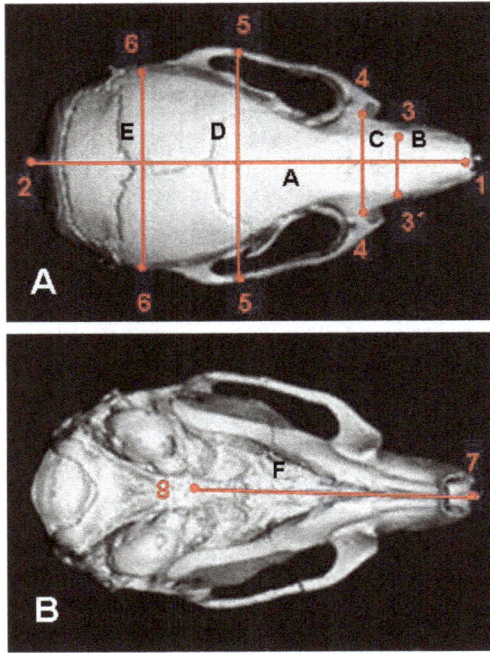

Fig. 2. Landmarks and measurements proposed for cephalometry in mice. A – Norma superior: 1: internasal point; 2: occipital point; 3: nasal points; 4: orbital point (right and left infraorbital foramina); 5: zygomatic points; 6: jugal process of squamosal bone; A: cranial length; B: internasal distance; C: interorbitary length; D: interzygomatic distance; E: bitemporal distance. B – Norma basalis: 7: interdental point; 8: posterior nasal spine; F: palatine length.

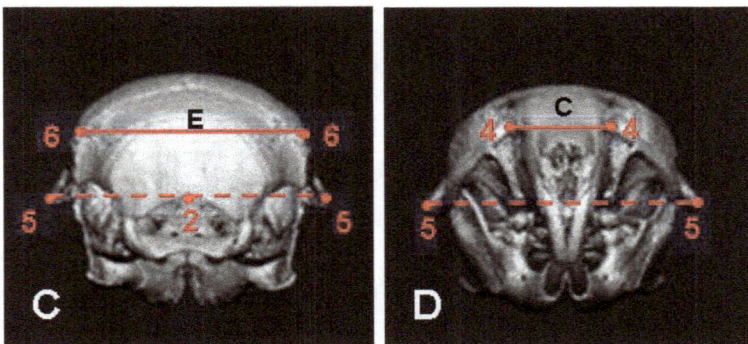

Fig. 2. Landmarks and measurements proposed for cephalometry in mice. C – Norma posterior: 2: occipital point; 5: zygomatic points; 6: jugal process of squamosal bone; E: bitemporal distance. D – Norma anterior: 4: orbital point (right and left infraorbital foramina); 5: zygomatic points; C: interorbitary length.

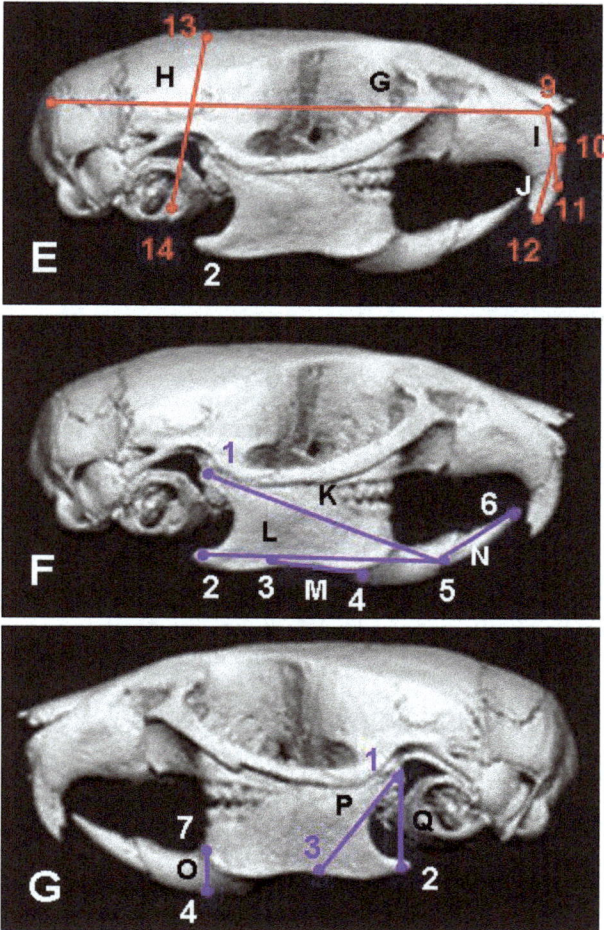

Fig. 2. Landmarks and measurements proposed for cephalometry in mice. E – Norma lateralis dextra: 9: naso-maxillary point; 10: superior incisor-alveolar point; 11: prostion; 12: superior incisor point; 13: parietal point; 14: tympanic point; G: sagittal cranial distance; H: posterior cranial height; I: anterior cranial height; J: upper incisor height. F – Norma lateralis dextra (mandible measurements): 1: condilion point; 2: gonion; 3: antegonion; 4: menton; 5: inferior incisor-alveolar point; 6: incisor inferior point; K: effective mandible length; L: mandible plain; M: mandible axis; N: inferior incisor axis. G – Norma lateralis sinistra (mandible measurements): 1: condilion point; 2: gonion; 3: antegonion; 4: menton; 7: mandible alveolar (or diastema) point; O: anterior mandible height; P: condilar axis; Q: posterior mandible height.

we purpose are based on other studies carried out in mice showing skull phenotypes caused by gene mutation (see Olafsdottir et al., 2007), and were homologous to those used for standard orthodontic cephalometry in humans (Burkhardt et al., 2003).

Accuracy of measurements should be a primary goal of scientists to prevent statistical errors and therefore to promote the comparison of the results obtained from various research groups. Therefore they must be vigilant during data collection and use the appropriate device/method. Skull measurements in mice require an accurate localization of landmarks and measurements, since errors can lead to inappropriate valuation of an experimental situation. The accuracy of cephalometric landmark identification it is not related to technical characteristic of the used 3D-μCT (Olszewski et al., 2008) but rather with the ability and training of the researchers. Moreover, 3D imaging allows for overall improved interobserver and intraobserver reliability in certain landmarks in vivo when compared with two-dimensional images, and intraexaminer and interexaminer reliabilities are high for most landmarks (Chien et al., 2009).

The following parameters are proposed (Figure 2):

Craniometric measurements:

1. Cranial length (A): measured between the internasal (top of the nose) and the occipital (the most distal point of the occipital bone) points.
2. Inter-nasal distance (B): measured between both nasal lateral points.
3. Inter-orbitary length (C): measured between right and left infraorbital foramina.
4. Inter-zygomatic distance (D): measured between both zygion points.
5. Bi-temporal distance (E): measured in the more distant point of the jugal process off squamosal with respect to the sagittal plane.
6. Sagittal cranial distance (G): measured between the occipital and the naso-maxillary point.
7. Posterior cranial height (H): measured between the tympanic and the parietal point.
8. Anterior cranial height (I): measured between the upper incisor and the prostion points.
9. Upper incisor height (J): measured between the upper incisor-alveolar bone and upper incisor edge.
10. Palatine length (F): measured between the posterior nasal spine and the inter-dental point.

Mandible measurements:

1. Posterior mandible height (Q): measured between the gonion and condilion points.
2. Condiloid axis (length of the ascending ramus) (P): measured between the condilion and antegonion points.
3. Anterior mandible height (O): measured between the menton and the mandibular alveolar (or diastema) points.
4. Effective mandible length (K): measured between the lower alveolar incisor (infradentale) and the condilyon points.
5. Mandible plain (L): measured between the gonion and the lower incisor-alveolar bone.
6. Mandible axis (M): measured between the antegonium and menton points.
7. Inferior incisor height (N): measured between the lower incisor-alveolar bone and the lower edge.

This method consent a complete quantitative evaluation of the length, height and, in a lesser extent, width of the skull. The results of the measurements we have performed in adult C57B1/6 mice using 3D-μC are summarized in table 1. In comparing these values with those obtained using simple radiography it can be observed that they are almost identical. However, some key measurements cannot be performed using plane radiography because landmarks cannot not be precisely localized (see table 1), thus reinforcing the usefulness of 3D-μCT in these studies. On the other hand, some measurements that may be of interest (i.e. Inter-molar maxillary distance, hemi-mandible length or inter-molar mandible length; see de Carlos et al., 2008) can be performed only if the mandible is isolated and detached off the skull.

Cranial measurements	µCT	SimpleRX
Line A: CL	22,61 ± 0,31	22,44 ± 0,46
Line B: Internasal D	3,85 ± 0,13	n.d
Line C: Inter-orbitary L	4,21 ± 1,1	3,96 ± 0,12
Line D: Interzygomatic D	12,12 ± 0,30	11,96 ± 0,22
Line E: Bi-temporal D	10,31 ± 0,17	10,41 ± 0,16
Line F: Palatine L	14,03 ± 0,11	n.d
Line G: Sagittal CD	21,22 ± 0,41	21,33 ± 0,42
Line H: Posterior CH	10,31 ± 0,21	10,04 ± 0,40
Line I: Anterior CH	2,69 ± 0,11	2,67 ± 0,16
Line J: Upper incisor H	4,02 ± 0,18	3,99 ± 0,16
Mandible measurements		
Line K: Effective ML	11,21 ± 0,20	n.d
Line L: M plain	10,39 ± 0,71	n.d
Line M: M axis	5,32 ± 0,33	n.d
Line N: Inferior incisor axis	4,30 ± 0,11	4,15 ± 0,21
Line O: Anterior MH	2,09 ± 0,09	2,09 ± 0,12
Line P: Condiloid axis	5,18 ± 0,10	n.d
Line Q: Posterior MH	4,13 ± 0,16	n.d

C = cranial; D = distance; H = height; L = length; M = mandible
n.d: not done

Table 1. Results of the cranium and mandible measurements in the mouse using µCT and simple radiography. Data were obtained from 10 adult C57Bl/6 mice

So, the values of measurements of the mice skull on conventional radiographs are comparable with measurements on 3D-µCT, but 3D-µCT allows for the demonstration of structures and landmarks that are impossible to identify by conventional radiographic methods.

A computational atlas of the mice skull using 3D-µCT has been developed by Olafsdottir et al. (2009) to automatically asses the variations in skull morphology and size of a mice model of Crouzon's syndrome. Although this atlas is a powerful method due to its plasticity and the results obtained with this system are the measurements they perform (skull length, height and width and interorbital distance) are not sufficient to completely evaluate the skull, since the mandible is not considered, and there are gene mutations that specifically affect to this bone.

4. Advantages and disadvantages of µCT for cephalometric measurements in mice

In the 1970 decade clinical imaging was radically changed by the introduction of computed tomography (CT). Until then, the examination of small animals in research, especially of mice and rats, was limited by the resolving capacity of clinical CT scanners (see central image of figure 1). However, over the past three decades 3D-µCT imaging has rapidly advanced with higher quality spatial and temporal resolution, the introduction of the cone beam reconstruction algorithm, and the availability of scanners specific for non-invasive small animal imaging research. These technical advancements have allowed researchers to capture detailed anatomical images and precisely localize landmarks (see Cavanaugh et al., 2004; Nalçaci et al., 2010; Schambach et al., 2010).

The limitations of plain film radiographs in skull evaluation are well documented in different classical texts and the introduction of 3D visualization of the bony skeleton has been a breakthrough (Papadopoulos et al., 2002). There are numerous studies reporting that measurements obtained by 3D methods, especially µCT, are more reliable than the conventional method (see Ozsoy et al., 2009; Zamora et al., 2011). Nevertheless, in our hands both simple radiography and 3D-µCT offer similar results for most of the cranial measurements, but not for the mandible.

So, 3D-µCT is actually the best method for noninvasive imaging of mouse cranial anatomy. The principle advantages of 3D-µCT technology for evaluation of the skull are: first, the ability to easily view and manipulate images in any plane; second, the ability to repeat the measure on the same individual animal over time; and third, the ability to minimize tissue and/or animal sacrifice. 3D-µCT however has the following main limitations: first, the image acquisition time is somewhat long; second, extensive hands-on data manipulation of the raw data is required before the final images can be rendered; third, it is expensive. But any case, surely this method is the present and the future.

5. References

Burkhardt DR, McNamara JA Jr, Baccetti T. 2003. Maxillary molar distalization or mandibular enhancement: a cephalometric comparison of comprehensive orthodontic treatment including the pendulum and the Herbst appliances. Am J Orthod Dentofacial Orthop 123: 108-116.

Cavanaugh D, Johnson E, Price RE, Kurie J, Travis EL, Cody DD. 2004. In vivo respiratory-gated micro-CT imaging in small-animal oncology models Mol Imaging 3: 55–62.

Chien PC, Parks ET, Eraso F, Hartsfield JK, Roberts WE, Ofner S. 2009. Comparison of reliability in anatomical landmark identification using two-dimensional digital cephalometrics and three-dimensional cone beam computed tomography in vivo. Dentomaxillofac Radiol 38:262-273.

Coleman RM, Phillips JE, Lin A, Schwartz Z, Boyan BD, Guldberg RE. 2010. Characterization of a small animal growth plate injury model using microcomputed tomography. Bone 46:1555-1563.

de Carlos F, Varela I, Germanà A, Montalbano G, Freije JM, Vega JA, López-Otín C, Cobo JM. 2008. Microcephalia with mandibular and dental dysplasia in adult Zmpste24-deficient mice. J Anat 213:509-519.

Enomoto A, Watahiki J, Yamaguchi T, Irie T, Tachikawa T, Maki K. 2010. Effects of mastication on mandibular growth evaluated by microcomputed tomography. Eur J Orthod 32:66-70.

Guldberg RE, Lin AS, Coleman R, Robertson G, Duvall C. 2004. Microcomputed tomography imaging of skeletal development and growth. Birth Defects Res C Embryo Today 72: 250-259.

Morriss-Kay GM, Wilkie AOM. 2005. Growth of the normal skull vault and its alteration in craniosynostosis: insights from human genetics and experimental studies. J Anat 207: 637–653.

Nalçaci R, Oztürk F, Sökücü O. 2010. A comparison of two-dimensional radiography and three-dimensional computed tomography in angular cephalometric measurements. Dentomaxillofac Radiol 39:100-106.

Nishimura I, Drake TA, Lusis AJ, Lyons KM, Nadeau JH, Zernik J. 2003. ENU large-scale mutagenesis and quantitative trait linkage (QTL) analysis in mice: novel technologies for searching polygenetic determinants of craniofacial abnormalities. Crit Rev Oral Biol Med 14:320-330.

Olafsdottir H, Darvann TA, Hermann NV, Oubel O, Ersboll BK, Frangi AF, Larse P, Perlyn CA, Morriss-Kay GM, Kreiborg S. (2007) Computational Mouse atlases and their application to autosomic assessment of craniofacial dysmorphology caused by the Crouzon mutation Fgfr2C342Y. J Anat 211, 37-52.

Olszewski R, Reychler H, Cosnard G, Denis JM, Vynckier S, Zech F. 2008. Accuracy of three-dimensional (3D) craniofacial cephalometric landmarks on a low-dose 3D computed tomograph. Dentomaxillofac Radiol 37:261-267.

Ozsoy U, Demirel BM, Yildirim FB, Tosun O, Sarikcioglu L. 2009. Method selection in craniofacial measurements: Advantages and disadvantages of 3D digitization method. J Cran Max Surg 37: 285-290.

Papadopoulos MA, Christou PK, Athanasiou AE, , Boettcher P, Zeilhofer HF, Sader R, Papadopulos NA.2002. Three-dimensional craniofacial reconstruction imaging. Oral Surg Oral Med Oral Pathol Oral Radiol Endod 93: 382–93.

Paulus M, Gleason S, Easterly M, Foltz C. 2001. A review of high-resolution X-ray computed tomography and other imaging modalities for small animal research. Laboratory Anim 30:36–45.

Perlyn CA, DeLeon VB, Babbs C, Govier D, Burell L, Darvann T, Kreiborg S, Morriss-Kay G. 2006. The craniofacial phenotype of the Crouzon mouse: analysis of a model for syndromic craniosynostosis using three-dimensional MicroCT. Cleft Palate Craniofac J 43:740-748.

Purushothaman R, Cox TC, Muga AM, Cunningham ML. 2011. Facial suture synostosis of newborn Fgfr1(P250R/+) and Fgfr2(S252W/+) mouse models of Pfeiffer and Apert syndromes. Birth Defects Res A Clin Mol Teratol doi: 10.1002/bdra.20811

Recinos R, Hanger C, Schaefer R, Dawson C, Gosain A. 2004. Microfocal CT: a method for evaluating murine cranial sutures in situ. J Surg Res 116: 322–329.

Saito F, Kajii TS, Sugawara-Kato Y, Tsukamoto Y, Arai Y, Hirabayashi Y, Fujimori O, Iida J. 2011a. Three-dimensional craniomaxillary characteristics of the mouse with spontaneous malocclusion using micro-computed tomography. Eur J Orthod 33:43-49.

Saito F, Kajii T, Sugawara-Kato Y, Tsukamoto Y, Arai Y, Hirabayashi Y, Fujimori O, Iida J. 2011b. Morphological evaluation of cranial and maxillary shape differences of the brachymorphic mouse with spontaneous malocclusion using three-dimensional micro-computed tomography. Orthod Craniofac Res 14:100-106.

Schambach SJ, Baga S, Schillingb L, Grodena C, Brockmanna. 2010. Application of micro-CT in small animal imaging. Methods, 50: 2-13.

Song X, Frey E, Tsui B. 2001. Development and evaluation of a MicroCT system for small animal imaging. IEEE Nuclear Sci Symp Med Imaging Conference 3: 1600–1604.

Tobita K, Liu X, Lo CW. 2010. Imaging modalities to assess structural birth defects in mutant mouse models. Birth Defects Res C Embryo Today 90: 176-184.

Verdyck P, Wuyts W, Van Hul W. 2006. Genetic defects in the development of the skull vault in humans and mice. Crit Rev Eukaryot Gene Expr 16:119-142.

Wilkie AO, Morriss-Kay GM (2001) Genetics of craniofacial development and malformation. Nat Rev Genet 2, 458-468.

Zamora N, Llamas JM, Cibrián R, Gandia JL, Paredes V. 2011. Cephalometric measurements from 3D reconstructed images compared with conventional 2D images. Angle Orthod.

9

X-Ray Fluorescence Microtomography in Biological Applications

Gabriela R. Pereira[1] and Ricardo T. Lopes[2]
[1]Non-destructive Testing, Corrosion and Welding Laboratory,
Department of Metallurgical and Materials Engineering COPPE/UFRJ
Federal University of Rio de Janeiro, Rio de Janeiro/RJ
[2]Nuclear Instrumentation Laboratory, Department of Nuclear Engineering
COPPE/UFRJ, Federal University of Rio de Janeiro, Rio de Janeiro/RJ
Brazil

1. Introduction

Since tomographic techniques were developed, X-ray transmission tomography has been used in nondestructive testing for investigating the internal structure of samples, and with the advent of intense synchrotron radiation sources the resolution of the tomography was improved into μm regime.

Other complementary tomographic techniques have been developed based on the detection of the scattered (Golosio et al., 2003) and fluorescent photons (Cesareo & Mascarenhas, 1989.) in other to get some properties that also depend upon the distribution of individual elements within the sample. The X-ray fluorescence associate with tomographic techniques can supply important information of the sample chemical properties and to produce high contrast in conditions where transmission tomography is not adjusted.

One of the drawbacks of X-ray fluorescence tomography is the reconstruction calculation that is more complex than X-ray transmission tomography's algorithm (Hogan et al., 1991). Hogan et al. proposed adapting one of the algorithms used in X-ray transmission tomography (Brunetti & Golosio, 2001). The simplest algorithm is based on the classical back projection algorithm used In X-ray transmission tomography. An algorithm more accurate applies corrections for absorption before and after the fluorescence point.

In recent years, there has been growing interest in understanding the exact role played by trace elements in several diseases. The biological function of some metal ions in combination with an investigation of element distribution patterns in malignant and in normal human tissues of cancer patients can give some indication of the effect of metal ions on carcinogenesis (Raju et al., 2006). Both excess and deficiency of trace elements have been associated with many diseases including cancer. Even though extensive work has been carried out to find an association between trace elements and cancer, and to understand the mechanisms involved in carcinogenesis, no definite conclusions are drawn so far (Rocha et al., 2007).

Although trace elements Fe, Cu, and Zn are extremely common, assessment of their amounts is crucial for disease diagnostics. Both excess and deficiency of trace elements have been associated with many diseases including cancer (Pereira et al., 2010). Iron, copper and zinc can not only be associated with functions that protect the body against to illness, but also with processes that facilitate its propagation.

Copper acts as catalytic for enzymes that have to defend the human organisms. In the other hand, the copper can act as catalyst for production of hydroxyl radicals that are related with cells destruction.

Changes in the concentration of iron must be associates to the vascularization and the increase of the supplement of blood for the tumors growth. Moreover, the iron is an essential element for the organism because it is part integrant of some proteins. The iron influences the process of cancer because it plays a vital role in the regulation of the cells growth and its differentiation (Pereira et al., 2008).

Zinc participates of many reactions in cellular metabolism including physiological processes, such as immune function, growth and development, acting as a structural and functional component of many enzymes and proteins. Studies show that the prostate has the capacity to secrete high zinc level and that the concentration of this metal it is directly related to the prostate cancer, therefore a deepened study on the behavior of zinc in the prostate it makes necessary.

X-ray fluorescence microtomography technique has enabled us to determine the elemental distribution of the elements inside of the sample without destructed it. It is a useful tool in qualitative and quantitative analysis of biological tissues (Pereira et al., 2010). The great advantage of this technique is the visualization in tree-dimension of the elemental distribution without material damages.

2. X-ray fluorescence microtomography

X-ray transmission computed tomography is a well established diagnostic technique in Medicine. It is a non-destructive testing and allows reconstructing the image of the cross-sections of a sample starting from a set of X-ray "radiographic" measurements taken at different angles. It is performed by placing an X-ray source and an X-ray detector aligned at opposite sides of the sample. The detector records the part of the radiation emitted by the X-ray source that crosses the sample without interacting with it. The reconstructed image represents a map of the cross section in terms of linear attenuation coefficient of the material, which is a function of the mean atomic number (Z) and density in each single volume element (voxel) (Pereira et al., 2009).

X-ray fluorescence tomography is based on detection of photons from fluorescence emission from the elements in the sample. These photons are acquired by an energy dispersive detector, placed at 90° to the incident beam direction, and they are used as additional information for sample characterization. Figure 1 shows a schematic diagram of X-Ray Fluorescence Tomography.

According to Hogan et al. 1991, the X-ray fluorescence radiation at each point in the sample can be obtained through the following equations.

For a particular element i and an atomic level v, the fluorescence radiation hitting the energy dispersive detector can be obtained through integration along the path du:

$$I_{iv}(\theta,s) = I_0 \int\limits_{-\infty}^{\infty} du \; f(\theta,s,u)p(s,u)g(\theta,s,u) \tag{1}$$

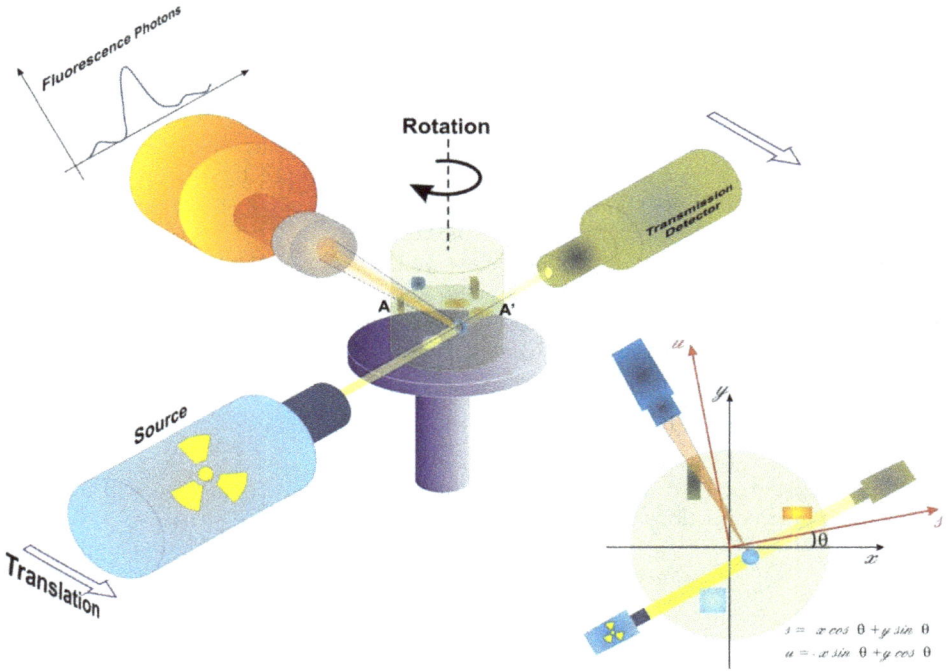

Fig. 1. Schematic diagram of X-ray fluorescence tomography.

where I_0 is the intensity of the incident beam; f is the survival probability of a photon from the source to the point (s,u), which is related to the sample absorption coefficient, μ_B, at the beam energy:

$$f(\theta,s,u) = e^{-\int_{-\infty}^{u} du' \mu_B(s,u')}$$
(2)

and g is the probability that a fluoresce photon emitted from the point (s,u) reaches the detector:

$$g(\theta,s,u) = \frac{1}{4\pi} \int_{\Omega_D} d\Omega \exp\left(-\int_{s,u}^{Det} \mu_F(l)dl\right)$$
(3)

where μ_F is the absorption coefficient of the sample at the fluorescence energy and Ω_D is the solid angle from the fluorescence point to the detector surface.

The function p is the probability that a fluorescence photon is produced from an incident photon along the path du:

$$p(s,u)du \propto N_{elem}$$
(4)

where, the concentration of the element at the point (s, u) is Nelem. If the solid angle defined by the detector surface is almost constant and the attenuation is small ($\mu_B \approx \mu_F \approx 0$) then:

$$I_{iv}(\theta,s) \propto I_0 \int_{-\infty}^{\infty} du \, N_{elem} \tag{5}$$

That means that the concentration of the element is proportional to the experimental projections and the usual algorithms of X-ray transmission tomography (Kak et al., 1988) can be used for reconstructed the images of X-ray fluorescence tomography. Otherwise, beam attenuation must be taken into account and new algorithms for tomographic reconstruction are indispensable (Brunetti & Golosio, 2001)
Self-absorption corrections are described below and it were implement in the Brunetti & Golosio 2001 algorithm. The algorithm is divided into two stages: MKCORR (that generates the matrix correction) and SCTOMO (backprojection algorithm).
Approximating the integral over du with a discrete sum, Eq. (1) can be expressed as

$$I(\theta,s) = \sum_{u=-\infty}^{+\infty} I_0 f(\theta,s,u) \, p(s,u) \, g(\theta,s,u) du \tag{6}$$

Following Hogan et al. 2001 it can be considering the total count, i.e. the sum of the counts from all those beam directions passing through the point (s_0, u_0)

$$I_{total}(s_0,u_0) = I\,(\theta_1,s_1) + I\,(\theta_2,s_2) + ... + I\,(\theta_n,s_n) \tag{7}$$

with can be expanded in terms of p and of the absorption factors f and g as:

$$\begin{aligned}
I_{total}(s_0,u_0) &= \sum_{u_1} I_0 f(\theta_1,s_1,u_1) \, p(s_1,u_1) \, g(\theta_1,s_1,u_1) \\
&+ \sum_{u_2} I_0 f(\theta_2,s_2,u_2) \, p(s_2,u_2) \, g(\theta_2,s_2,u_2) \\
&+ ... + \sum_{u_n} I_0 f(\theta_n,s_n,u_n) \, p(s_n,u_n) \, g(\theta_n,s_n,u_n).
\end{aligned} \tag{8}$$

Separating, in this sum, the contribution due to the point (s_0,u_0):

$$\begin{aligned}
I_{total}(s_0,u_0) &= I_0 f_0(\theta_1,s_1,u_1) \, p(s_0,u_0) \, g_0(\theta_1,s_1,u_1) \\
&+ I_0 f_0(\theta_2,s_2,u_2) \, p(s_2,u_2) \, g_0(\theta_2,s_2,u_2) \\
&+ ... + I_0 f_0(\theta_n,s_n,u_n) \, p(s_n,u_n) \, g_0(\theta_n,s_n,u_n) \\
&+ \sum_{u_1 \neq u_0} I_0 f(\theta_1,s_1,u_1) \, p(s_1,u_1) \, g(\theta_1,s_1,u_1) \\
&+ \sum_{u_2 \neq u_0} I_0 f(\theta_2,s_2,u_2) \, p(s_2,u_2) \, g(\theta_2,s_2,u_2) \\
&+ ... + \sum_{u_n \neq u_0} I_0 f(\theta_n,s_n,u_n) \, p(s_n,u_n) \, g(\theta_n,s_n,u_n).
\end{aligned} \tag{9}$$

where the subscripts zero on f and g signify the appropriate absorption factors for the point (s_0, u_0). Solving for $p(s_0,u_0)$, Eq. (9) yields:

$$p(s_0, u_0) = \frac{I_{total}(s_0, u_0)}{I_0 \sum\limits_{i=1}^{n} {}_0 f_0(\theta_i, s_i, u_i) \, g_0(\theta_i, s_i, u_i)} + \sum (outros \ termos). \qquad (10)$$

According to Hogan, the "other terms" are noise that can be regarded as an artifact of backprojection. Such noise can thus be removed by convolution of the projections with a filter suitable for backprojection. Therefore p(s₀,u₀) can be approximated as

$$p(s_0, u_0) = \frac{\tilde{I}_{total}(s_0, u_0)}{I_0 \sum\limits_{i=1}^{n} {}_0 f_0(\theta_i, s_i, u_i) \, g_0(\theta_i, s_i, u_i)}, \qquad (11)$$

where the tilde above I_{total} represents the operation of filterd backprojection.
A common approach is to determine the absorption coefficient distribution μ_B and μ_F using two conventional transmission tomographies.

3. Crystal monochromator

Multilayer crystals are part of a new generation of optical components based on X-ray diffraction of synthetic crystals.
Sometimes referred to as layered synthetic microstructures (LSM) or simply as multilayers, these optical components consist of layered depositions of materials A and B, having a significant difference in their indices of refraction. Most commonly, n layer pairs are fabricated to form a structure of uniform period by depositing alternating thin layers on top of smooth substrate. Material A is low-Z material such as carbon or silicon and B is a high-Z material such as tungsten or platinum. The efficiency of diffraction can be as high as 50 to 80% over bandwidths of 0.005 to 0.1, making feasible a new class of high-power, large bandwidth X-ray optics (Ebashi et al., 1991).
The performance of multilayer crystals are mainly influenced by the refractive index of materials and the number and thickness of individual layers.
The Figure 2 shows the reflectivity curve from a crystal monochromator made of tungsten and carbon (W-C) and it has 75 layer pairs, $\Delta E/E = 0,03$.

4. Sample preparation

The main advantage of X-ray Fluorescence Microtomography (XRFμCT) resides in being a non-destructive technique, allowing the use of the same sample for further characterization with other kind of techniques like X-ray diffraction (Rocha et al., 2007). In comparison with conventional micro X-ray fluorescence analysis, the XRFμCT does not require any sample preparation such as embedding or fixing the samples in paraffin to get an ultrafine and accurate slices (approximately 15 microns). The XRFμCT does not require this kind of sample preparation; it is not necessary to cut the sample to analyze the tomographic plane.
It is possible to analyze small samples without destroying them, biopsies for example. It is not necessary frozen and dried the samples. Sometimes, the samples can be frozen and dried before being analyzed to reduce the attenuation of X-ray fluorescence and the measurement time in biological samples, for example.

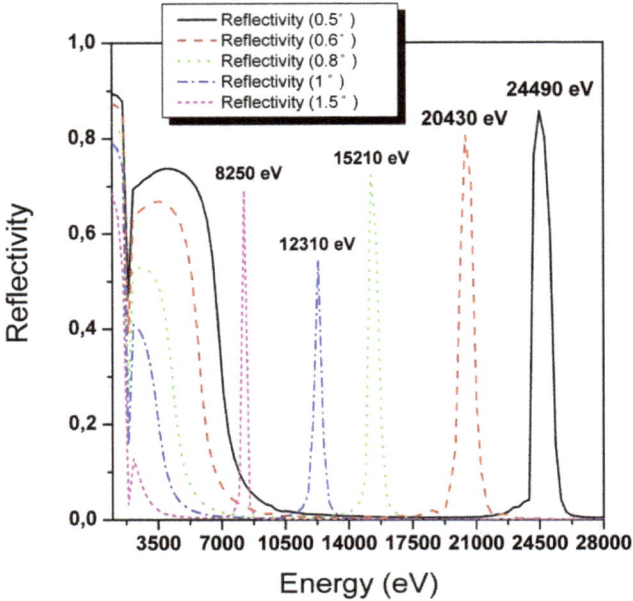

Fig. 2. Reflectivity curve.

5. Methods

There are many methods that can be implement to develop X-ray fluorescence microtomography. It can be use conventional X-ray tube, synchrotron radiation, X-ray microfocus and other sources. Also in many cases it is used a confocal geometry.

The excellent properties of synchrotron radiation sources, such as the possibility of setting a specific energy (monochromatic beam); high coherency beam; high photon flux; broad energy spectrum and natural collimation allow the use of X-ray fluorescence microtomography techniques. The use of synchrotron radiation reduces a lot the acquisition time and the noise in X-ray fluorescence images.

It will be present a development of a system to study X-ray fluorescence microtomography at the X-Ray Fluorescence Facility (D09B-XRF) at the Brazilian Synchrotron Light Laboratory (LNLS), Campinas, Brazil. A white beam (4-23 keV), a monochromatic beam produced by a Si (111) at 9.8 keV and a quasi-monochromatic beam produced by a multilayer monochromator at 12 keV, $\Delta E/E = 0.03$ collimated to a 200 x 200 μm^2 area with a set of slits, were used to sample excitation. The crystal multilayer monochromator is made of W-C and it has 75 layer pairs.

The intensity of the incident beam was monitored with an ionization chamber placed in front of it, before the sample. A schematic of the experimental setup for an X-ray fluorescence microtomography using a multilayer monochromatic beam is shown in Figure 3. The setup using white beam is the same setup of figure 3 but without the multilayer crystal and to obtain the monochromatic setup we change the multilayer system by two crystal of Si(111).

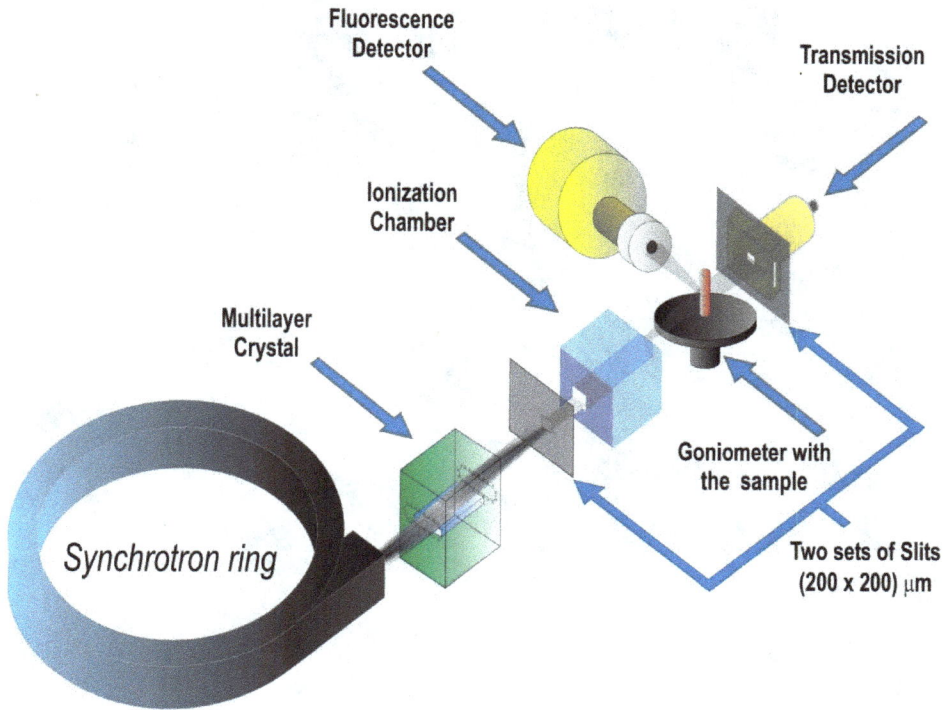

Fig. 3. The experimental arrangement for an X-ray fluorescence microtomography measurement using a multilayer monochromator beam.

The sample was placed on a high precision goniometer and translation stages that allow rotating as well as translating it perpendicularly to the beam. The fluorescence photons were collected with an energy dispersive HPGe detector placed at 90° to the incident beam, while transmitted photons were detected with a fast NaI (Tl) scintillation counter placed behind the sample on the beam direction. This detector geometry allows reducing the elastic and Compton X-ray scattering from the sample due to the high linear polarization of the incoming beam in the plane of the storage ring, thus improving the signal to background ratio for the detection of trace elements (Naghedolfeizi et al., 2003).

The quality of the reconstruction is a compromise between the measuring time required for an acceptable counting statistic of the X-ray fluorescence peaks and the step size necessary to linearly move and rotate the samples. In one projection, samples were positioned in steps of 200μm (actual beam size) perpendicularly to the beam direction covering the whole transversal section of the sample proof. The number of translations was about 20 according to the sample.

Each single value in a projection is obtained by measuring the fluorescence radiation emitted by all pixels along the beam. The object is then rotated, and another projection is measured. Projections are obtained in steps of 3° until the object has completed 180°. The number of rotations was 60. The selected measuring time was about 10s for each scanned point according to the sample.

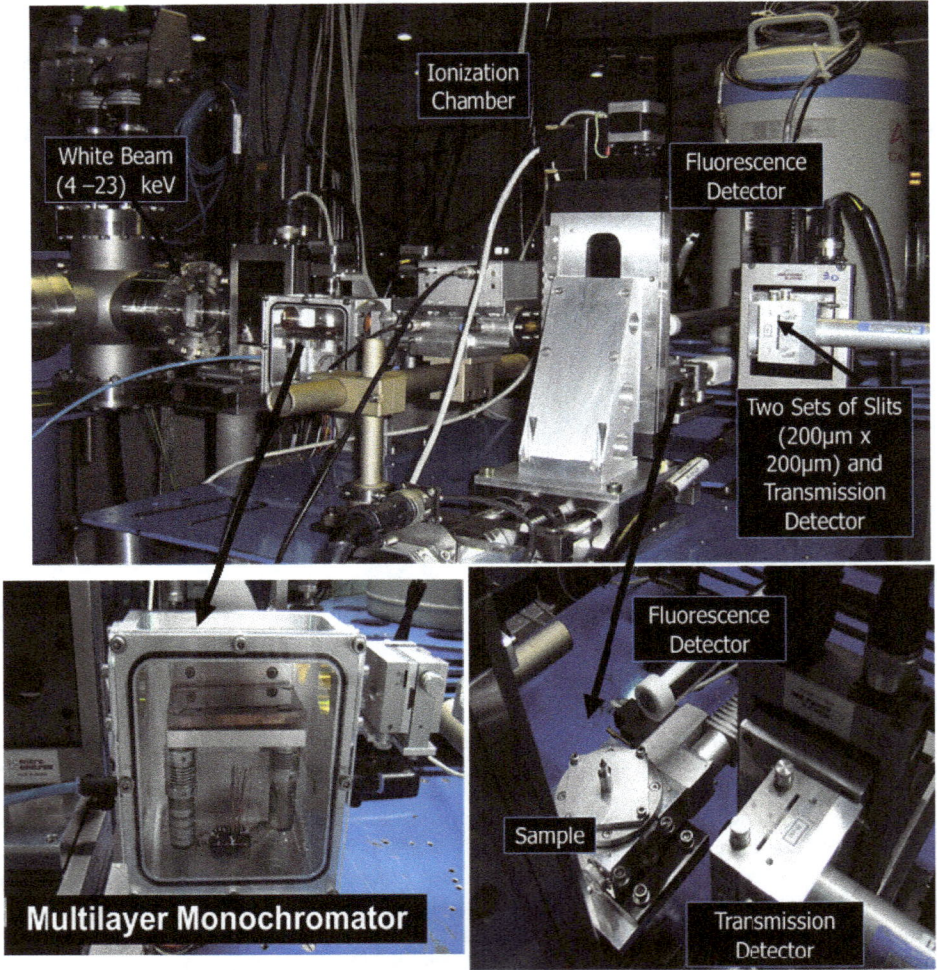

Fig. 4. A photo of an X-ray fluorescence microtomography measurement using a multilayer monochromator beam at LNLS/Brazil.

A reference sample made of filter paper was first analyzed and used as a test sample. One piece of the filter was impregnated with a solution containing 500 ppm of zinc while the other remained untouched. Both pieces of filter paper were rolled up until it reached a cylindrical shape. The filter paper thickness was approximately 130 μm.

Another reference sample mades of polyethylene filled with a standard solution of copper was analyzed and used as a test sample too. That reference sample is made of a polyethylene cylinder with two millimeters diameter with an internal cylinder with one millimeter diameter filled a standard solution of copper, 100 parts per million (100 ppm).

As a second part of the experiments, X-ray fluorescence microtomographies were performed on human breast, lung and prostate tissue samples. The component tissues were identified by the pathologist who made the sample available. The tissues were cut in cylindrical form with 1.5 mm to 2.0 mm thickness by 4.0 mm to 5.0 mm of height and were frozen and dried before being analyzed.

The Figure 4 shows a photograph of the experimental setup for an X-ray fluorescence microtomography measurement using a multilayer monochromator beam. .

After the data from X-ray fluorescence microtomography were obtained, the spectra were analyzed using the software QXAS (Quantitative X-ray Analysis System)(Bernasconi et al,1996). The QXAS makes the analysis of the X-ray fluorescence peaks and generates an output file with all the intensity of X-ray fluorescence for each element in each point in the sample.

The X-ray transmission and the X-ray fluorescence images were reconstructed using a in-house program developed using MATLAB® applying filtered-back projection algorithm. The absorption corrected matrix was obtained using MKCORR, a program developed by Brunetti & Golosio, 2001. The 3D images were reconstructed using the 3D-DOCTOR software.

6. Results and discussion

The X-ray transmission and X-ray fluorescence microtomography of test samples are shown in Fig. 5-8. In Figure 5, it can be observed that while X-ray transmission microtomography shows all layers of the filter paper, X-ray fluorescence microtomography shows only those regions where the element of interest (Zn) was localized. These tomographies show the viability of XRFμCT and confirm that this technique can be used to complement other techniques for sample characterization.

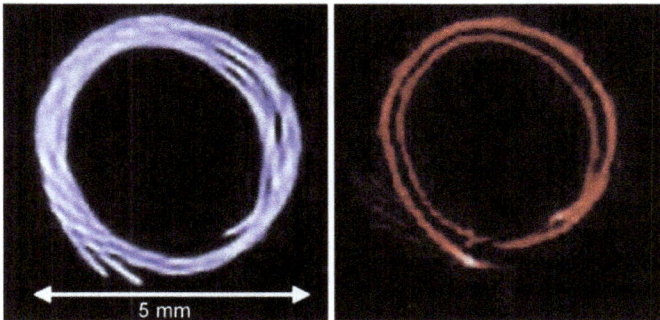

Fig. 5. Tomography images of paper filter (left: transmission and right: X-rayfluorescence).

The results for the test samples made of a polyethylene are shown in Figures 6-8. Analyzing the images it can be seen that the X-ray transmission images show the polyethylene matrix and the internal cylinder while the X-ray fluorescence images show only those regions where the elements of interest (copper) were localized. The results for the test samples made of polyethylene using a white beam, a monochromatic beam at 9.8 keV and a quasi-monochromatic beam at 12 keV are shown in Figure 6, 7 and 8, respectively.

In the figures, the left image shows the X-ray transmission microtomography and the right shows the X-ray fluorescence microtomography of copper reconstructed with filtered-back projection algorithm without absorption corrections. These tomographies show the viability of X-ray fluorescence microtomography and confirm that this technique can be used to complement others techniques for sample characterization.

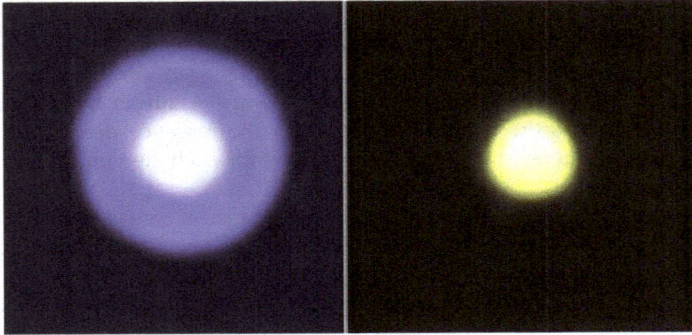

Fig. 6. Tomographic images using a white beam (left: Transmission microtomography; right: X-ray fluorescence microtomography of Cu).

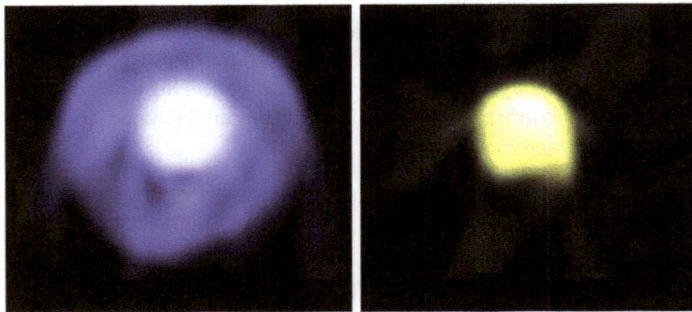

Fig. 7. Tomographic images using a monochromatic beam at 9.8 keV (left: Transmission microtomography; right: X-ray fluorescence microtomography of Cu).

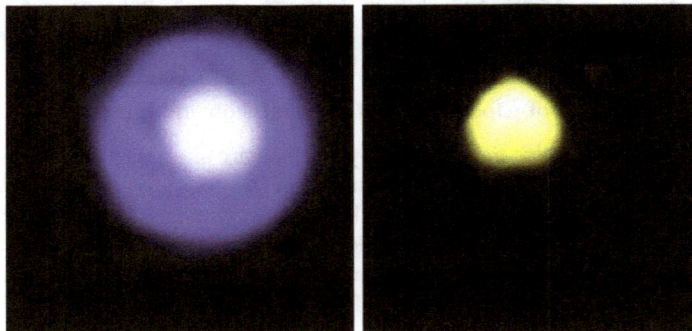

Fig. 8. Tomographic images using a quasi-monochromatic beam at 12 keV (left: Transmission microtomography; right: X-ray fluorescence microtomography of Cu).

Analyzing the test samples images, it can be observed that the images do not have differences; the images have the same characteristics. The biggest advantage of the analysis with a monochromatic beam or quasi-monochromatic beam is the possibility to determine the attenuation coefficients for the fluorescence energy and for beam energy and with these coefficients make the absorptions corrections and accurately determining the concentration in each point of the sample. The advantage of the quasi-monochromatic beam at 12 keV is the bigger photon flux than the monochromatic beam at 9.8 keV. Using a quasi-monochromatic beam at 12 keV, with lesser time it could be obtained an image with a better statistic value and lesser radial artefacts.

The results that will be presented are part of a study about elemental distribution and concentration of iron, copper and zinc in breast, lung and prostate samples.

Before the tissues tomographic measurements were initiated, the X-ray beam was centered on each tissue sample to determine the detectable trace elements. The measured fluorescence spectrum from a breast cancer sample is shown in Figure 9.

X-ray fluorescence microtomographies were performed on prostate tissue, human breast, embryo lung and adult lung samples and the results can be shown in Figures 10, 11, 12, 13, 14 and 15.

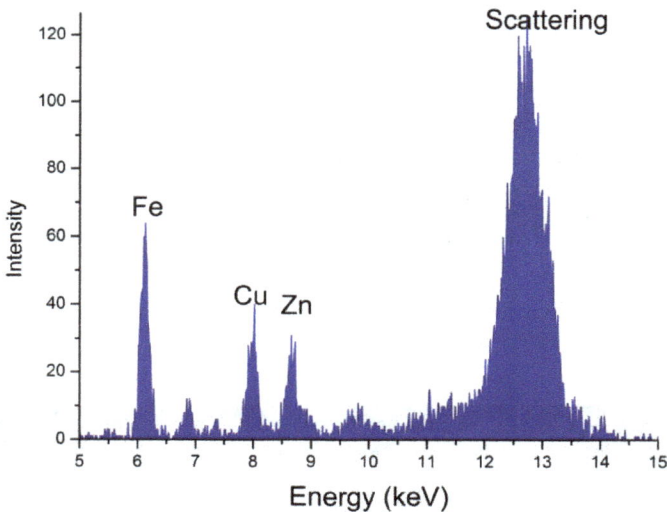

Fig. 9. An X-ray fluorescence spectrum from the breast cancer sample.

X-ray fluorescence microtomographies were performed on human prostate tissue samples. It was analyzed three prostate samples with BPH for tree different patients.

The result for human prostate samples is shown in Figure 10. Each line in the Figure 10 shows the X-ray transmission microtomography and the X-ray fluorescence microtomographies of Fe, Cu and Zn with absorption corrections for each prostate tissue.

Analyzing the X-ray fluorescence microtomographies of human prostate tissue sample fragments, it was possible to see the elemental distribution of iron, copper and zinc. It was verified that these tissues have a less concentration of copper and iron than zinc and the mean concentration of zinc in the BPH samples is about 150 to 300 μg/g.

In Figure 10f it can be seen that there is a flaw in the iron X-ray fluorescence distribution image. There is not iron in the entire sample.

Figure 11 also shows the 3D images of a prostate sample with Benign Prostatic Hyperplasia (BPH). It was not possible reconstruct the 3D X-ray Fluorescence Microtomography (XRFμCT) copper because the concentration of this element in that sample are very small, less than 3 μg/g.

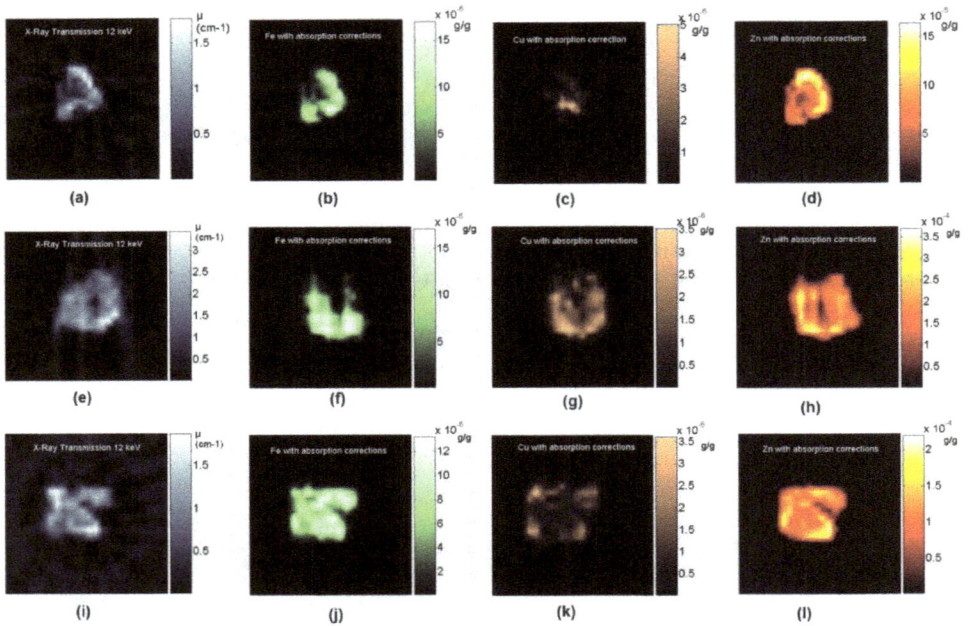

Fig. 10. X-ray transmission microtomographies and XRF microtomographies of iron, copper and zinc in human prostate BPH samples.

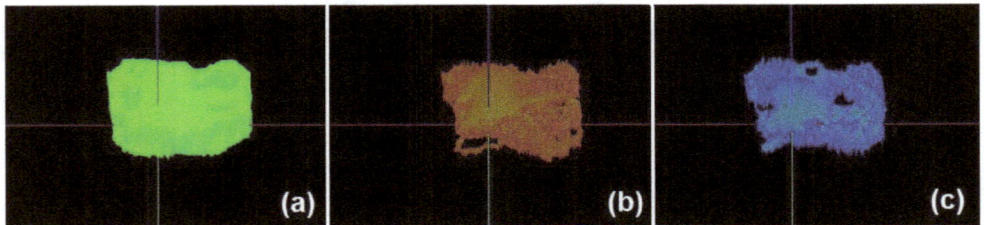

Fig. 11. 3D Tomographic images of a prostate sample with Benign Prostatic Hyperplasia (BPH), (a) CT, (b) XRFμCT of iron, (c) XRFμCT of zinc.

X-ray fluorescence microtomographies were performed on human breast tissue samples. Malignant breast tumor (ductal carcinoma) and healthy tissues were analyzed for the same patient. The component tissues were identified by the pathologist who made the sample available. The result for a breast samples are shown in Figure 12. In the first line at Figure 12 it can be seen the results for a cancer sample and the second one, it can be observed the results for a healthy breast tissue sample.

Analyzing the images, it can be observed that the two samples have a bigger concentration of iron comparing with the concentration of copper and zinc and for this patient; the concentration of iron and zinc is bigger in the cancer sample than in the healthy sample.

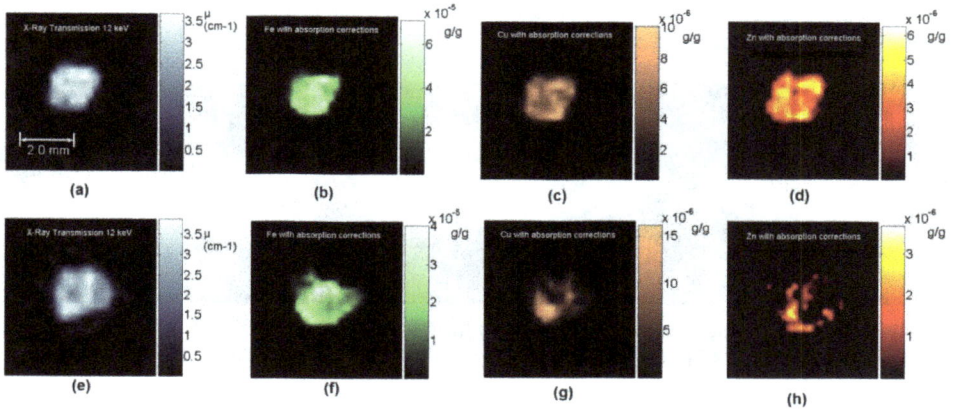

Fig. 12. X-ray transmission microtomographies and X-ray fluorescence microtomographies of iron, copper and zinc in human breast tissue samples.

The mean concentration of iron is about 50 $\mu g/g$, for copper the mean concentration is about 6 $\mu g/g$ and for zinc is about 7 $\mu g/g$ in healthy tissue. Comparing these mean values for healthy tissue with the mean values for cancer tissue for the same patient, it can be seen that for iron the mean value is forty percent greater in cancer sample, for copper there is no significant difference and for zinc the mean concentration doubling in cancer sample. These results are in accordance with the literature (Geraki et al., 2004). But it is necessary to measure more samples and quantify the difference in concentration in one sample and between normal and abnormal tissues to use the X-ray fluorescence microtomography as an analytic tool to analyze biological tissues.

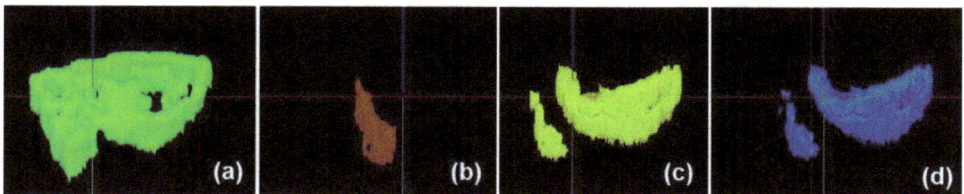

Fig. 13. 3D Tomographic images of healthy breast sample, (a) CT, (b) XRFµCT of iron, (c) XRFµCT of copper, (c) XRFµCT of zinc.

In Figure 13 it can be also observed the 3D visualization of a healthy breast sample. The distribution of iron, copper and zinc in the healthy breast tissue is different and heterogeneity. There are some regions with no concentration of these metals. It can be seen in figure 13b that there is no iron in the entire sample but only in a small part of that sample. Analysis of healthy and cancer breast sample led us to discovery that the concentration of Fe is bigger in the tumor compared with healthy breast tissues for the same patient (Pereira et al., 2006).

Figure 14 and 15 show the 3D images of lung samples. The figure 14 shows an embryo lung samples and Figure 15 shows an adult lung sample. In these 3D images, it was not possible reconstruct the 3D X-ray transmission tomography because the sample and the attenuation coefficient are very small. On the other hand, it was possible to visualize the 3D XRFμCT for the elements iron, copper and zinc.

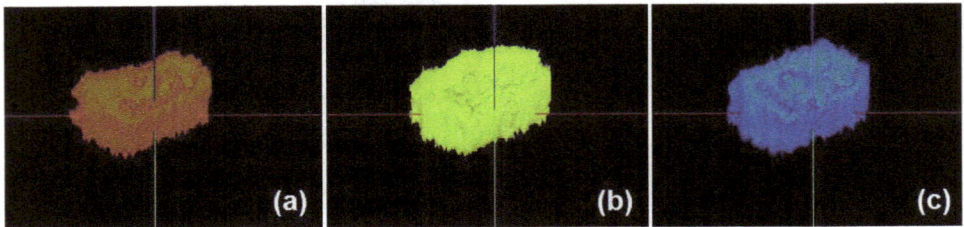

Fig. 14. 3D Tomographic images of an embryo lung samples , (a) XRFμCT of iron , (b) XRFμCT of copper, (c) XRFμCT of zinc.

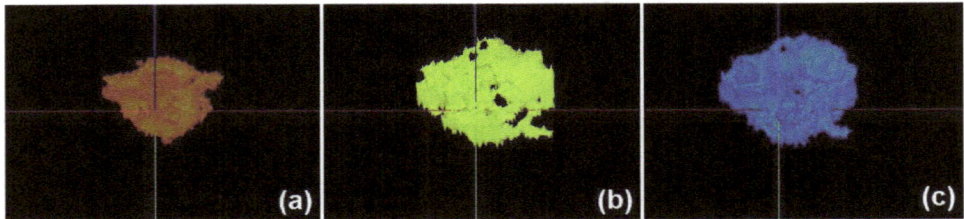

Fig. 15. 3D Tomographic images of an adult lung samples , (a) XRFμCT of iron , (b) XRFμCT of copper, (c) XRFμCT of zinc.

Comparing the elemental distribution images of an embryo and an adult lung, it can be observed that the embryo sample is denser than the adult lung sample. This fact can be explained because the embryo lung was not totally developed.

Although trace elements Fe, Cu, and Zn are extremely common, assessment of their amounts is crucial for disease diagnostics. Both excess and deficiency of trace elements have been associated with many diseases including cancer. However, until now, the evidence linking iron, copper and zinc to cancer is far from being conclusive (Rocha et al., 2007) and further research is needed. Using XRFμCT the elemental map can be obtained. Pathologist-oncologist cooperation would be most advantageous for future research in this area.

Analyzing the 3D visualization, it can be observed that the distribution of iron, copper and zinc are different and heterogeneity in those samples. Unfortunately, so far with these samples was not possible to determine the influence of heterogeneous concentrations in the same sample. Greater cooperation with pathologist is required to evaluate these irregular distributions.

The radial streak effects that can be visualized in tomographic reconstructions are because of the low counting statistic in each projection. The images were not processed.

7. Conclusion

XRFμCT technique has enabled us to determine the elemental distribution of the elements inside of the sample without destroying it. It is a useful tool in qualitative and quantitative analysis of light materials including biological tissues. The great advantage of this technique is the visualization in tree-dimension visualization of the elemental distribution without damaging the material.

The test samples show the viability of X-ray fluorescence microtomography and confirm that this technique can be used to complement other techniques for sample characterization. It is very important to use the algorithm with absorption corrections to get the corrected value of concentration if a quantitative analysis is necessary.

It is necessary to measure more samples and quantify the difference in concentration in one sample and between normal and abnormal tissues to use the X-ray fluorescence microtomography as an analytic tool to analyze biological tissues.

The better definition of the interfaces in X-ray fluorescence images was striking and the spatial resolution of the system can be optimized as a function of the application. In this work, it is used 200 μm, but it is possible to work with a resolution higher until 20 μm using capillary optics. The experimental set up at XRF-LNLS has shown to be very promising and this effort at implementing X-ray fluorescence microtomography was justified by the high quality of the images obtained.

8. Acknowledgment

This work was partially supported by National Council for Scientific and Technological Development (CNPq), Research Foundation of the State of Rio de Janeiro (FAPERJ) and Brazilian Synchrotron Light Laboratory(LNLS).

9. References

Bernasconi, G. & Tajani, A. (1996) Quantitative X-Ray Analysis System (QXAS) Software, Package: Documentation Version 1.2. International Atomic Energy Agency, Vienna.

Brunetti, A. & Golosio, B.(2001). Software for X-ray Fluorescence and scattering Tomographic Reconstruction.*Comput. Phys. Commun.*, Vol. 141(3), pp. 412-425.

Cesareo, R. & Mascarenhas, S. (1989). A New Tomographic Device Based on the Detection of Fluorescent X-rays. *Nuclear Instruments and Methods*, Vol. A277, pp. 669-672.

Ebashi S., Koch M. & Rubenstein E. (1991) Handbook on Synchrotron Radiation, 4 ed., Elsevier Science Publishers.

Geraki K.; Farquarson, M.J.; Bradlet, A. (2004) X-ray Fluorescence and Energy Dispersive X-ray Diffraction for the Quantification of Elemental Concentrations in Breast Tissue, *Physics in Medicine and Biology, Vol* 49, pp. 1-12.

Golosio, B. et al.(2003). Internal Elemental Microanalysis Combining x-RayFluorescence, Compton and Transmission Tomography, *Journal of applied Physics*, Vol.94, pp. 145-156.

Hogan, J. P. et al. (1991) Fluorescent Computer Tomography: A Model for Correction X-Ray Absorption, *IEEE Transactions on Nuclear Science*,Vol. 38, pp.1721-1727.

Kak, A. C. & Slaney,M. (1988) Principles of Computerized Tomographic Imaging, *IEEE Press*, New York.

Naghedolfeizi, M. et al. (2003). X-ray Fluorescence microtomography study of Trace elements in a SiC Nuclear Fuel Shell. *Journal of Nuclear Materials*, Vol. 312, pp. 146-155.

Pereira, G. R. et al. (2010). Biological tissues analysis by XRF microtomography. *Applied Radiation Isotopes*, Vol. 68(4-5), pp. 704–708.

Pereira, G. R. et al. (2009). X-Ray fluorescence microtomography under various excitation conditions. *X-Ray Spectrometry*, Vol. 38, pp. 244-249.

Pereira, G. R. et al. (2008). Elemental distribution mapping on breast tissue samples. *European Journal of Radiology*, Vol. 68S, pp. S104–S108.

Pereira, G. R. et al. (2006). *Journal of Radioanalytical and Nuclear Chemistry*, G. R. et al. (2008). Vol. 269, pp. 469-.

Rocha, H. S. et al. (2007). Diffraction enhanced imaging and X-ray fluorescence microtomography for analyzing biological samples. *X-Ray Spectrometry*, Vol. 36, pp. 247–253.

Raju, G. J. N. et al. (2006). Trace elemental correlation study in malignant and normal breast tissue by PIXE technique.*Nucl. Instr. and Meth. B*, Vol. 247, pp. 361–367.

Effect of Buoyancy on Pore-Scale Characteristics of Two-Phase Flow in Porous Media

Tetsuya Suekane and Hiroki Ushita
The University of Tokushima
Japan

1. Introduction

Carbon dioxide (CO_2) is the most important anthropogenic greenhouse gas. The global atmospheric concentration of CO_2 has increased from a pre-industrial value of approximately 280 ppm to 379 ppm in 2005. The warming of the climate system is unequivocal, as is now evident from observations of increasing global average air and ocean temperatures, widespread melting of snow and ice and rising global average sea level (IPCC, 2007a). To stabilize the concentration of CO_2 in the atmosphere, emissions need to peak and then decline thereafter. In the long term, energy conservation, efficiency improvements in energy conversion, lower carbon fuels such as natural gas and renewable energy sources are the most promising alternatives. For lower stabilization targets, scenarios put more emphasis on the use of low-carbon energy sources, such as renewable energy and nuclear power, and the use of CO_2 capture and storage (CCS; Pacala & Socolow, 2004; IPCC, 2007b); however, the transition from the current dependence on fossil fuels would take many decades. The capture of CO_2 from fossil fuel power plants and other large-scale stationary emission sources and storage in geologic formations is the only option that permits a transition from current high-intensity carbon-based energy sources to low-carbon energy sources.

The safety of geologic storage of CO_2 is obviously a central concern in planning carbon sequestration on a large scale. The current concept of geologic storage involves the injection of CO_2 into deep formations, which typically contain brine. CO_2 is supercritical at temperatures and pressures above the critical values of 304 K and 7.38 MPa. In typical geologic formations, the critical condition of CO_2 is reached at a depth of approximately 740 m. Because of geologic pressure, the density of CO_2 dramatically increases with depth; however, the density of CO_2 is approximately 0.9 times that of water, so when CO_2 is injected into the subsurface, buoyancy tends to bring CO_2 upward in geologic formations. On the other hand, CO_2 will be retained by physical and geochemical mechanisms, such as physical trapping (IPCC 2005), capillary trapping (Suekane et al. 2008, 2010a; Al Mansoori et al. 2010; Pentland et al. 2010; Zhou et al. 2010; Wildenschild et al. 2010; Saadatpoor 2010), solubility trapping (Lindeberg & Wessel-Berg 1997; McPherson & Cole 2000; Ennis-King et al. 2003; Gilfillan et al. 2009; Iding & Blunt 2010) and mineralization (Gunter et al. 1993).

Capillary trapping is sometimes referred to as residual gas trapping or relative permeability hysteresis trapping. When CO_2 is injected into the subsurface, it spreads in geologic formations in a continuous phase, displacing brine. As it migrates through a formation, the saturation of CO_2 decreases and some of it is retained in pore space by capillary forces. In the case of Berea sandstone, residual CO_2 saturation ranges from 24.8 to 28.2% at supercritical conditions (Suekane et al. 2008). Once the gas bubbles are trapped, they are stable against water flow, because the capillary forces acting on the gas bubbles are much higher than buoyancy and viscous sheer stress (Suekane et al. 2010a; Zhou et al. 2010).

Saturation of CO_2 trapped by capillarity also depends on numerous factors, such as how the wetting fluid gets in (either by forced or spontaneous imbibition), the rate of imbibition, CO_2 saturation at flow reversal and the properties of porous media (Holtz 2002; Suekane et al. 2010b). In the case of the Sleipner project, CO_2 was injected into a point approximately 200 m below the caprock. The CO_2 plume spreads upward by buoyancy before accumulating below the caprock (IPCC 2005; Arts et al. 2008). On the other hand, in the case of oil production by gas-assisted gravity drainage (GAGD) processes, crestal gas injection uses wells in higher structural positions close to the top of the reservoir. GAGD has been considered to be a very attractive oil recovery process because of its higher efficiency (Hagoort 1980; de Mello et al. 2009; Rostami et al. 2010). When gas is injected vertically downward into the formations, the higher sweep efficiency could be achieved with the aid of stabilization of a displacement front by buoyancy. For upward displacement of fluids by buoyant gas, however, fingering and instability of a displacement front reduces the sweep efficiency and gas saturation. The gas saturation at the flow reversal has strong influence on the residual gas saturation.

In this study, the effect of the stability of a displacing front in gravity drainage on the initial gas saturation is discussed using dimensionless parameters and the relationship between initial gas saturation and residual gas saturation is explored. Gas injection experiments were carried out with packed beds of glass beads using a nitrogen and water system in laboratory conditions. The three-dimensional structure of the distribution of gas in the packed beds was visualized by means of a microfocused X-ray CT scanner. Water was injected into the packed beds to evaluate the residual gas saturation. Finally, gas was injected vertically upward into the packed bed to study the effect of the direction of gas injection with respect to gravity on the gas saturation.

2. Experiments

2.1 Experimental apparatus and procedure

Glass beads with a diameter of 100 μm, 200 μm or 400 μm were packed in an acrylic resin tube with an interior diameter of 10 mm and a height of 40 mm (Fig. 1a). First, the packed bed was soaked in water. After gas contained in the packed bed was evacuated by a vacuum pump, water was forced into pore spaces during the recovery of ambient pressure to atmospheric pressure. Next the packed bed, aligned vertically, was connected by Teflon tube to a gas reservoir containing nitrogen at a pressure of 0.12 MPa and a syringe pump filled with water (Fig. 1b). Nitrogen was injected into the packed bed vertically downward or upward at a constant flow rate, by withdrawing water into the syringe pump at a constant flow rate. Five units of pore volume (PV) of nitrogen were injected into the packed bed. This condition is often referred to as an irreducible water condition, where the remaining water in a porous media is immobile. In this paper, we define the gas saturation at this condition to be the initial gas saturation. Then, the packed bed was disconnected from the tubing systems and placed in an X-ray CT scanner

(Comscantechno Co. ScanXmate-RB090SS) to observe the distribution of gas and water. Following the CT scan, the packed bed was connected again to the syringe pump (Fig. 1c). Five PV of water was injected vertically upwards into the packed bed at a constant flow rate. The resulting condition is referred to as the residual gas condition, where gas bubbles are trapped by capillarity in porous media. The saturation at this condition is referred as residual gas saturation. The packed bed was scanned by the X-ray CT scanner again. An X-ray CT scan was performed at the steady state of the packed bed after each gas or water injection.

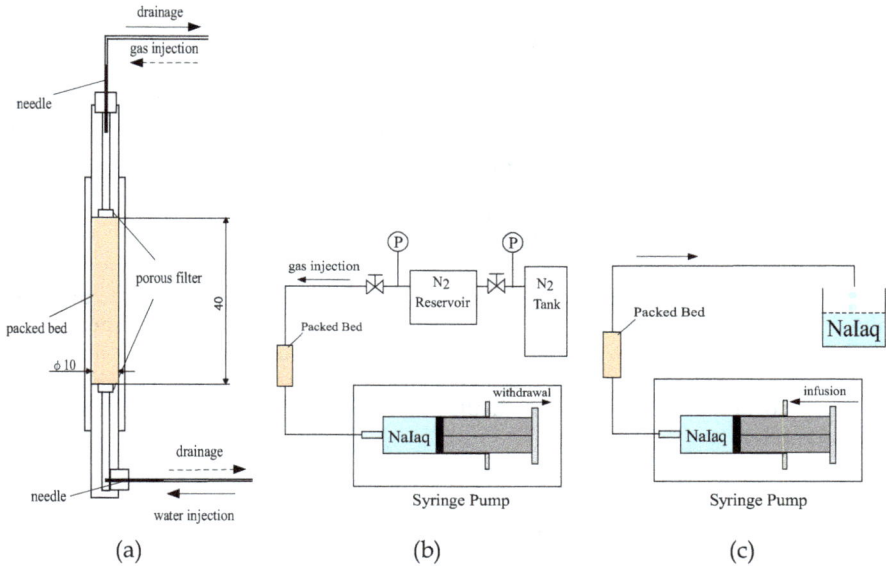

Fig. 1. Schematic views of (a) the packed bed of glass beads, (b) experimental setup for the drainage process and (c) experimental setup for the imbibition process.

2.2 Dimensionless parameters and experimental conditions
2.2.1 Dimensionless parameters
Two-phase flows in porous media are influenced by interfacial tension, buoyancy and viscous sheer stress. The Bond number (Bo) and capillary number (Ca) are defined as

$$Bo = \frac{(\rho_w - \rho_n)gR^2}{\sigma} \tag{1}$$

$$Ca = \frac{\mu_w v}{\sigma}, \tag{2}$$

where ρ is the density, g is the acceleration due to gravity, R is the particle radius, σ is interfacial tension, μ is the viscosity, v is the displacing fluid velocity and subscripts w and n denote the wetting phase and non-wetting phase, respectively. Bo and Ca represent the ratio of buoyancy force and of viscous sheer stress to the capillary force, respectively. Instead of

Equation 1, the Dombrowski–Brownell number, which is the ratio of the pore scale hydrostatic pressure drop to the capillary pressure (Rostami et al. 2010), is defined as

$$N_{DB} = \frac{(\rho_w - \rho_n)g(k/\phi)}{\sigma},$$ (3)

where k is the absolute permeability and ϕ is the porosity. The semi-heuristic Carman-Kozney model of permeability predicts the permeability of packed beds as follows (Kaviany 1995):

$$k = \frac{\phi^3}{45(1-\phi)^2}R^2.$$ (4)

For gravity drainage processes, which correspond to vertically downward injections of gas into the packed bed in the current experiments, the critical gravity drainage velocity is defined by Blackwell and Terry (1959) and Dumore (1964) as

$$v_c = \frac{(\rho_w - \rho_n)gk}{\mu_w}.$$ (5)

The critical gravity drainage velocity depends on the difference in the density, the viscosity of drained fluid and the permeability of porous media. In the current experiments, because we used the nitrogen and water system in laboratory conditions, the critical gravity drainage velocity depends only on the radius of glass beads from equation 5. The ratio of the critical gravity drainage velocity to the displacing fluid velocity, vc/v, is referred to as the stability parameter.

2.2.2 Experimental conditions

All experiments were performed for the nitrogen and water system in laboratory conditions. The fluid properties of the nitrogen and water system and the supercritical CO_2 and water system at a typical reservoir condition, which corresponds to the depth of approximately 850 m, are summarized in Table 1.

		Viscosity, μ (μPa s)	density, ρ (kg/m³)	interfacial tension, σ (mN/m)	Ca	Bo
Reservoir condition (318 K, 8.5 MPa)	sc CO_2	20	259.6	35.7	1.681×10^{-2} $\times$ v	2.017×10^5 $\times R^2$
	H_2O	600	993.9			
Laboratory condition (293 K, 0.1 MPa)	gas N_2	17.87	1.123	72.6	1.463×10^{-2} $\times$ v	1.345×10^5 $\times R^2$
	H_2O	1062	996.7			

Table 1. Fluid properties under experimental conditions and typical reservoir conditions.

We used nitrogen as a non-wetting phase instead of CO_2 for these experiments to reduce the dissolution in water. Interfacial tension between supercritical CO_2 and water is approximately half of that between nitrogen and water in laboratory conditions. Because of the high density of supercritical CO_2 with respect to nitrogen, buoyancy is also lower for supercritical CO_2. As a result, the Bond number falls in a similar range.

The water used in the experiments was doped with sodium iodide (NaI) at 7.5 wt% to enhance the X-ray attenuation. Henceforth, for simplicity, this aqueous phase is referred to as water. During drainage processes, the injection flow rate of nitrogen was controlled by a syringe pump to cause the capillary number to be in the range between 3.72×10^{-7} and 1.86×10^{-5}. Depending on the radius of the glass beads, the stability parameter vc/v ranges from 0.05 to 37.9. In imbibition processes, the injection flow rate of water was controlled such that the capillary number was 1.00×10^{-6}.

Reconstructed three-dimensional images are $608 \times 608 \times 610$ pixels at a resolution of 25.048 μm/pixel in all directions.

3. Results and discussion

3.1 Stability effect of gravity drainage on gas saturation
3.1.1 Stable gravity drainage
Nitrogen was injected vertically downward into the packed bed filled with water at various flow rates to investigate the effect of the instability of a displacing front on gas saturation. Figure 2 shows vertical cross-sectional images around the axis of the packed bed. For drainage at stability parameters of 9.2 and 1.8, high initial gas saturations, Sg^*, of 91 and 85%, respectively, are achieved without the effect of gas fingering with the aid of a stable interface of displacement. When the displacement velocity is above the critical gravity drainage velocity, large fractions of water remain in the packed bed. At stability parameters lower than 0.36, fingering of injected gas results in gas saturations below 25%. The distribution of gas shown in Fig. 2 suggests that the critical gravity drainage velocity defined by equation 5 gives an appropriate criterion for the stability of a drainage interface.

3.1.2 Fingering
Figure 3 shows vertical cross-sectional images after the unstable drainage of vc/v = 0.36 for four independent experimental runs under the same conditions, where the capillary number is 9.30×10^{-6} and the Bond number is 5.38×10^{-3}. Because the drainage is unstable, fingering has a great influence on gas distributions. Reflecting the nature of instability, the initial gas saturation varies widely from 22 to 67%. Because the glass beads on the surface of cylindrical tube tend to be sorted, the porosity at the region adjacent to the surface is higher than that at the centre of the packed bed. Figure 3c suggests that heterogeneity in porosity enhances the effect of fingering and reduces the displacement efficiency.

3.1.3 Effect of capillary number on initial gas saturation
The effect of capillary number on the initial gas saturation is shown in Fig. 4 for packed beds of glass beads with the diameters 100 μm, 200 μm and 400 μm. With an increase in capillary number, the initial gas saturation decreases, as has been reported by many researchers (Morrow & Songkran, 1982; Chatzis et al. 1983; Morrow et al. 1988; Rostami et al. 2010). At a capillary number of 9.30×10^{-6} with 200-μm diameter glass beads, the initial gas saturation varies widely due to fingering of the interface (Fig. 3). At a low capillary number of 3.72×10^{-7}, an initial gas saturation of more than 70% can be achieved, even for the fine glass beads.

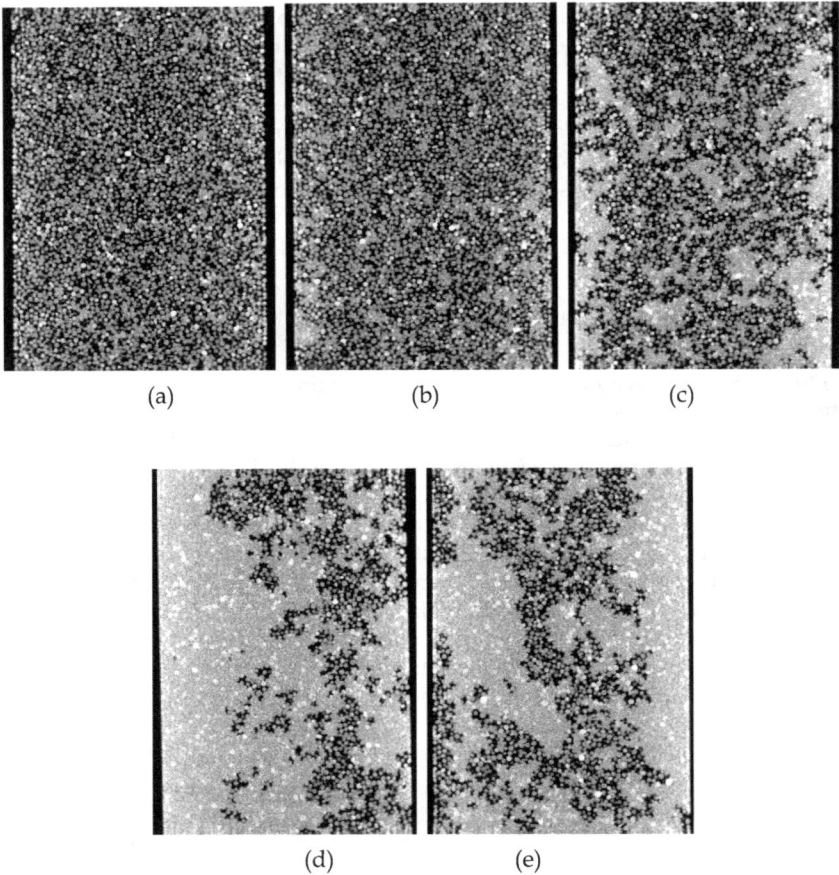

Fig. 2. Effect of the stability parameter vc/v on gravity drainage by gas injection. (a) Ca = 1.86×10^{-7}, vc/v = 9.2, Sg* = 91% (b) Ca = 3.72×10^{-7}, vc/v = 1.8, Sg* = 85% (c) Ca = 1.86×10^{-6}, vc/v = 0.92, Sg* = 69% (d) Ca = 9.30×10^{-6}, vc/v = 0.36, Sg* = 25% (e) Ca = 1.86×10^{-5}, vc/v = 0.18, Sg* = 24%. Glass beads with a diameter of 200 μm were packed in a tube with an inner diameter of 10 mm, shown as black regions at the image edge.

3.1.4 Bond number effect on initial gas saturation

The effect of Bond number on the initial gas saturation is shown in Fig. 5 for packed beds of glass beads with various diameters at a constant injection flow rate corresponding to a capillary number of 3.72×10^{-7}. Because the higher Bond number results in a more stabilized displacement front, higher displacement efficiency could be achieved for high Bond numbers (Fig. 4).

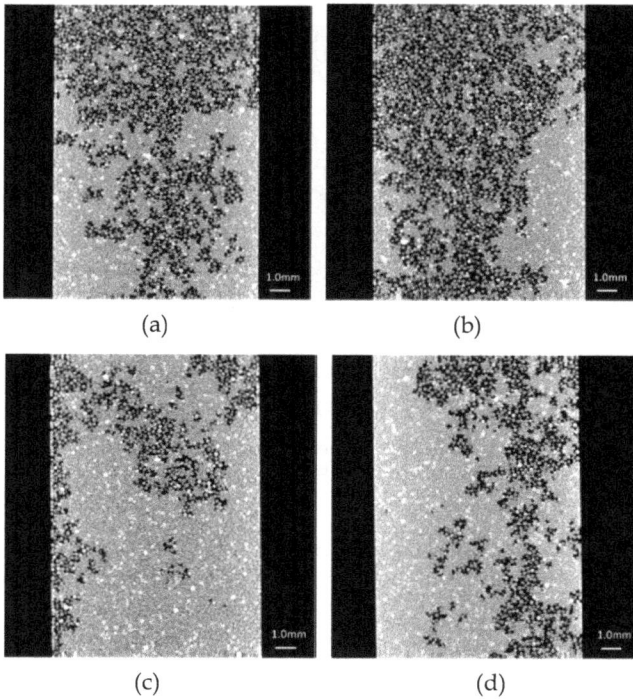

Fig. 3. Reproducibility of gravity drainage in the unstable condition where Ca = 9.30×10^{-6} and Bo = 5.38×10^{-3}.

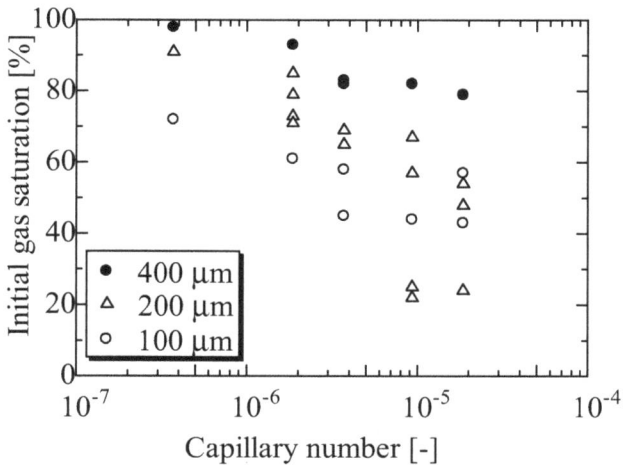

Fig. 4. Effect of capillary number on the initial gas saturation for drainage processes with downward gas injection.

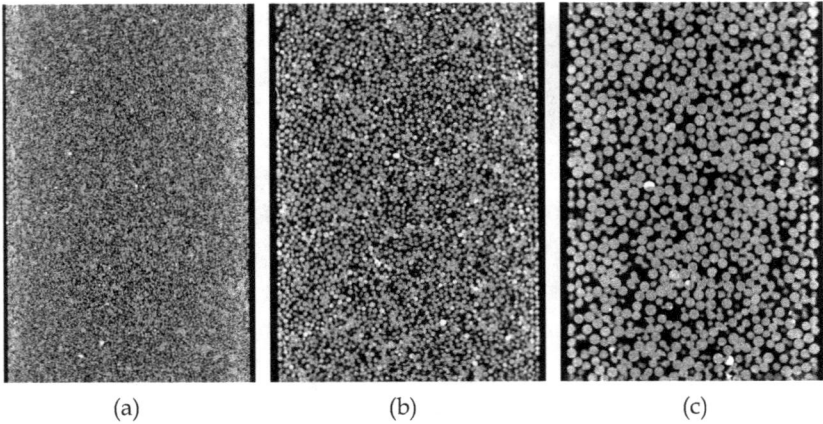

(a)   (b)   (c)

Fig. 5. Bond number effect on gravity drainage by gas injection at the capillary number of
3.72×10^{-7}. (a) Bo = 3.36×10^{-4}, R = 50 µm (b) Bo = 1.35×10^{-3}, R = 100 µm
(c) Bo = 5.38×10^{-3}, R = 200 µm.

The Bond number effect on the initial gas saturation for drainage processes is shown in Fig.
6 for various capillary numbers. With an increase in Bond number, the initial gas saturation
increases. With higher diameter glass beads, the higher critical gravity drainage velocity
results in the higher displacement efficiency associated with the reduction in capillary force
(Rostami et al. 2010). The displacement front of drainage is stable for all experimental runs
shown in Fig. 5. Therefore, for the large, 400 µm glass beads, an extremely high gas
saturation of 98% can be achieved at a high Bond number. This is an attractive fact that
suggests high oil recovery of GAGD.

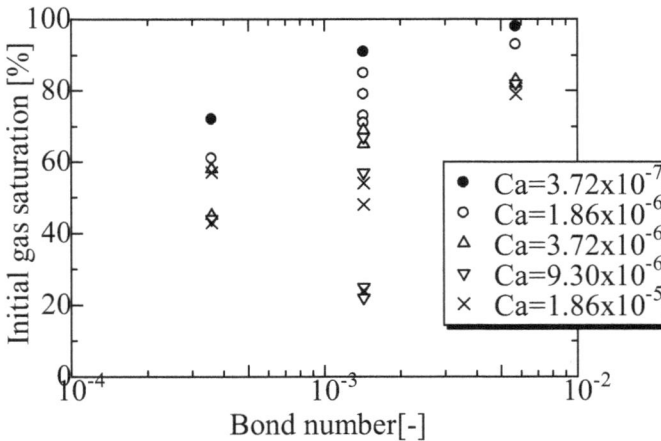

Fig. 6. Bond number effect on the initial gas saturation for drainage processes with
downward injection of gas.

3.2 Effect of initial gas saturation on residual gas saturation
3.2.1 Morphology of trapped gas bubbles

Water is injected vertically upward into the packed bed of glass beads at a constant flow rate, which corresponds to a capillary number of 1.0×10^{-6}, after gravity drainage processes. Figure 7 shows the distributions of gas after drainage processes and the distributions of trapped gas bubbles after the imbibition processes for each diameter of glass beads. Because of low gas-injection flow rate at a capillary number of 3.72×10^{-7}, high initial gas saturations are achieved for each packed bed after the drainage processes (Fig. 7a–c). Into these packed beds, 5 PV of water was injected vertically upwards at a capillary number of 1.0×10^{-6}. Distributions of trapped gas bubbles are shown in Fig. 7d–f for each diameter of glass beads. As the diameter of glass beads decreases, residual gas saturation increases because the capillary force becomes high compared with buoyancy. Gas is perfectly non-wetting to glass beads. Therefore, gas bubbles with low volume are trapped at the centre of pore spaces. Gas bubbles with a volumetric scale of several pores are trapped in the packed beds spreading over several pores without surface contact of glass beads by thin water films.

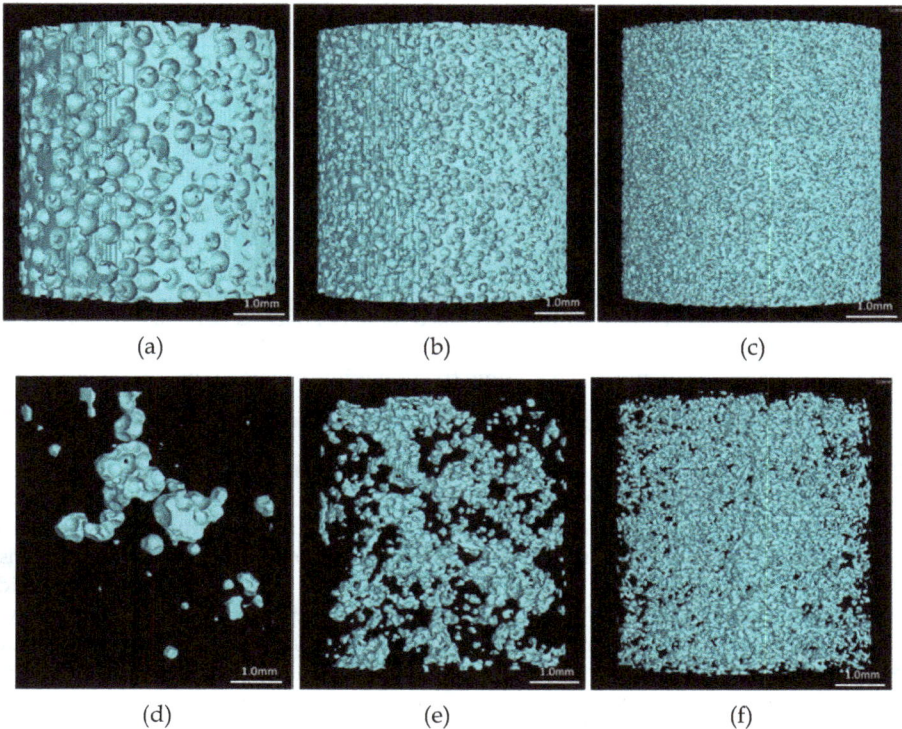

Fig. 7. Distributions of injected gas after stable drainage (a–c) and trapped gas bubbles after water imbibition (d–e) for the packed bed of glass beads with a diameter of (a, d) 400 μm, (b, e) 200 μm and (c, f) 100 μm. Surface of the gas in the cylindrical domain with a diameter of 5 mm and a length of 5 mm is visualized.

Distributions of the volume of trapped gas bubbles are shown in Fig. 8. The volume of gas bubbles were analysed using the image processing software ImageJ (Abramoff et al. 2004; Rasband 1997–2008) with some plug-ins for the cylindrical domain at a diameter of 9 mm and length of 2.5 mm. The volume of bubbles is normalized with that of packed glass beads. For lower diameter glass beads, the largest gas bubble tends to be large compared to the glass bead. The volume of the largest bubble in the packed bed of 400 μm glass beads is approximately one order of magnitude larger than that of the glass bead. On the other hand, in a packed bed of 100 μm glass beads, the volume of the largest bubble is approximately 73,000 times as large as that of a glass bead. This largest gas bubble contains approximately 98% of all trapped gas.

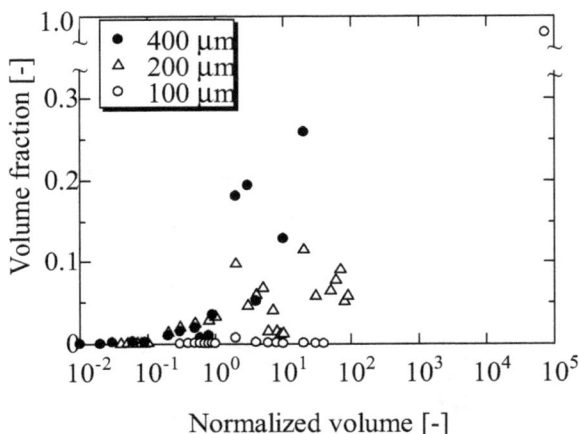

Fig. 8. Distribution of the volume of trapped gas bubbles in packed beds of glass beads with various diameters. The volume of gas bubbles is normalized with that of a glass bead in the packed bed. Vertical axis denotes the volume fraction with respect to the total volume of trapped gas.

3.2.2 Relationship between initial and residual gas saturations

An increase in the injection flow rate of gas results in a decrease in the initial gas saturation (Fig. 4) because of the instability of displacing fronts. Residual gas saturation is affected by initial gas saturation, even for water injection at the same capillary number. The relationship between the initial gas saturation and residual gas saturation is shown in Fig. 9. The residual gas saturation peaks against the initial gas saturation at approximately 50%. An inverse trend between initial gas saturation and residual gas saturation has been found in unconsolidated sandstone (Holtz 2002) and in the packed bed (Suekane et al. 2010b). During imbibition processes, the migration of gas is assisted by buoyancy, because water is injected vertically upward. For higher initial gas saturations, gas in a continuous phase is hardly disconnected from the continuum. Because the displacing front of water is stabilized by buoyancy, the branch of gas jutting from the continuum into water retreats due to buoyancy before being disconnected by capillary forces (Setiawan et al. 2010). From a viewpoint of the safety of geologic storage of CO_2, the difference between initial and residual gas saturations, which denotes the fraction of CO_2 escaping through a porous media, would be reduced by the design of injection strategy to adjust the initial gas saturation.

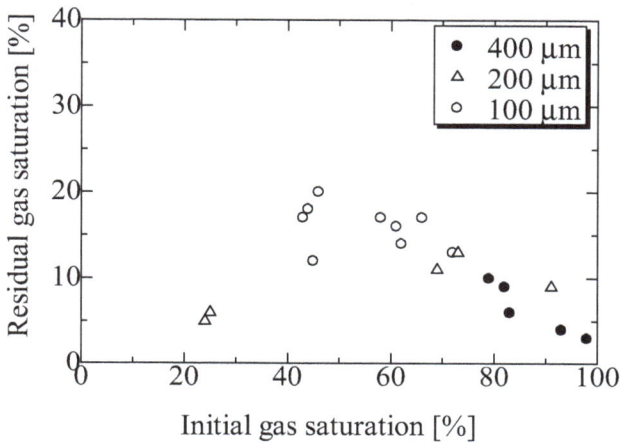

Fig. 9. Relationship between the initial and residual gas saturations.

3.2.3 Stability of gravity drainage and gas trapping

The initial gas saturation for the packed bed of 400 μm glass beads after drainage at stability parameters vc/v of 37.9 and 0.76, was 98 (Fig. 7a) and 79%, respectively. After water imbibition, the residual gas saturation was 3 and 10%, respectively, and the trapped gas bubbles are shown in Figs. 7d and 10, respectively. Distribution of the volume of trapped gas bubbles is shown in Fig. 11. In the case of unstable drainage, even though the initial gas saturation is lower than that in the case of stable drainage, residual gas saturation is high, because large bubbles with the scale of several pore sizes remain in porous media.

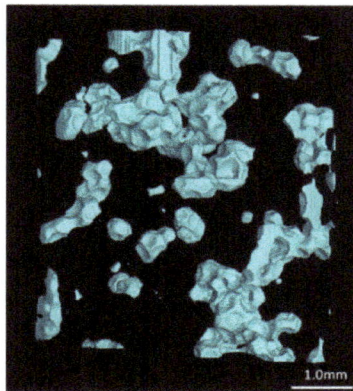

Fig. 10. Trapped gas bubbles in the packed bed of 400 μm glass beads at a residual gas saturation of 10%, after unstable drainage at a stability parameter vc/v of 0.76.

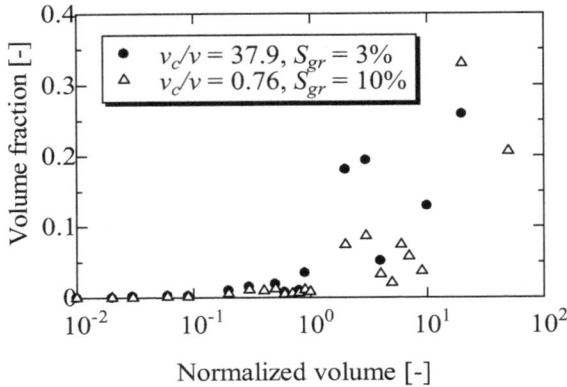

Fig. 11. Distribution of the volume of trapped gas bubbles in packed beds of 400 μm glass beads. After drainage at stability parameters vc/v of 37.9 and 0.76, water was injected at a capillary number of 1.0×10^{-6}. The volume of gas bubbles is normalized with that of a glass bead in the packed bed.

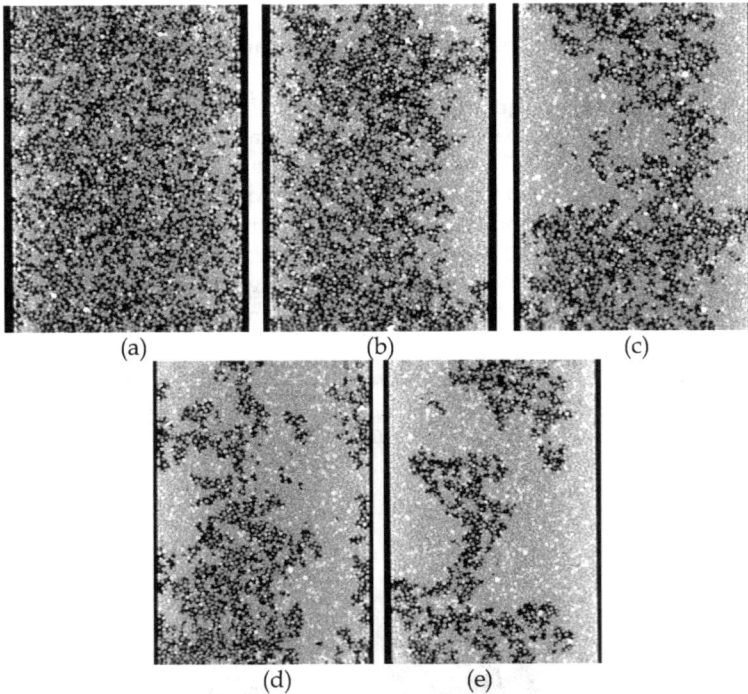

Fig. 12. Vertically upward drainage by gas injection at a capillary number of (a) Ca = 1.86 × 10^{-7}, (b) Ca = 3.72 × 10^{-7}, (c) Ca = 1.86 × 10^{-6}, (d) Ca = 9.30 × 10^{-6}, (e) Ca = 1.86 × 10^{-5}. Glass beads with a diameter of 200 μm were packed in tube with an inner diameter of 10 mm, shown as black regions at the image edges.

3.3 Upward drainage

In this section, we injected gas vertically upward as is often the case in actual CCS projects. The packed bed of glass beads and experimental setup used in the experiments were the same as that shown in Fig. 1, except for the direction of gas injection.

Figure 12 shows vertical cross-sectional images at various injection flow rates of gas. Except for the direction of gas injection, gas injection flow rates in Fig. 12a–e are the same as those in Fig. 2a–e, respectively. The initial gas saturations are compared for the direction of gas injection in Fig. 13. In the case of the upward injection of gas, gravitational force and capillary pressure let water remain in porous media against gas migration. With a decrease in the gas injection flow rate, the initial gas saturation increases; however, the initial gas saturation at the upward gas injection is lower than that at the downward gas injection at the same capillary number because of instability of displacing front.

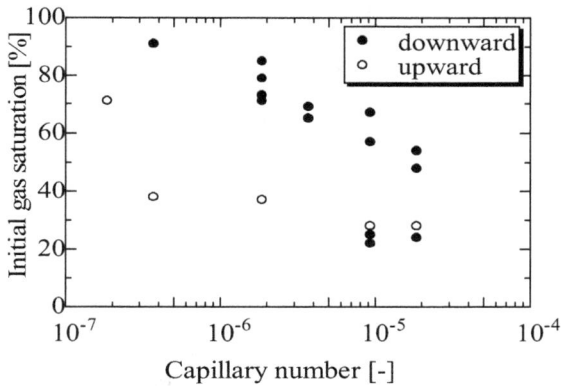

Fig. 13. Effect of the direction of gas injection on the initial gas saturation at various capillary numbers.

4. Conclusion

Gas injection experiments were carried out using packed beds of glass beads with a nitrogen and water system in laboratory conditions. The three-dimensional structure of the distribution of gas in the packed beds was visualized by means of a microfocused X-ray CT scanner.

First, the effect of the stability of a displacing front in gravity drainage on the initial gas saturation was discussed with dimensionless parameters. For gravity drainage in stable conditions, high initial gas saturation is achieved without the effect of gas fingering with the aid of a stable interface of displacement. When the displacement velocity is above the critical gravity drainage velocity, large fractions of water remain in the packed bed. Reflecting the nature of instability, the initial gas saturation varies widely from drainage to drainage. Heterogeneity in porosity enhances the effect of fingering and reduces the displacement efficiency. With an increase in Bond number and a decrease in capillary number, the initial gas saturation increases. In the packed bed of 400μm glass beads, an extremely high gas saturation of 98% can be achieved at a capillary number of 3.72×10^{-7}.

Next, water was injected in the packed beds to evaluate the residual gas saturation. The residual gas saturation has a peak against the initial gas saturation at approximately 50%.

During imbibition processes, migration of gas is assisted by buoyancy because water is injected vertically upward. For higher initial gas saturations, gas in a continuous phase is hardly disconnected from the continuum.

Finally, gas was injected vertically upward into the packed bed to study the effect of the direction of gas injection with respect to gravity on gas saturation. In the case of the upward injection of gas, gravitational forces and capillary pressure let water remain in porous media against gas migration. With a decrease in the gas injection flow rate, the initial gas saturation increases; however, the initial gas saturation due to upward gas injection is lower than that due to downward gas injection at the same capillary number because of instability of the displacing front.

5. References

Abramoff, M. D.; Magelhaes, P. J. & Ram, S. J. (2004). Image processing with image. *J. Biophotonics Int.*, Vol. 11, pp. 36-44

Al Mansoori, S.K.; Itsekiri, E.; Iglauer, S.; Pentland, C.H.; Bijeljic, B. & Blunt, M.J. (2010). Measurements of Non-Wetting Phase Trapping Applied to Carbon Dioxide Storage. *International Journal of Greenhouse Gas Control*, Vol. 4, pp. 283-288

Arts, R.; Chadwick, A.; Eiken, O.; Thibeau, S. & Nooner, S. (2008). Ten Year's Experience of Monitoring CO_2 Injection in the Utsira Sand at Sleipner, Offshore Norway. first break, Vol. 26, (January 2008) pp. 66-72

Blackwell, J.T. & Terry, M.W. (1959). Factors Influencing the Efficiency of Miscible Displacement. Transactions of AIME. Vol. 216, pp. 1-8

Chatzis, I.; Morrow, N.R. & Lim, H.T. (1983). Magnitude and Detailed Structure of Resiual Oil Saturation. Society of Petroleum Engineers Journal, (April 1983), pp. 311-326

de Mello, S.F.; Trevisan, O.V. & Schiozer D.J. (2009) Review on Gravity Dreainage Performance, Presented at 20th International Congress of Mechanical Engineering, Grambado, RS, Brazil, November 15-20, 2009

Dumore, J.M. (1964). Stability Consideration in Downward Miscible Displacement. Society of Petroleum Engineers Journal. Vol. 4, pp. 356-362

Ennis-King, J; Gibson-Poole, C.M.; Lang, S.C. & Paterson, L. (2003). Long Term Numerical Simulation of Geological Storage of CO_2 in the Petral Sub-Basin, North West Autralia. Proceeding of 6th Internationl Conference on Greenhouse Gas Control Technologies, J. Gale & Y. Kaya (eds.) Vol. 1, Kyoto, Japan, Octover 1-4, 2002

Gilfillan, S.M.V.; Lollar, B.S.; Holland, G.; Blagburn, D.; Stevens, S.; Schoell, M.; Cassidy, M.; Ding, Z.; Zhou, Z.; Lacrampre-Couloume, G. & Ballentine, C.J. (2009). Solubility Trapping in Foramtion Water as Dominant CO_2 Sink in Natural Gas Fields. Nature, Vol. 458, (April 2009), pp. 614-618

Gunter, W.D.; Perkins, E.H. & McCann, T.J. (1993). Aquifer Dsposal of CO_2-Rich Gases: Reaction Design for Added Capacity. Energy Conversion and Management. Vol. 34, pp. 941-748

Hagoort, J. (1980) Oil Recovery by Gravity Drainage. Society of Petroleum Engineers Journal. (June 1980) pp. 139-150

Holtz, M.H. (2002). Residual Gas Saturation io Aquifer Influx: A Calculation Method for 3-D Computer Reservoir Contruction. Presented at the SPE Gas Technology Symposium, Alberta, Canada, April 30–May 2, 2002 SPE 75502

Iding, M. & Blunt, M.J. (2010) Enhanced Solubility Trapping of CO_2 in Fractured Resrvoirs, Presented at 10th International Conference on Greenhouse Gas Control Technologies, Amsterdam, The Netherlands, September 19-23, 2010

IPCC, (2005). IPCC Special Report on Carbon Dioxide Capture and Storage. Metz, B.; Davidson, O.; de Coninck, H.C.; Loos, M. & Meyer, L.A. (eds.), Cambridge University Press, Cambridge, UK and USA pp. 195-276

IPCC, (2007a). Climate Change 2007: The Physical Science Basis. Contribution of waroking Group I to the Frouth Assessment Report of the Intergovernmental Panel on Climate Change. S. Solomon; D. Qin; M. Manning; Z. Chen; M. Marquis; K.B. Averyt; M. Tignor & H.L. MIller (eds.), Chambridge University Press, ISBN 978-0-521-70597-7 New York, USA

IPCC, (2007b). Climate Change 2007: Mitigation of Climate Change. Contribution of waroking Group III to the Frouth Assessment Report of the Intergovernmental Panel on Climate Change. B. Metz; O.R. Davidson; P.R. Bosch; R. Dave & L.A. Meyer (eds.), Chambridge University Press, ISBN 978-0-521-70598-1 New York, USA

Kaviany, M. (1995). Principles of Heat Transfer in Porous Media. Springer-Verlag New York, Inc., ISBN 0-387-94550-4, New York, USA

Lindeberg, E. & Wessel-Berg, D. (1997). Vertical Convection in an Aquifer Column under a Gas Cap of CO_2. Energy Conversion and Management. Vol. 38 No. Suppl. pp. S229-S234

McPherson, B.J.O.J. & Cole, B.S. (2000). Multiphase CO_2 Flow, Transport and Sequestration in the Powder River Basin, Wyoming, USA. Journal of Geochemical Exploration, Vol. 69-70, No.6, pp. 65-70

Morrow, N.R. & Songkran, B. (1982). Effect of Viscous and Buoyancy Forces on Nonwetting Phase Trapping in Porous Media, In: Surface Phenomena in Enhanced Oil Recovery, D.O. Shah (ed.), 287-411, Plenum Press, New York City

Morrow, N.R.; Chatzis, I. & Taber, J.J. (1988). Entrapment and Mobilization of Residual Oil in Bead Packs. SPE Reservoir Engineering, (August 1988), pp. 927-934

Pacala, S. & Socolow, R. (2004). Stabilization Wedge: Solving the Climate Problem for the Next 50 Years with Current Technolgies. Science, Vol. 305, No. 5686, (August 2004), pp. 968-972

Pentland C.H.; El-Maghraby, R.; Georgiadis, A.; Iglauer, S. & Blunt, M.J. (2010) Immiscible Displacement and Capillary Trapping in CO_2 Storage. Presented at 10th International Conference on Greenhouse Gas Control Technologies, Amsterdam, The Netherlands, September 19-23, 2010

Rasband, W. S. (1997-2008) ImageJ [Internet]. Bethesda (Maryland, USA): US National Institute of Health. Available from: http://rsbweb.nih.gov/ij/.

Rostami, B.; Kharrat, R.; Pooladi-Darvish, M. & Ghotbi, C. (2010). Identification of Fluid Dynamics in Forced Gravity Drainage Using Dimensionless Goups. Trasport in Porous Media, Vol. 83, pp. 725-740

Saadatpoor, E., Bryant, S.L. & Sepehrnoori, K. (2010). Effect of Upscaling Heterogeneous Domain on CO_2 Trapping Mechanisms. Presented at 10th International Conference on Greenhouse Gas Control Technologies, Amsterdam, The Netherlands, September 19-23, 2010

Setiawan, A.; Nomura, H. & Suekane, T. (2010). Pore-scale visualization of imbibition process in porous media by using X-ray CT scanner, *presented at 7th International Conference of Flow Dynamics*, Sendai, Japan, November 1-3, 2010

Suekane, T.; Nobuso, T.; Hirai, S. & Kiyota, M. (2008) Geological Storage of Carbon Dioxide by Residual Gas and Solubility Trapping. International Journal of Greenhouse Gas Control, Vol. 2, No.1, pp. 58-64

Suekane, T.; Zhou, N.; Hosokawa, T. & Matsumoto, T. (2010a) Direct Observation of Gas Bubbles Trapped in Sandy Porous Media. Transport in Porous Media, Vol. 82, No. 1, pp. 111-122

Suekane, T.; Zhou, N. & Hosokawa, T. (2010b) Maximization of Capillary Trapping Ratio to Injected CO_2 by Means of Co-injection. Presented at 10th International Conference on Greenhouse Gas Control Technologies, Amsterdam, The Netherlands, September 19-23, 2010

Wildenschild, D.; Armstrong R.T.; Herring, A.L.; Young, I.M. & Carey, J.W. (2010) Exploring Capillary Trapping Efficiency as a Function of Interfacial Tension, Viscosity, and Flow Rate. Presented at 10th International Conference on Greenhouse Gas Control Technologies, Amsterdam, The Netherlands, September 19-23, 2010

Zhou, N.; Matsumoto, T.; Hosokawa, T. & Suekane, T. (2010) Pore-Scale Visualization of Gas Trapping in Porous Media by X-ray CT Scanning. Flow Measurement and Instrumentation, Vol. 21, pp. 262-267

Differential Cone-Beam CT Reconstruction for Planar Objects

Liu Tong
Singapore Institute of Manufacturing Technology
Singapore

1. Introduction

1.1 Industrial CT system

All commercially available industrial CT systems share some similarity in both machine structure that, as illustrated in Figure 1, generally consists of a tube, a digital flat panel detector and a manipulator, and the CT inspection process which includes scanning, reconstruction and visualization. Figure 2 is the flowchart showing a typical CT examination process:

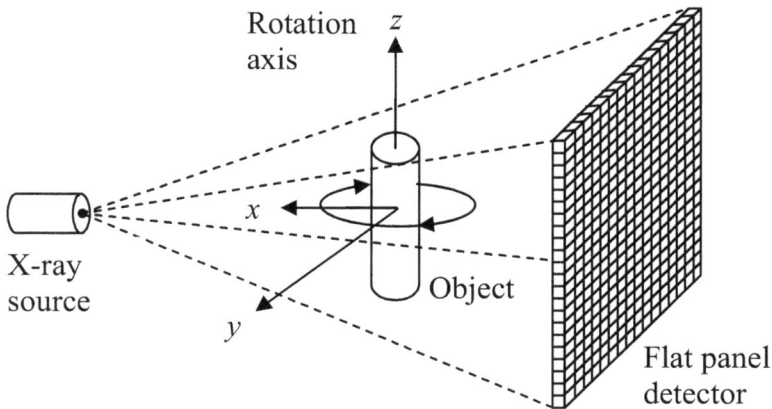

Fig. 1. Illustration of a modern industrial CT system

1.2 Central ray determination

Central ray is the projected position of the centre-of-rotation on the detector (Figure 3). This parameter must be known before starting the reconstruction and its accuracy has a direct impact on the reconstruction quality.

```
┌─────────────────────────────────┐
│          Mount sample           │
└─────────────────────────────────┘
                 ↓
┌─────────────────────────────────┐
│      Set system parameters      │
└─────────────────────────────────┘
                 ↓
┌─────────────────────────────────┐
│     Change sample to wire-      │
│          phantom (WP)           │
└─────────────────────────────────┘
                 ↓
┌─────────────────────────────────┐
│       Scan wire-phantom         │
└─────────────────────────────────┘
                 ↓
┌─────────────────────────────────┐
│       Change WP to sample       │
└─────────────────────────────────┘
                 ↓
┌─────────────────────────────────┐
│           Scan sample           │
└─────────────────────────────────┘
                 ↓
┌─────────────────────────────────┐
│       Determine central ray     │
│          with WP data           │
└─────────────────────────────────┘
                 ↓
┌─────────────────────────────────┐
│       Reconstruct of object     │
└─────────────────────────────────┘
                 ↓
┌─────────────────────────────────┐
│     Visualization and analysis  │
└─────────────────────────────────┘
                 ↓
       ┌───────────────────┐
       │       Report      │
       └───────────────────┘
```

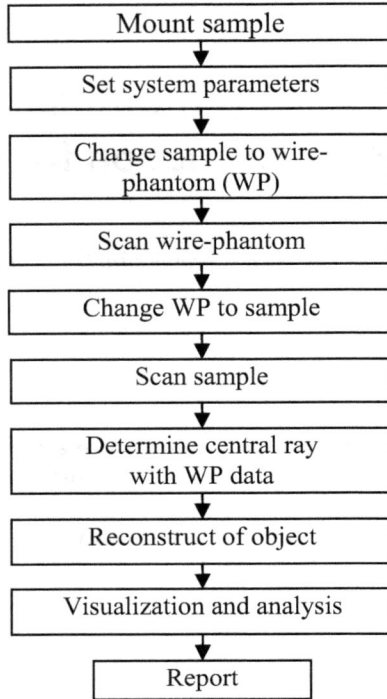

Fig. 2. Flowchart of a type CT examination process

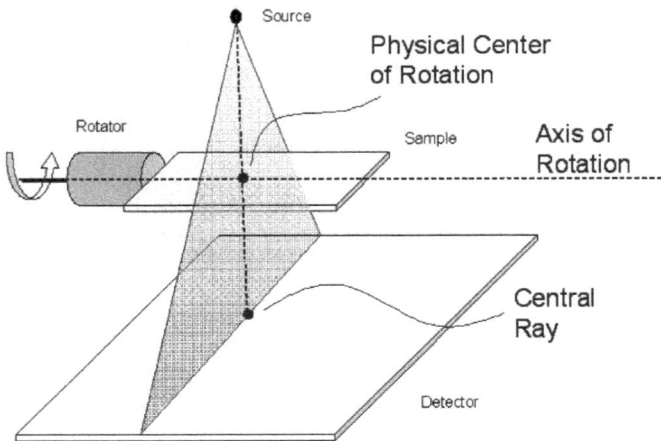

Fig. 3. Illustration of centre-of-rotation and central ray

There are many studies about the impact of the central ray error[1-5]. Figure 4 shows the simulation results of introducing a 10-pixel error to the true value of the central-ray used for CT scans of a dot, a circle and a square[1].

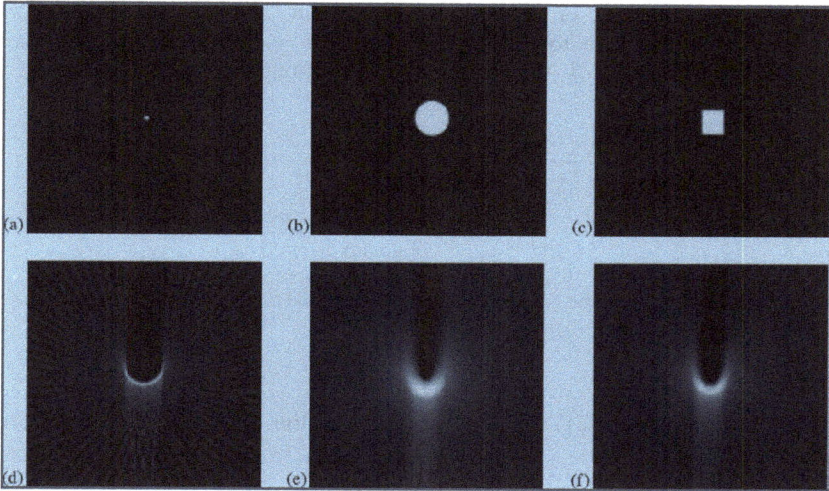

Fig. 4. The simulated reconstructions results of a dot, a circle and a square with (a)-(c) the true value of the central-ray; and (d)-(f) A 10 pixel offset.

The impact of the central-ray error is also demonstrated with a real IC chip. As shown in Figure 5(a), when the IC chip is reconstructed with an accurate central-ray, its features can be clearly presented on the image; however, when we introduce a small error to the central ray and redo the reconstruction of the same cross-section, it becomes very difficult to interpret, as shown in Figure 5(b).

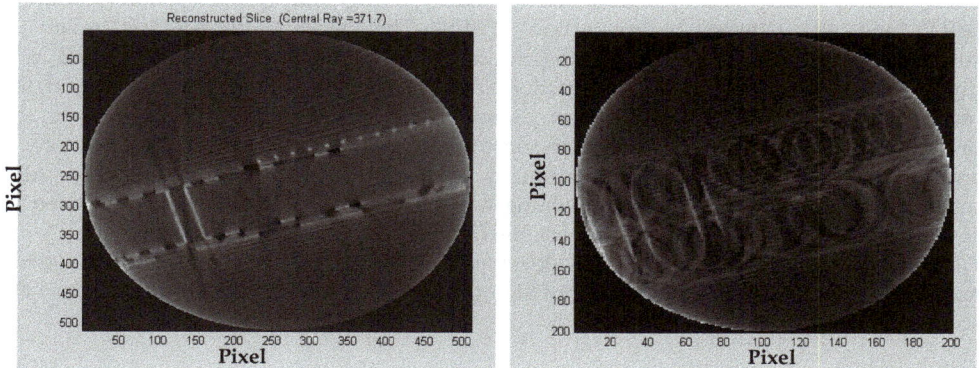

Fig. 5. Impact of the central ray error: (a) A reconstructed cross-section of a IC chip; (b)The reconstruction result of the same cross-section with a small error introduced to the central ray

1.2.1 Conventional central-ray determination theory and practice

Conventional central-ray determination is based on the centre-of-mass theory[4]. This theory works well with parallel-beam sinogram data. However, for fan-beam system it only works when the object approximates a delta function.

Figure 6 shows the schematic of the fan-beam projection CT geometry. Let $f(x,y)$ be the cross-sectional object function to be reconstructed and $g_f(t,\beta)$ the fan-beam projection data, for each projection angle β, the projection centre-of-mass can be defined as

$$\bar{t}(\beta) = \frac{\int_{-\infty}^{\infty} t \times g_f(t,\beta) dt}{g_f(t,\beta) dt}$$

$$= \frac{1}{M} \int_{-\infty}^{\infty} \int_{-\infty}^{\infty} f(x,y) \frac{l(\tau' + x\cos\beta + y\sin\beta)}{l' + x\sin\beta - y\cos\beta} dxdy \qquad (1)$$

where M is the total mass of the object and is calculated as

$$M = \int_{-\infty}^{\infty} \int_{-\infty}^{\infty} f(x,y) dxdy \qquad (2)$$

If the center-of-rotation is $(\bar{x}, \bar{y})$, the sinusoid traced by the centre-of-mass in the projection can also be found:

$$t_{(\bar{x},\bar{y})}(\beta) = \frac{l(\tau' + \bar{x}\cos\beta + \bar{y}\sin\beta)}{l' + \bar{x}\sin\beta - \bar{y}\cos\beta} \qquad (3)$$

One can prove that equivalence exists between $\bar{t}$ and $\bar{t}_{(\bar{x},\bar{y})}$ only when $f(x,y)$ is a delta function. This is exactly why in the past almost all commercial industrial CT systems use a pin (wire) phantom for central-ray calibration before the real scan of the object.

1.3 Filtered backprojection CT reconstruction

There are two widely used reconstruction approaches[6-9]: algebraic reconstruction techniques (ART) and the filtered backprojection (FBP)[6]. The concept of ART is relatively straightforward: the 2-dimensional cross-section to be reconstructed is represented as a digital image, i.e., as a linear combination of a finitely many basis functions. And the reconstruction task is to find the best digital matrix that would give an error to the projections for all angles not greater than some non-negative small number. ART basically is an iterative approach and computationally very demanding. Because of this, ART reconstruction is up to date still remaining as an academic topic and is seldom used in commercial CT systems. Instead, they use the filtered backprojection approach.

Filtered backprojection algorithm was developed from parallel-beam projection; however, nowadays only fan-beam and cone-beam algorithms have actual applications in modern CT scanners.

1.3.1 Fourier slice

As illustrated in Figure 7, we have an object with attenuation distribution $f(x,y)$. Its parallel projection taken at angle θ, $p_\theta(t)$, is related to the original function by the following equation:

$$p(t,\theta) = \int_{(\theta)} f(s,t)ds = \int_{-\infty}^{\infty} \int_{-\infty}^{\infty} f(x,y)\delta(x\cos\theta + y\sin\theta - t)dxdy \tag{4}$$

and inversely, the object density distribution function can be obtained from the measurements of projections by

$$f(x,y) = \int_0^\pi d\theta \int_{-t_m}^{t_m} p(t,\theta)h(t'-t)dt \tag{5}$$

where $h(t)$ is convolution kernel, written in discrete form as

$$h(n\delta) = \begin{cases} \dfrac{1}{4\delta^2} & n = 0 \\ 0 & n \text{ even} \\ -\dfrac{1}{(n\pi\delta)^2} & n \text{ old} \end{cases} \tag{6}$$

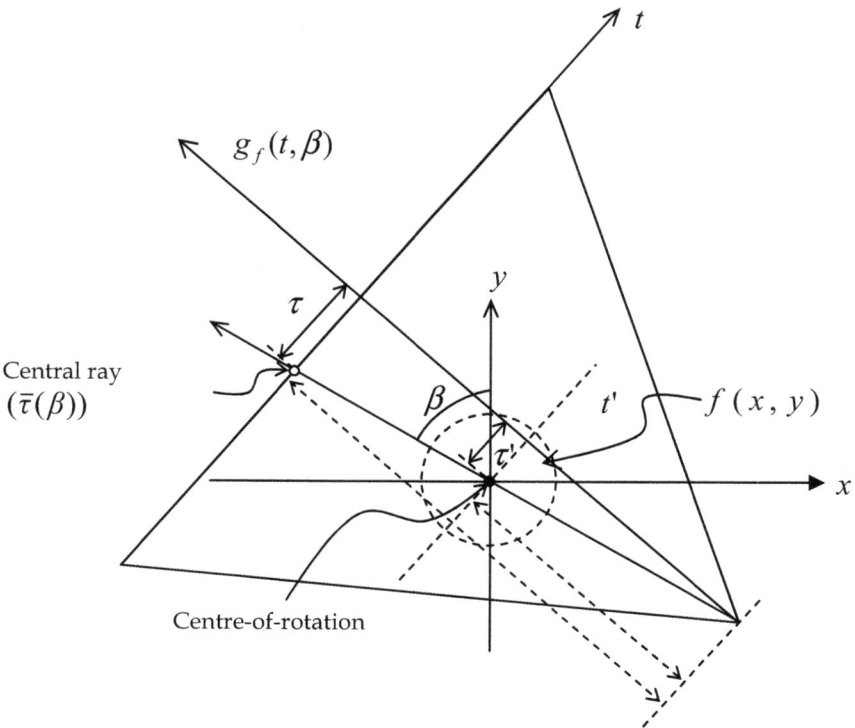

Fig. 6. Schematic of fan-beam projection CT geometry

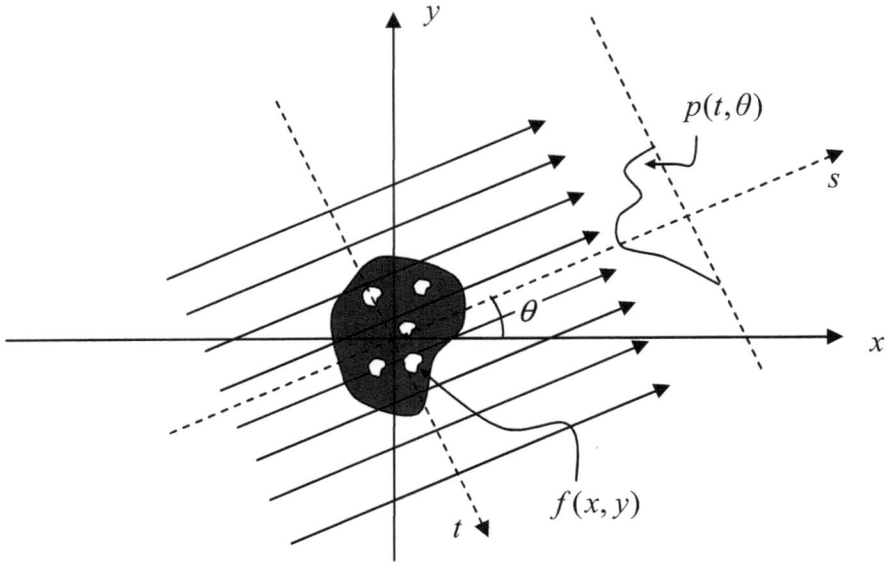

Fig. 7. Illustration of a parallel-beam projection

1.3.2 Fan-beam algorithm

Fan-beam reconstruction algorithm was developed for the 3rd and 4th generation of CT systems which employed a line detector. With this configuration, the line detector is so placed that the plane formed by it and the source is perpendicular to the rotation axis, leading to the fact that the cross-section of the object intersecting with this plane remains on the line detector during the scanning.

Figure 8 illustrate the geometrical relationship of the fan-beam projection. Let $R_\beta(s)$ be the fan-beam projection at pixel s and projection angle β. The cross-sectional intensity of the object can be reconstructed as

$$f(x,y) = \int_0^{2\pi} \frac{D^2}{(D + r\sin(\beta - \varphi))^2} \int_{-\infty}^{\infty} R_\beta(s) g(s' - s) \frac{D}{\sqrt{D^2 + s^2}} ds\, d\beta \qquad (6)$$

where g is the modified convolving kernel and takes the following form:

$$g(na) = \begin{cases} \dfrac{1}{8a^2}, & n = 0 \\ 0, & n \text{ even} \\ -\dfrac{1}{2n^2\pi^2 a^2}, & n \text{ old} \end{cases} \qquad (7)$$

and s' is calculated as

$$s' = \frac{Dr\cos(\beta - \varphi)}{D + r\sin(\beta - \varphi)} \qquad (8)$$

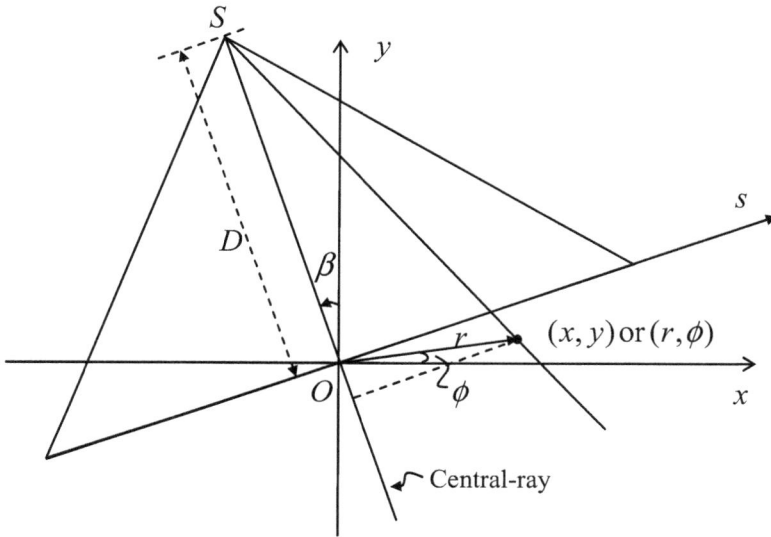

Fig. 8. Geometrical relationship of a fan-beam projection

1.3.3 Cone-beam algorithm

Figure 9 illustrates the definitions of the reconstruction slices and the associated coordinate systems involved in the development of the traditional cone-beam reconstruction algorithm. With these definitions, any point on the ith slice of the object is calculated as[7]

$$f(x,y,z_i) = \frac{1}{2}\int_{-\gamma}^{2\pi-\gamma}(\frac{D}{D+y'})^2 d\beta \int_{-\gamma_m}^{\gamma_m} q(s,v,\beta)h(s'-s)\frac{D}{\sqrt{(D^2+s^2+v^2)}}\,ds^\beta \qquad (9)$$

where h is the convolving kernel; D is the source-to-object distance, i.e., the distance from the source to the global coordinate centre; and $q(s,v,\beta)$ is the projection data at pixel (s,v) at projection angle β, with (s,v) being calculated as

$$\begin{pmatrix} s \\ v \end{pmatrix} = \frac{D}{D-(x\sin\beta+y\cos\beta)}\begin{pmatrix} x\cos\beta - y\sin\beta \\ z_i \end{pmatrix} \qquad (10)$$

1.4 Two issues with conventional CT inspection
1.4.1 Central ray determination with wire phantom

This method simply means that one needs an extra scan just for the determination of the central ray parameter. This is not only a waste of human and system resources and effort, but also a cause of uncertainty in the determination of central ray due to the mounting and dismounting process of the wire-phantom and the object. To minimize the effect of these problems, many techniques have been developed[4, 5]. These methods adopt similar ideas of either integrating the wire-phantom into the rotary system or scanning object and wire-

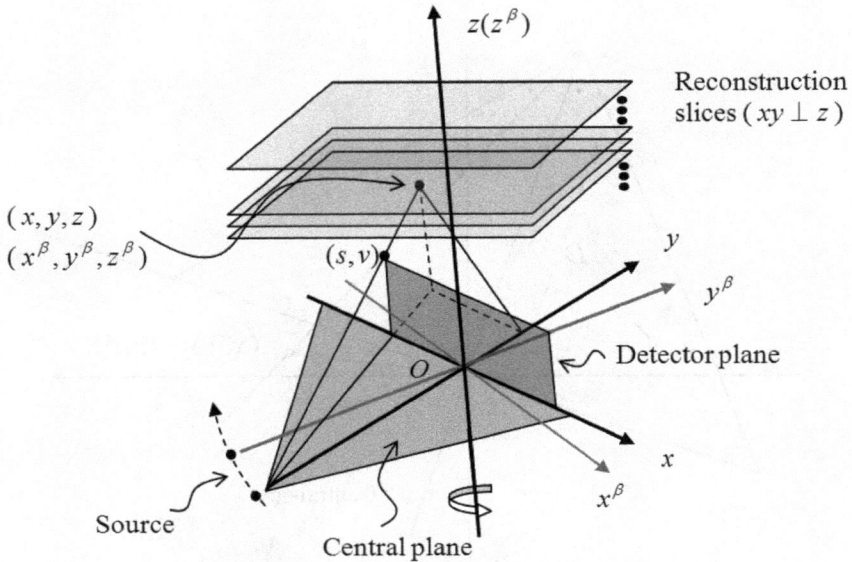

Fig. 9. Geometric relationship of a cone-beam projection

phantom together with a special fixture and then extracting the wire-phantom's projection information for central ray determination before reconstruction. These methods have been proven to be non-satisfactory because either complex sample fixture is required, or artifacts are introduced by the combined scanning.

1.4.2 Low efficiency of reconstruction with planar objects

The second problem of traditional CT is its low-efficiency for reconstructing planar objects such as stacked IC chips. These objects usually have a large area-to-thickness ratio. The low efficiency of the traditional CT mainly comes from two ways. First, due to a generally unavoidable imperfect mounting, the object would be scanned with a start orientation that may have tilt angles with both the rotation axis and the detector plane. As a result the reconstructed object will be obliquely reconstructed inside the reconstruction volume. As we know, the reconstructed data will only become interpretable through the visualization process. A tilted orientation will generally lead to a time-consuming visualization process, particularly for multilayered objects. Second, traditional CT always reconstructs an object with a cubic reconstruction volume (or a series of square slice) regardless of its particular shape. This is reasonable for general objects, however, for planar objects that have a large aspect ratio, the majority of the resources and computation time will be wasted on reconstructing the meaningless air. Besides, for most electronic devices, the resolution in the thickness dimension is generally more important than that on the transverse directions. However, the traditional CT reconstruction method is unable to conduct a discriminate reconstruction to enhance the resolution on the thickness dimension without significantly increasing the computation time and the requirement for computer specifications.

2. Automatic centre determination

2.1 Dual-boundary-point approach

Figure 10 describes the geometrical relationship between several important parameters of the micro-CT system and the basic idea of the dual-boundary-point approach[11, 12]. In this illustration, an object with several balls of different radius is used for the CT inspection. With a 360° scan, only the ball with the longest radius generates the widest projection on the detector. In other words, the left and right outermost boundaries of the sinogram of a selected slice actually come from the longest-radius ball on that slice of object. Therefore, once the position of the center-of-rotation is given, the angle of $\angle MSN$ is determined only by the radius of this longest-radius ball. This means, by finding the corresponding scan angles of the left and right boundaries of the projection, the angle of $\angle MSN$ can be calculated, which in turn leads to the determination of the central ray which must bisect the angle of MSN.

Although this is true theoretically, it is not easy to identify accurately the corresponding projection angles in practice because the two boundary points are actually the two tangential points on the circular trajectory of the longest-radius ball. As a result, the central ray is hard to be accurately determined too. A practical way is to make use of the vertical channel which is defined as the pixel on which the ray is perpendicular to the detector plane. With this consideration, the central ray can be determined by

$$\overline{OC}(=\frac{\overline{SC}}{P}*tg\left\{\left[tg^{-1}\left(\frac{\overline{LC}*p}{\overline{SC}}\right)-tg^{-1}\left(\frac{\overline{CR}*p}{\overline{SC}}\right)\right]/2\right\} \tag{11}$$

where $\overline{SC}$ is the source-to-detector distance (unit: μm); p is the pixel size of the detector; $\overline{OC}$, $\overline{LC}$, $\overline{RC}$ are vector distances from the central ray point O, the left end of projection L and the right end of projection R to the vertical channel point C respectively (unit: pixel).

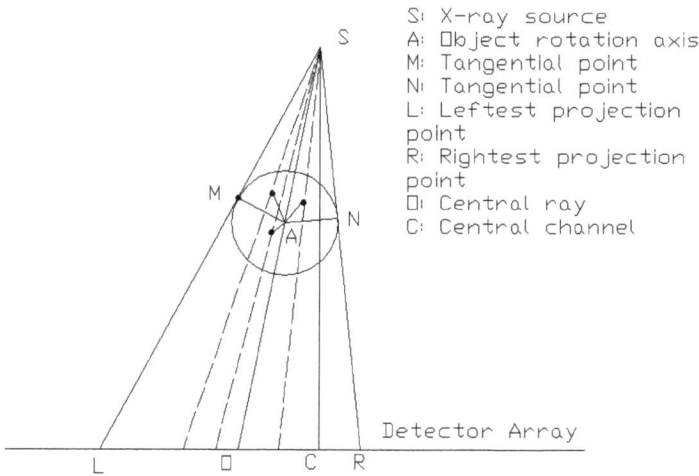

S: X-ray source
A: Object rotation axis
M: Tangential point
N: Tangential point
L: Leftest projection point
R: Rightest projection point
O: Central ray
C: Central channel

Detector Array

Fig. 10. The geometrical relationship of the CT system

The vertical line C is a fixed parameter and only need to be recalibrated when some movement conducted to the detector in possible system maintenance or detector repair. If both $\overline{LC}$ and $\overline{RC}$ are small compared to $\overline{SC}$ so that $\tan x \approx x$ is true, the central ray can be simply determined as the center of $\overline{LR}$, that is,

$$\overline{LO} = \frac{1}{2}\left|\overline{LC} + \overline{CR}\right| \qquad (12)$$

2.1.1 Case studies
We demonstrate this method with two different samples. The first one is a hearing-aid die that is scanned with a 693m source-to-image distance (SID) and a 15.58mm source-to-object distance (SOD). Figure 11(a) and 11(b) show respectively one of the 2D projections and its central beam sinogram. Note that this sample contains many mental pads, discretely distributed on the low-density substrate material. Compared to the substrate material which is polymer, the contrast of these metal dots is much easier for us to perform automatic edge detection. In this case the metal dot that has the longest rotation radius to the centre-of-rotation is selected for central ray determination and is calculated as 705.55 (in pixel) with Equation (11), as shown as white line in Figure.11(b). Because there is no reliable way to calibrate the true value of the central-ray, the accuracy is evaluated by reconstructing the object with the determined central ray (Figure 11(c)). We found it is at least comparable to the result reconstructed with the wire-phantom method

The second sample is a metal wire bundle. It is scanned with a 10mm SOD. Unlike the first sample, this time the boundary points of the entire object were used for central-ray calculation. Figure 12 shows one of its 2d projections, the determined boundary positions and central ray, and the reconstruction result of the middle cross-section. For this study the central ray is determined as 713.07 (in pixel).

2.2 Direct COR determination with the scanning data of the object
The reliability and accuracy of the dual-boundary-point method relies on the proper detection of the edge points of a particular feature, either being the surface point of the sample that has the longest distance to the centre-of-rotation, or a high-density point-feature inside the sample. However, there are some cases under which this method may not work properly. For example, when a high-magnification scan is conducted, one cannot obtain a complete sinogram of the entire object because part of it would rotate out of the field of view. This makes outermost boundary points detection impossible. Other cases include the situations of weak boundary contrast or no clear high-density feature for boundary detection.

Direct central ray determination approach[13] is then developed to overcome the above drawbacks of the dual-boundary-point method.

2.2.1 Principle of universal central ray determination technique
As shown in Figure 13, with a fan-beam arrangement we suppose JK is an arbitrary straight line on the object slice and KJ is obtained by rotating JK an angle of $\angle MPN$. Actually, when we rotate an object over the rotation axis P, each line on the object slice only have two

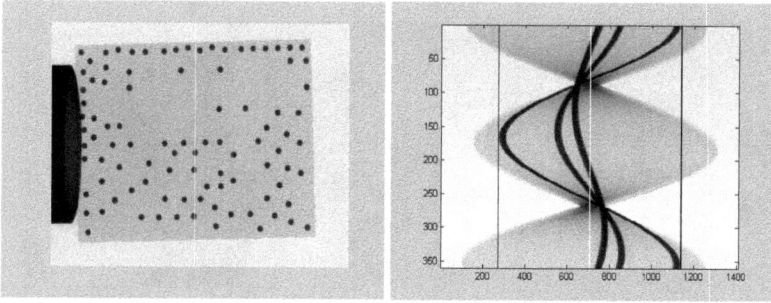

(a)   (b)

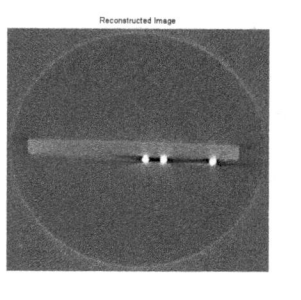

(c)

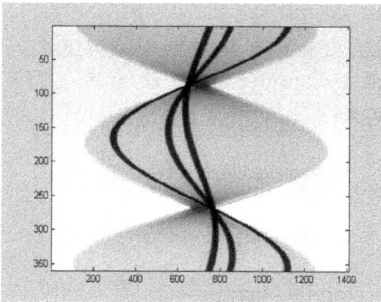

(d)

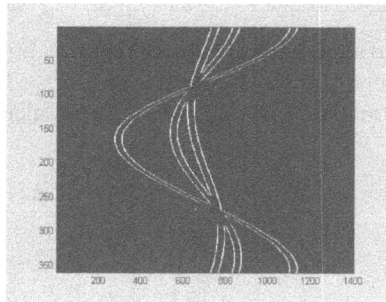

(e)

Fig. 11. CT scan of a hearing-aid die: (a) A 2D projection; (b) the sinogram of one slice with the two boundaries (black lines) and central ray (white line) identified; (c) the reconstructed image of the slice in (b)

(a)   (b)

(c)

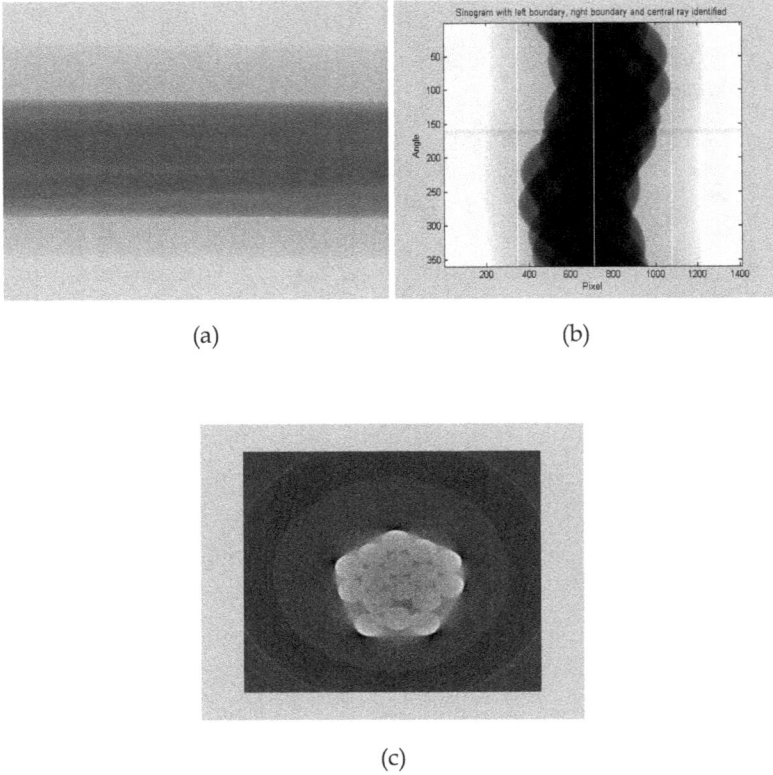

Fig. 12. CT scan of a segment of electric wire bundle: (a) A 2D projection; (b) the sinogram of one slice with the two boundaries and central ray (white lines) identified; (c) the reconstructed image of the slice in (b)

chances to align with the source point S. Supposing the two detector pixels that correspond respectively to the two alignments are s_1 (JK) at a scanning angle α and s_2 (KJ) at the scanning angle $\alpha + \beta$, β and s_2 can be calculated as

$$\beta(s_1) = \angle MPN = 180 - 2\angle ASC = 180 - 2\left(\arctan\frac{s_1}{h_0} - \arctan\frac{c_0}{h_0}\right) \tag{13}$$

$$s_2(s_1) = h_0 tg\angle BSO = h_0\left(2\arctan\frac{c_0}{h_0} - \arctan\frac{s_1}{h_0}\right) \tag{14}$$

where c_0 is the true central ray and h_0 is the source-to-image distance (SID).

Ignore the effect of the minor variation of the X-ray beam intensity over the detector pixels, we have

$$P_\alpha(s_1) = P_{\alpha+\beta}(s_2) \tag{15}$$

This property is the basis of our universal fan-beam central ray determination. In the practical implementation, we can assume a set of central ray values $\{c_i\}$ and for each c_i we calculate s_2 and β, and then perform the following measurement

$$M(c_i) = \sum_{\alpha=n_1}^{n_2} \sum_{s_1=t_1}^{t_2} [P_\alpha(s_1) - P_{\alpha+\beta(s_1)}(s_2(s_1))]^2 \tag{16}$$

Obviously M should reach a minimum value when $c_i = c_0$.

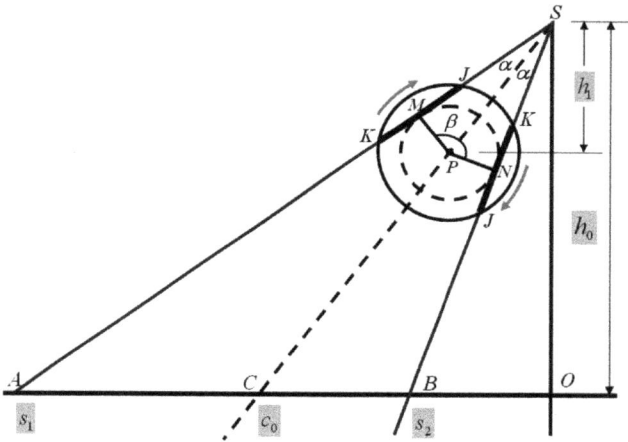

Fig. 13. Principle of the universal central ray determination method.

The computer implementation of the proposed algorithm is described as below:

Step 1. Calculate the angle of each pixel, $\gamma(i) = \arctan[s(i)/h_0]$, with respect to the middle ray SO, where i is the pixel index number, $s(i)$ is the distance of the ith pixel to point O.

Step 2. Calculate $\gamma(i) - \gamma_{c_i}$. Here $\gamma_{c_i} = \arctan(c_i / h_0)$ is the angle of the assumed central ray with respect to the middle ray SO.

Step 3. Calculate $\beta(i)$ and $s_2(i)$ using Equations (13) and (14) respectively.

Step 4. Calculate $M(c_i)$ using Equation (16). Because both $\beta(i)$ and $s_2(i)$ can be fractional numbers, bilinear interpolation is applied.

Step 5. For the next assumed central ray value, repeat step 2 to 5.

Step 6. The true central ray is then identified as the minimum value of measurement data (if necessary, a curve fitting can be applied).

2.2.2 Experimental demonstration and discussion

To evaluate the accuracy of the proposed method, an experiment was arranged to scan an electronic component used in a cashcard and a wire phantom at the same position. Figure 14(a) is a 2D image of the sample and Figure 14(b) shows a central slice sinogram of the scan. The sinogram of the wire phantom is shown in Figure 14(c), from which the central ray is determined as 688.0798 (in pixel) with the conventional method. Figure 14(d) shows the research curve of applying the new method and the central ray is determined as either the minimum of the curve or a curved fitted minimum of it. In this study, they are 687.9849 and 687.7449 respectively. The total computation time is about 20 second with a MATLAB programming. One can note that the central ray determined with the sample projection data agrees very well with that calibrated with the wire phantom.

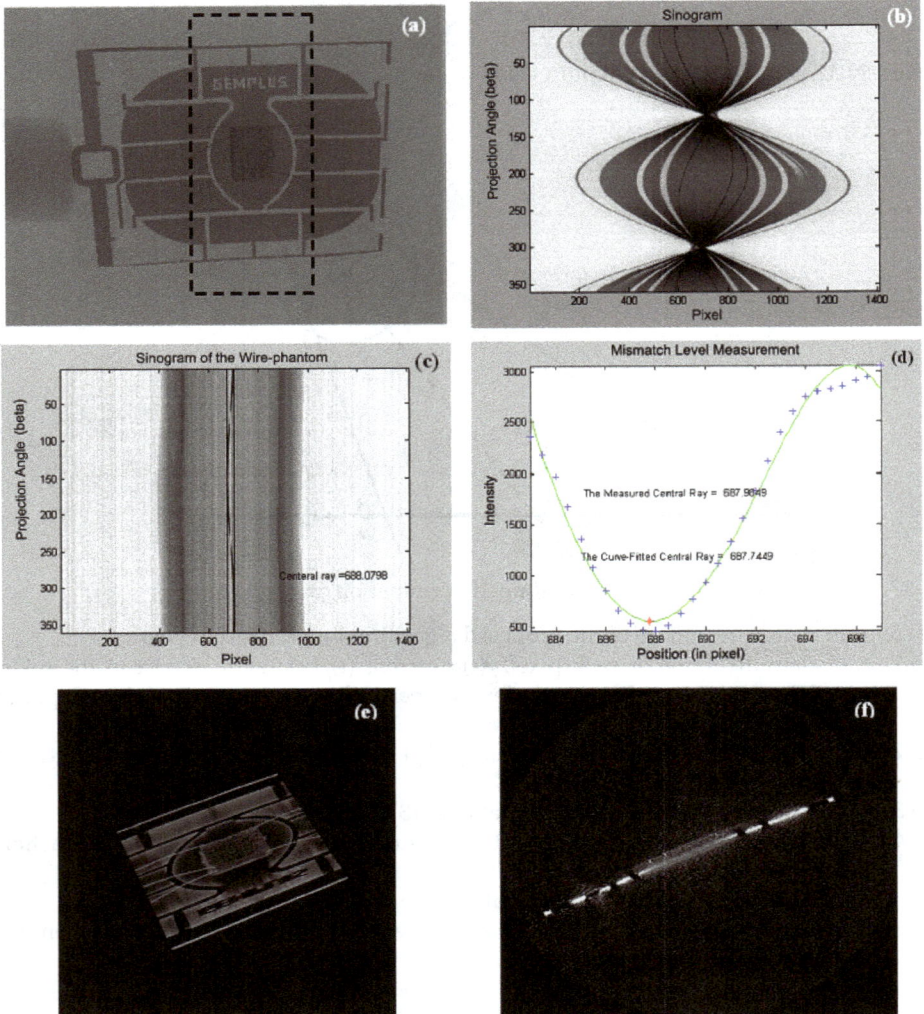

Fig. 14. Demonstration of the proposed method: (a) A 2D image of a cashcard electronic component; (b) A sinogram of the scan (a); (c) The wire-phantom sinogram; (d) The measurement curve obtained with the present method; (e) A reconstruction volume of part of the sample; (f) One slice from the volume reconstruction.

With the central ray determined, the central part of object (the dash line-box area in Figure 14(a) was reconstructed using a volume cone-beam algorithm, written by the author in Matlab. Figures 14(e) and 14(f) show respectively the 3D result and one of the slices, from which one can see that the small wires are clearly reconstructed. This is an indication that the reconstruction is performed with an accurate central ray value.

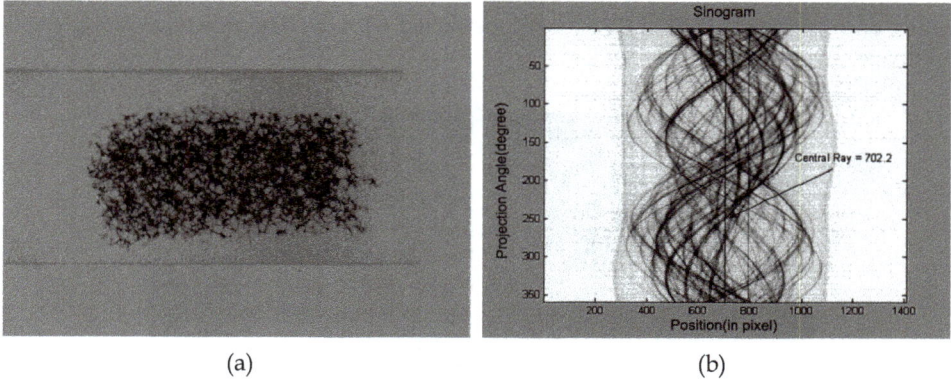

(a)   (b)

Fig. 15. A 2D image of the foam sample (a) and its sinogram of CT scan(b).

We then tested the performance of this method by scanning a foam sample. The sample was made of flexible polyurethane (PU) foam as matrix and carbonyl iron powders as fillers. It was laboratory synthesized through the fundamental polymerization reaction between polyols and isocyanates. The iron powders originally are several microns to several tens of microns in size. However, when synthesized, some of them may form much larger clusters. Figure 15 shows one 2D image of a foam sample and its sinogram. Obviously due to the weak boundary contrast, the reliable detection of the boundary points would be challenging without user's interaction. Figure 16 shows the measurement curve obtained with the proposed method, from which the central ray is determined as 702.2 (in pixel). Its

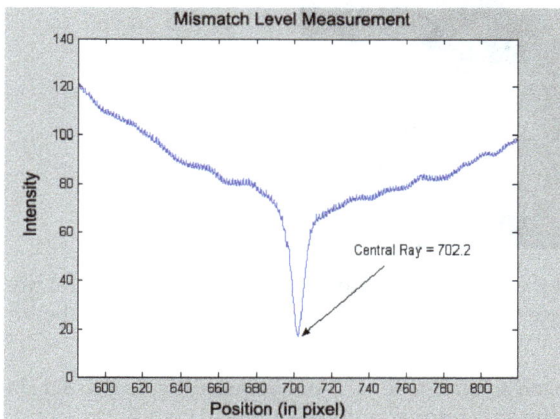

Fig. 16. The measurement curve obtained with Eq.(16) for the foam sample and the determined central ray.

corresponding position in the sinogram is also indicated in Figure 15(b), shown as the bold line. One may notice that in this sinogram there is also a smaller line to the right of the central ray line. This line is actually formed by a spoiled detector cell and has no meaning in our experiment. To evaluate its performance, we deliberately introduce different errors to the central ray and redo the reconstruction of the same slice. Figure 17(a) to 17(e) are those reconstructed results obtained with $702.2, 702.2 \pm 1$ and 702.2 ± 3. From the blur level of the images, one can notice that the CT slice reconstructed with the determined central ray is the best image.

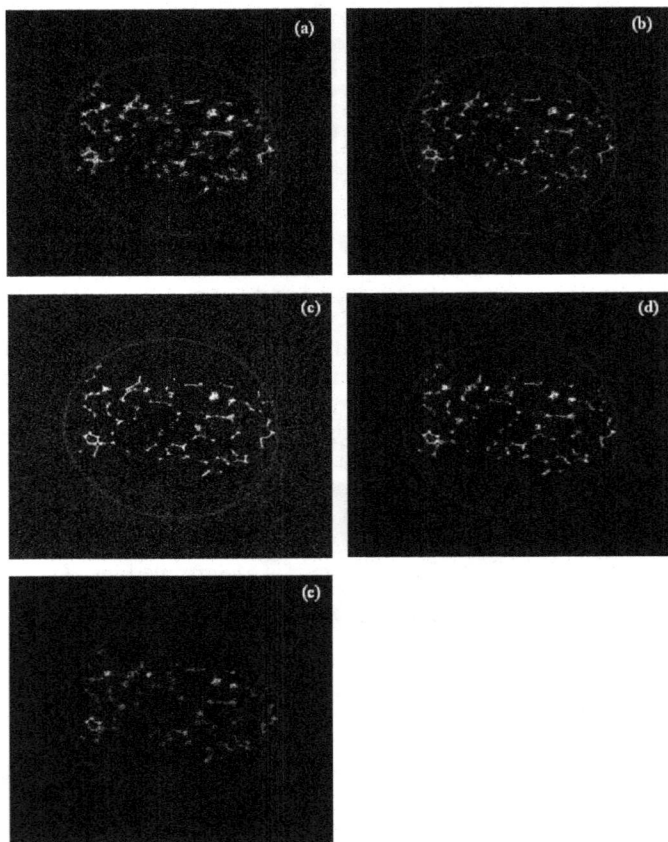

Fig. 17. The results of the same slice reconstructed at different central ray values.(a) 699.2; (b) 701.2; (c) 702.2 (the determined value with the present method, as shown in Fig.4) ; (d) 703.2; (e)705.2.

Note that this approach in principle will not require the whole set data of the sinogram; instead, a portion of the sinogram around the guessed central-ray point is generally enough for a good determination. This feature makes it still valid for high-magnification scan where incomplete sinogram of the object will be encountered.

3. Cone-beam CT reconstruction for planar objects

3.1 CT scan efficiency problems for planar object

As we discussed before, conventional CT always provides a reconstruction volume which is formed by a number of square slices. This is a natural selection for general CT applications because we may encounter objects that have totally different shape, regular or irregular. However, it indeed loses efficiency when reconstructing and visualizing planar objects such as stacked IC chips, MEMS devices and so on.

Figure 18 illustrates a typical reconstruction result of a planar object. There are two observations that one can make easily: First, the planar object only occupies a small portion of the reconstruction volume, meaning that the majority of the reconstruction is wasted on reconstructing the meaningless air; Second, the planar object has a tilt orientation with respect to the reconstruction volume, leading to a time-consuming visualization process, particular when multilayered objects are analyzed in a layer-wise manner.

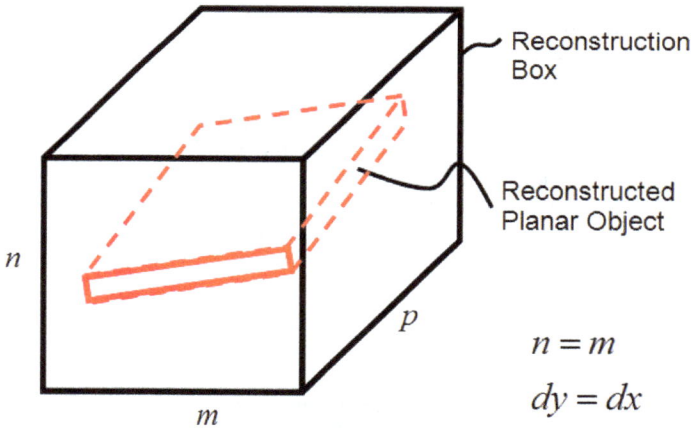

Fig. 18. Illustration of a planar object in the reconstruction volume

This tilted orientation of the planar object in the reconstruction volume is generally unavoidable because it is a direct consequence of the uncertainty in mounting object to the rotary system. As illustrated in Figure 19, there generally exist a non-default scan-start-angle and an axial-tilt-angle when mounting and scanning a planar object. Unfortunately this problem is hard to solve through good mechanical design of sample fixtures due to the variation in sample shape, size and surface features.

3.2 Differential cone-beam reconstruction for planar object [14-15]
3.2.1 Concept of differential reconstruction

Differential reconstruction is proposed based on the characteristics of scanning a planar object that has generally a large area-to-thickness ratio. To illustrate this idea, we first take a look at a special case when applying traditional CT on a planar object. For easier explanation, we also assume that the scan of the plane object is started with its cross-section being parallel to one of the detector dimensions. Consequently, the reconstruction image of this object cross-section would be also parallel to one dimension of the

(a)   (b)

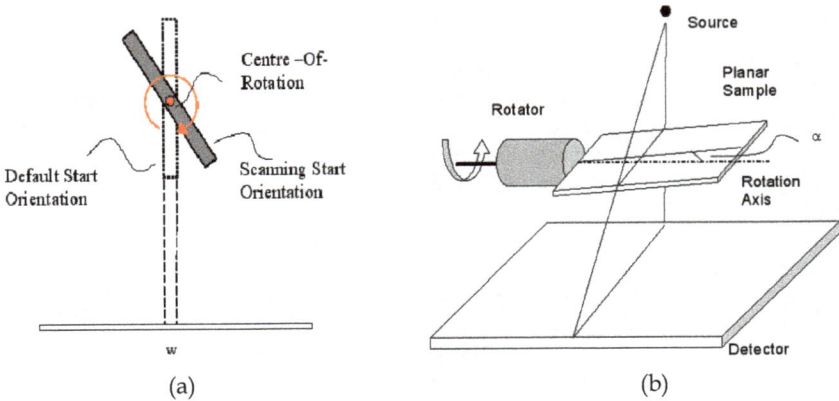

Fig. 19. Two issues that contribute to the tilted orientation of the reconstructed object: (a) The start orientation of the object does not match the default start angle of the reconstruction algorithm; (b) A tilt angle exists between the primary plane of the object and the rotation axis.

reconstruction matrix (Figure 20(b)). However, as described previously, due to the large aspect ratio, the object area only occupies a small part of the square matrix. Now imaging that if we know the thickness of the object and its position in the projection image, we would be available to define a reconstruction matrix that may just cover the object, as shown in Figure 19(c). Furthermore, we can even consider defining a higher reconstruction resolution in the generally more critical thickness dimension to obtain more fine features. This is exactly what the term 'differential reconstruction' means.

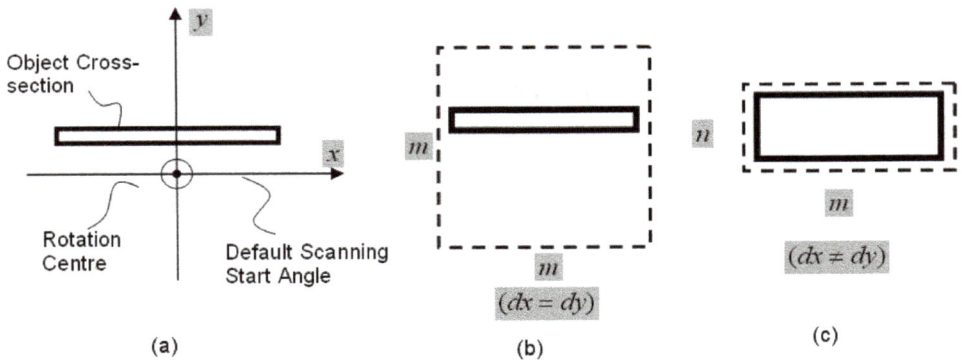

(a)   (b)   (c)

Fig. 20. Illustration of the concept of differential reconstruction: (a) the orientation of the object cross-section is aligned with the default object orientation of the reconstruction algorithm; (b)The reconstruction result of the object slice with a   reconstruction matrix; (c) Result with the proposed differential reconstruction.

3.2.2 Simulation of scanning a planar object
The key issue to materializing the planar CT reconstruction is the appropriate definition of the reconstruction matrix and volume, and this requires us to know the actual object orientation, position and thickness (the size of the object's lateral dimension is generally not

critical and can be ignored in this study. Instead, we will discuss it role later in the section of targeted planar CT reconstruction). In order to understand how these parameters are determined and applied in this new approach, we conduct a simulation of scanning a planar object with a parallel-beam arrangement. Because the determination of these parameters only involved the central-beam slice, using a parallel-beam arrangement is not a problem because it is nowadays a relatively trial work to convert a fan-beam sinogram to a parallel-beam sinogram without any ambiguity for the central-beam slice[7]. As illustrated in Figure 21, a planar object is scanned separately with parameter sets of (a=0, t=3mm, b1=10mm, b2=-10mm, α=33°) and (a=5mm, t=3mm, b1=15mm, b2=-5mm, α=-30°), Here α is the start angle of a scan and it is interpreted as, if we choose to start the scan at α=33°, it actually means we rotate the object an angle of 33° from the initial position and then start the scan. The results are shown in Figure 22 and Figure 23 correspondingly.

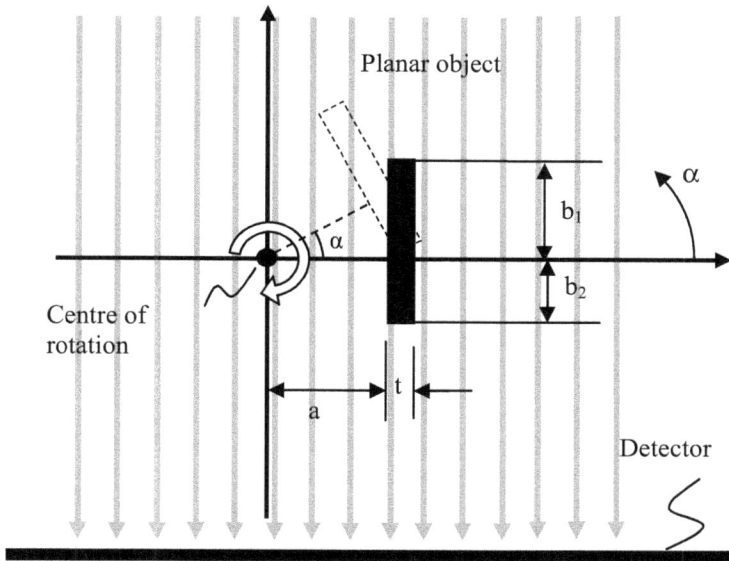

Fig. 21. Simulation of scanning a planar object with a parallel-beam configuration

One can note that when we scan the object at two different start positions, their sonograms have different shapes (Figure 22a and Figure 23a). However, the subtractions of the two edge curves are exactly the same except their different start point due to the different scan-start-angles used. One can also find from figures 22(c) and 23(c) that the data values near each tip point is approximately linearly approaching to the tip point. This characteristic will be used later for detecting the scan-start-angle in a real scan.

Another important observation with this simulation is the position variation of the narrowest shadow with the scan-start-angle. Because in this simulation, the two scans start at 33° and -30°, we find that their narrowest shadows occurs respectively at 147° (=180°-33°) and 30°(=0°-(-30°)). This means with a real scan, we can calculate the scan-start-angle, i.e., the orientation of the object for the first projection of the scan, by identifying the narrowest shadow position of the sinogram.

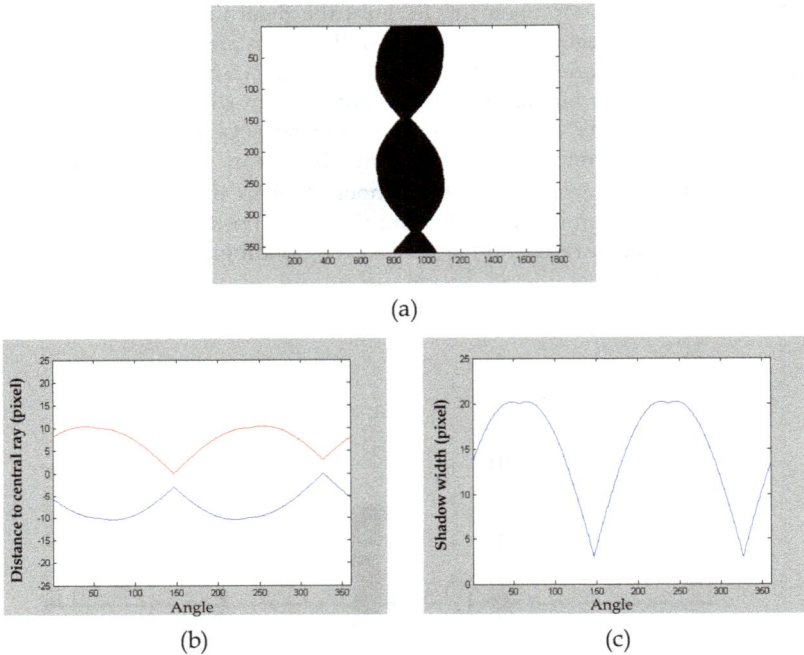

(a)

(b)

(c)

Fig. 22. Simulation results with parameter setting: a=0, t=3mm, b1=10mm, b2=-10mm, α=33°. (a) The sinogram; (b) The edge profiles; (c) Top edge curve minus bottom edge curve in (b).

With the actual scan start angle determined, we now can simplify our problem by assuming that we always start the scan with a zero scan-start-angle. Then we can focus on how to determine the possible axial-tilt-angle and the object's projected thickness and thickness centre location on the detector.

The projected thickness and centre location can be determined from the narrowest shadow, as illustrated in Figure 24 (which is a copy of Figure 23(b)). The projected thickness of the object, t, will be used to define the size of the reconstruction in the thickness dimension and distance between the thickness centre to the central-ray, d, required for defining the position of the reconstruction matrix in the field of view. If we consider to add a small margin to the determined thickness t, the height of the reconstruction matrix is calculated as.

$$l = t + 2s \qquad (17)$$

If there is an axial-tilt-angle, γ, Equation (17) becomes

$$l = t + \Delta z \times \tan \gamma + 2s \qquad (18)$$

(a)

(b)

(c)

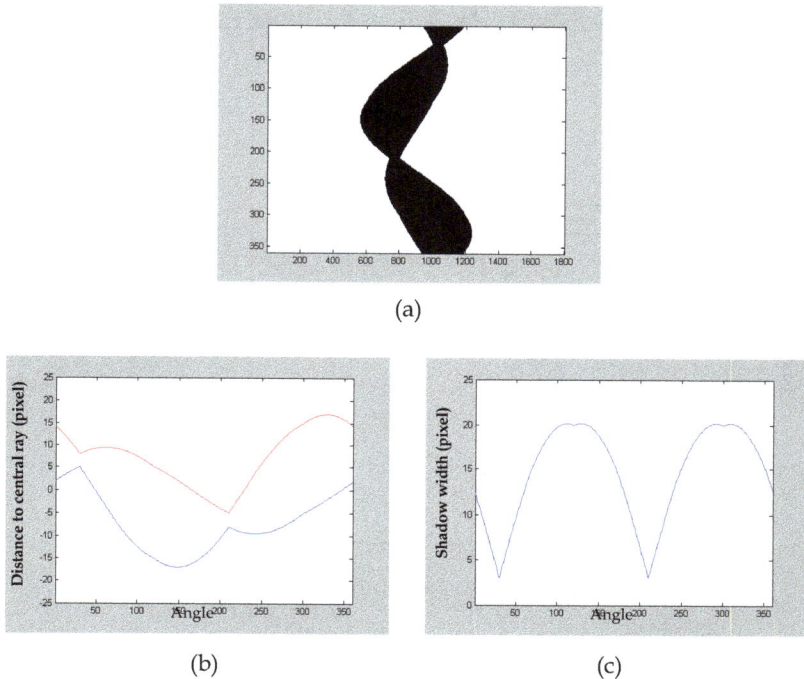

Fig. 23. Simulation results with parameter setting: a=5, t=3mm, b1=15mm, b2=-5mm, α=-30°. (a) The sinogram; (b) The edge profiles; (c) Top edge curve minus bottom edge curve in (b).

where Δz is the object's projected length on the detector.

The pixel number of the matrix in the thickness dimension, n, is then calculated with a given reconstruction resolution (or reconstruction pixel size) in this dimension, dy, as

$$n = l \, / \, dy \qquad (19)$$

It is worthy pointing out again that because the lateral size of the planar object is usually comparable to the size of the field-of-view, it is not very meaningful to determine the actual projected size of the object in this dimension. Instead, we simply leave it the same as that with the conventional method. However, this dimension may become useful in targeted planar CT reconstruction, which we will discuss later.

3.2.2.1 Reconstruction slice definition

Figure 25 shows the reconstruction matrix definition and the back-projection relation when $\theta_k = 0$ (1st projection) with the determined parameters. To compare with the traditional method, we draw the new definition directly on the traditional definition of the reconstruction matrix. The size and position of the new matrix are defined with the determined l and d.

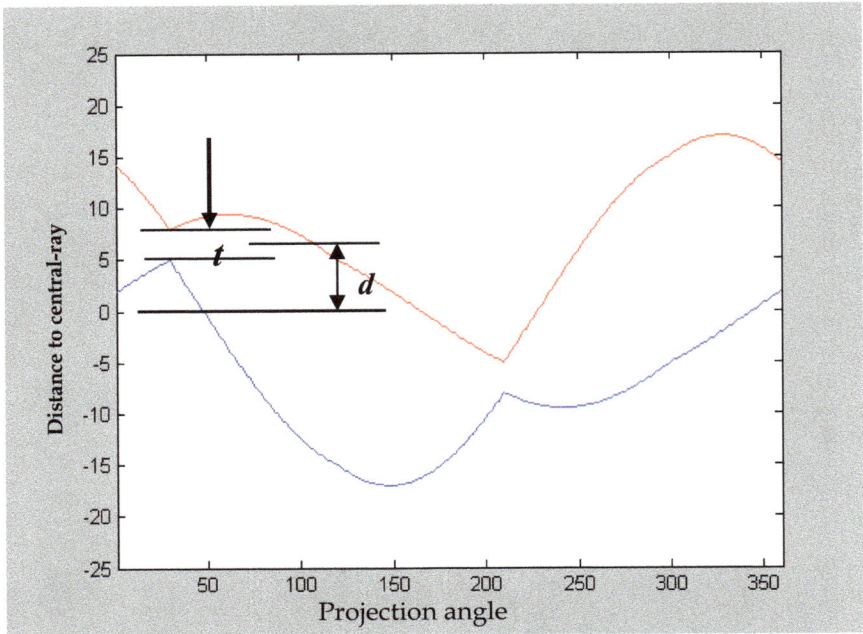

Fig. 24. Estimate the object thickness and its position to the centre-of-rotation (COR)

Suppose with conventional CT the reconstruction matrix is defined as $A(i,j), 1 < i < a, 1 < j < a$ (pixel size: $dx_a = dy_a$), and with the present method it is defined as $B(n,m), 1 < n < l, 1 < m < a$ ($dx_b \neq dy_b$), then in the FDK backprojection process we have
For conventional CT

$$
\begin{aligned}
&X_A(i,j) = (i - a/2)dx_a \\
&Y_A(i,j) = (j - a/2)dy_a \\
&\beta_k(i,j) = \tan^{-1}(Y_A(i,j)/X_B(i,j)) + \theta_k \\
&r_A = \sqrt{X_A(i,j)^2 + Y_A(i,j)^2} \\
&p_k = \frac{D \times r_A \times \cos(\beta_k(i,j)/d_p}{D - r_A \times \sin(\beta_k(i,j))}
\end{aligned}
\tag{20}
$$

For the present method,

$$
\begin{aligned}
&X_B(n,m) = (m - a/2)dx_b \\
&Y_B(n,m) = (n - b/2)dy_b + d \\
&\beta_k(n,m) = \tan^{-1}(Y_B(n,m)/X_B(n,m)) + \alpha + \theta_k \\
&r_B = \sqrt{X_B(n,m)^2 + Y_B(n,m)^2} \\
&p_k = \frac{D \times r_B \times \cos(\beta_k(n,m)/d_p}{D - r_B \times \sin(\beta_k(n,m))}
\end{aligned}
\tag{21}
$$

where β_k is the back-projection angle, α is the scanning start angle, θ_k is the projection (system rotation) angle for the kth projection, d_p is the pixel size of the imaginary detector, D is the source-to-object distance, and p_k is the back-projection position (in pixel) on the detector.

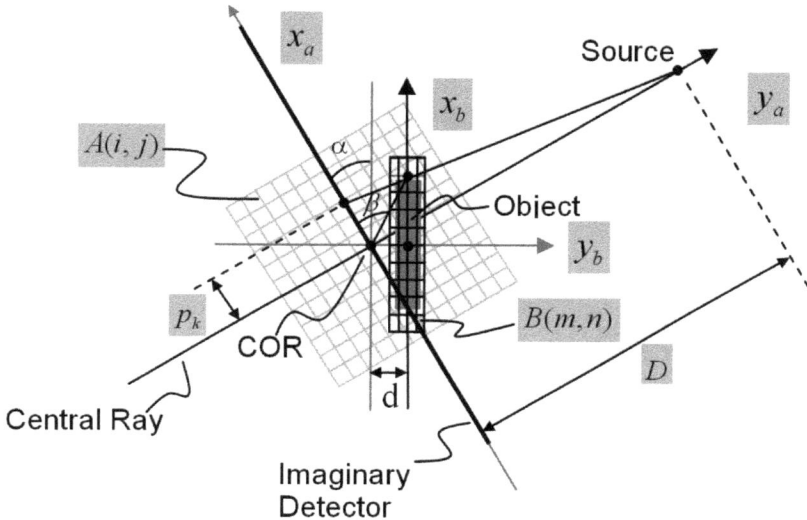

Fig. 25. Definition of reconstruction matrix with the present method in the backprojection process

3.2.3 Determination of key geometrical parameters with scanning data of object

Now we explain how to determine the key parameters required for proper reconstruction matrix definition with the present method in real CT inspection applications. Figure 26(a) is the central-slice sinogram of scanning a planar object (after a fan-beam to parallel-beam conversion). The black vertical line on the image is the central ray's position. With this sinogram, we first sum the intensities of pixels along the horizontal direction and obtain a summed intensity variation over the projection angle, as shown in Figure 26(b). Then we identify the two tips and perform curve fitting to the points on both sides of each tip. The intersection of the two fitted lines is the projection angle γ that gives us the narrowest projection shadow. Then the scan-start-angle (SSA) is calculated as $(90° - \gamma)$ with a 1-degree angular step in the scan.

Then the rest three parameters are determined with the 2d projection image that gives the narrowest shadow, as illustrated in figure 27. First we perform edge detection to both sides of the object shadow and then curve fittings to find the slopes of the edge lines. The axial-tilt-angle can be determined as either the average of the two slopes, or just one of them. If both surfaces of the planar object are flat and parallel to each other, these two choices don't give different results for the axial-tilt-angle determination; however, for cases where only one surface is flat, we chose the flat surface for axial-tilt-angle calculation.

(a)

(b)

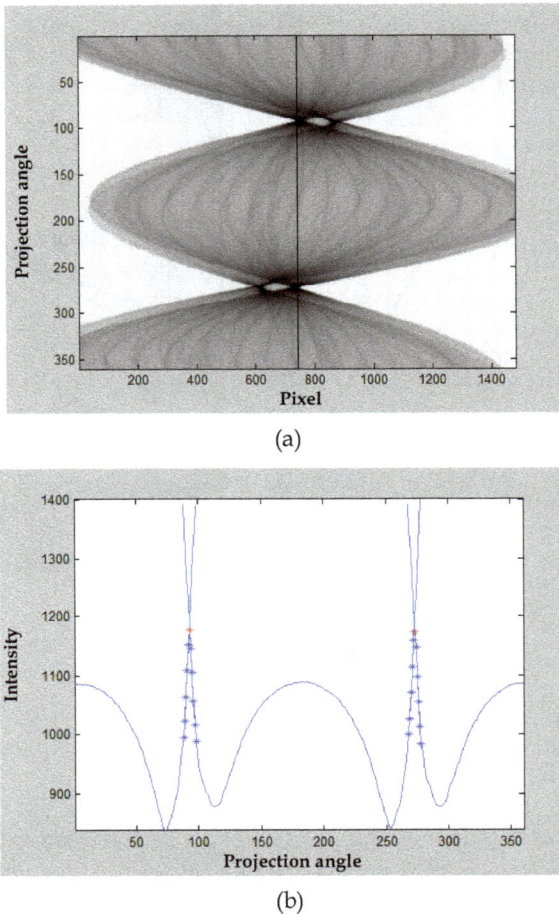

Fig. 26. A sinogram of scanning planar object (a) and the determination of the scan-start-angle with it (b)

The determination of the object's projection thickness, t, and its centre-position is straightforward with the obtained edge lines. The former is calculated as the distance between the two edge points intersecting with the central beam and the later is the distance between the thickness centre and the central-ray (not shown in the figure). The accuracy of these two parameters is not critical and one can actually consider adding a small margin to the determined thickness to accommodate possible bumps on the surfaces.

3.2.4 Image rotation for the 3rd dimension alignment

After we reconstruct the planar object with the matrix defined in Figure 25, we could have the object's cross-section well-oriented on each slice; however, due to the axial-tilt-angle (ATA) the location of the object's cross section would vary over the axis-of-rotation direction, as shown in Figure 28(a). To make the reconstructed object also aligned with the reconstruction volume in

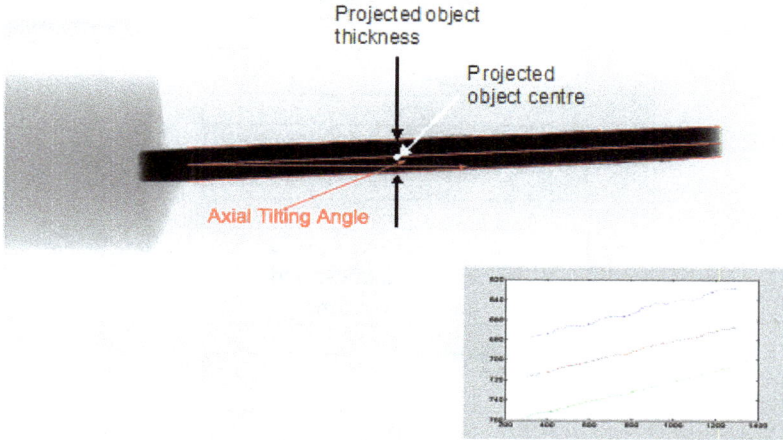

Fig. 27. Definition of the projected object thickness and centre

the axis-of-rotation direction, one needs to conduct an image rotation around the x axis. The final reconstruction result should be the case illustrated in Figure 28(b), which is an orientation that will make subsequent layer separation easy and reliable.

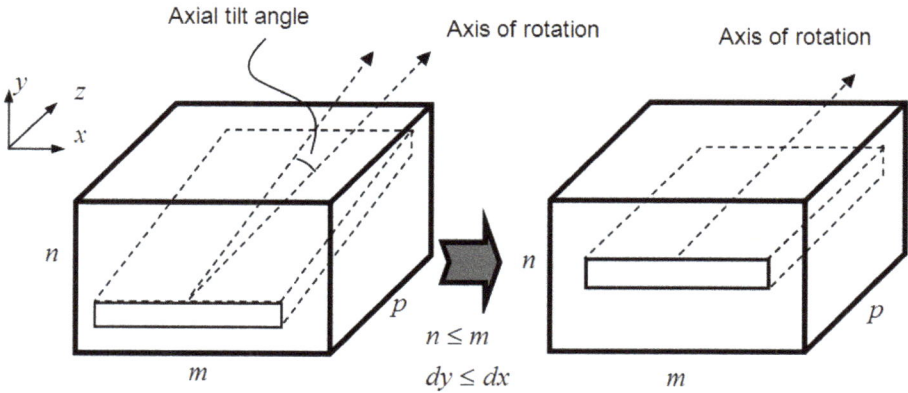

Fig. 28. Image rotation for aligning the planar object to the reconstruction volume in the rotation-of-axis direction

The whole data processing and reconstruction process is summarized in the flowchart shown in Figure 29.

```
┌─────────────────────────────────┐
│          Mount sample           │
└─────────────────────────────────┘
                 ↓
┌─────────────────────────────────┐
│       Set system parameters     │
└─────────────────────────────────┘
                 ↓
┌─────────────────────────────────┐
│              Scan               │
└─────────────────────────────────┘
                 ↓
┌─────────────────────────────────┐
│    Determine central ray with   │
│     central slice sinogram      │
└─────────────────────────────────┘
                 ↓
┌─────────────────────────────────┐
│   Determine SSA, ATA, object's  │
│     projected thickness and     │
│        thickness centre         │
└─────────────────────────────────┘
                 ↓
┌─────────────────────────────────┐
│   Define reconstruction volume  │
└─────────────────────────────────┘
                 ↓
┌─────────────────────────────────┐
│     Cone-beam reconstruction    │
└─────────────────────────────────┘
                 ↓
┌─────────────────────────────────┐
│    Image rotation by a ATA angle│
└─────────────────────────────────┘
                 ↓
┌─────────────────────────────────┐
│             Report              │
└─────────────────────────────────┘
                 ↓
┌─────────────────────────────────┐
│              End                │
└─────────────────────────────────┘
```

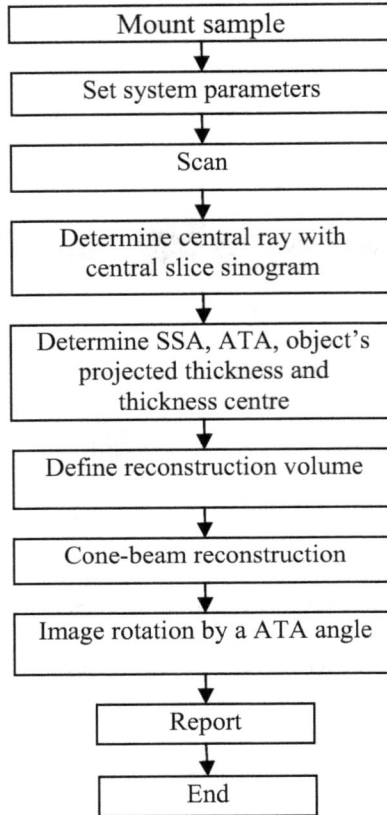

Fig. 29. Flowchart of differential cone-beam reconstruction

It should be pointed out that the definition of the reconstruction matrix will not suffer the reconstruction quality because for every pixel within the new matrix, it still goes through the reconstruction process as exactly the same as that for reconstructing a pixel in the conventional reconstruction matrix.

But the image rotation process would have some influence to the reconstruction result because it is basically an interpolation process. This influence might become meaningful when inspecting objects with very thin internal layers that have fine features on them.

3.3 Reconstruct object along its primary direction

The efficiency of reconstruction for planar objects can be further improved by defining and reconstructing the slices along the object's primary axis, instead of the axis-of-rotation. As we know that so far for all conventional cone-beam reconstruction algorithms, the slices are defined as being perpendicular to the axis-of-rotation. This is the root cause of the tilted reconstruction of a planar object which is scanned with an axial-tilt angle to the axis-of-rotation[16].

As illustrated in Figure 30(a), the dotted-line box represents a general orientation of a planar object at the start time of a CT scan, its primary plane is xz. z' is the axis of rotation, and $x'z'$ represents the equivalent detector plane. The axis x forms an angle (β, i.e., the scan-start-angle) with x' and z forms an angle (α) with z' (when $\beta = 0$, it is the axial-tilt-angle). The solid-line box is the reconstruction volume, defined in such a way that its slices (reconstruction matrices) are perpendicular to z (Figure 30(b)) and the lateral dimension of each slice (matrix) is parallel to the primary dimension of the object's cross-section.

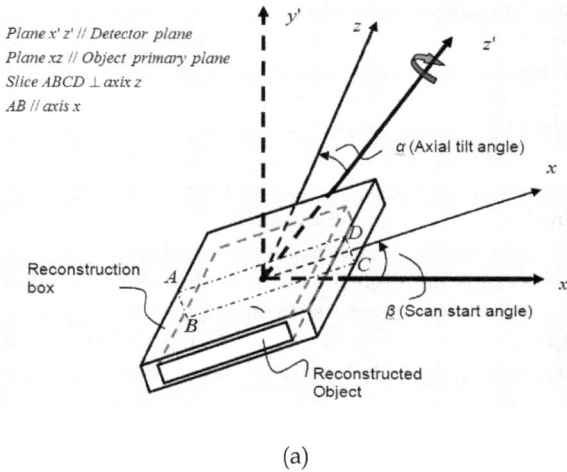

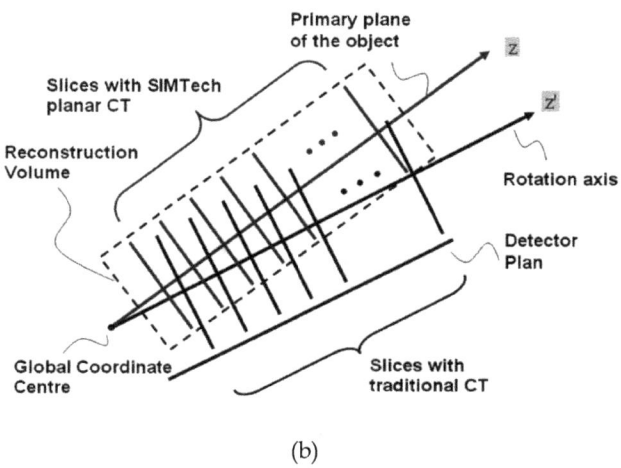

Plane $x'z'$ // Detector plane
Plane xz // Object primary plane
Slice $ABCD \perp$ axix z
AB // axis x

α (Axial tilt angle)

Reconstruction box

β (Scan start angle)

Reconstructed Object

(a)

Primary plane of the object

Slices with SIMTech planar CT

Reconstruction Volume

Rotation axis

Detector Plan

Global Coordinate Centre

Slices with traditional CT

(b)

Fig. 30. Illustration of defining reconstruction volume along the object orientation. (a) The geometrical relationship between the reconstruction volume and the object in the physical scanning space; (b) The side view of (a) showing the difference in reconstruction slice orientation between the proposed method and conventional method.

Although the concept of the present idea looks quite straightforward and simple, its implementation is definitely not so. Fortunately, it is possible for us to decouple the roles of the scan-start-angle and the axial-tilt angle in the reconstruction process. Considering the fact that we can always rearrange the projections to an equivalent scan that starts with a zero scan-start angle by assigning the actual scan-stat-angle to the first projection, we just need to consider a non-zero axial-tilt-angle situation in developing the reconstruction algorithm for the proposed method.

Figure 31 is the schematic of the four coordinate systems involved in the new method for a cone-beam reconstruction. Note that in this illustration we still use the convention that the object is stationary and the source-and-detector pair is rotated for a scan. Point O is the global center of all the coordinate systems. $x'y'z'$ is the initial scanner position with its x' being one of the equivalent detector dimensions, z' being the axis-of-rotation and y' being the line passing through O and the initial X-ray source point. xyz represents the object space, it can be obtained by rotating $x'y'z'$ system an angle α around the x' axis, with α corresponding to the axial-tilt-angle in a real scan. (To avoid congestion, the axes x and y are purposely drawn on the reconstruction slice, not from the global centre O). $x^\beta y^\beta z^\beta$ is the projection coordinate system, obtained by rotating $x'y'z'$ an angle of β around the z' axis. Obviously, $x'y'z'$ and $x^\beta y^\beta z^\beta$ are superimposed when β is zero. x'' is a line on the slice parallel to x'. The angle between x'' and x is the scan-start-angle. With traditional reconstruction method, when a non-zero scan-start-angle exists, one will obtain a tilted orientation of the object's cross-section with respect to the reconstruction matrix due to the use of a zero scan-start-angle in default. Finally, sv is called the image coordinate system. It can be thought of as a particular plane in the $x^\beta y^\beta z^\beta$ coordinate system when $y^\beta = 0$.

One can note that in this illustration, slices $(x',y')_{z'=1,2,...}$ correspond to conventional reconstruction volume definition and that $(x,y)_{z=1,2,...}$ are the slices defined with the present method. When there is no axial tilt (α is zero), they become the same.

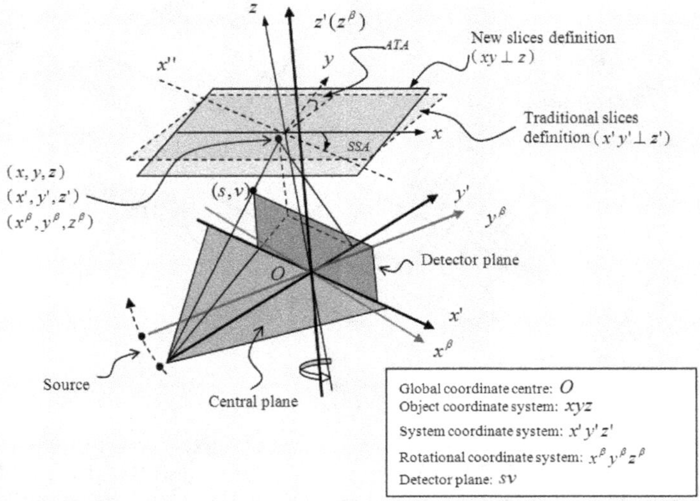

Fig. 31. Schematic of the four coordinate systems used in the new method

Similar to deriving the conventional algorithm[7], the key job here is to establish the relationship between an object point (x,y,z) and its projection position (s^β, v^β) at each projection angle β. With the proposed method, (s,v) is calculated as

$$\begin{pmatrix} s^\beta \\ v^\beta \end{pmatrix} = \frac{D}{D - (x\sin\beta + \cos\beta(y\cos\alpha + z\sin\alpha))} \begin{pmatrix} x\cos\beta - \sin\beta(y\cos\alpha + z\sin\alpha) \\ -y\sin\alpha + z\cos\alpha \end{pmatrix} \quad (22a)$$

And the object function can be reconstructed as:

$$f(x,y,z) = \frac{1}{2} \int_{-\gamma}^{2\pi-\gamma} (\frac{D}{D+y'})^2 d\beta \int_{-\gamma_m}^{\gamma_m} q(s^\beta, v^\beta, \beta) h(s' - s^\beta) \frac{D}{\sqrt{(D^2 + (s^\beta)^2 + (v^\beta)^2)}} ds^\beta \quad (22b)$$

3.4 Targeted CT reconstruction for planar object[17]

Targeted reconstruction is adopted in CT inspection practice to achieve high-resolution reconstruction to a small region-of-interest(ROI). This is particularly useful when scanning a large IC chip on which only a small region is interesting to us. Instead of reconstructing the whole IC chip in the field of-view, only the ROI is reconstructed. In conventional targeted reconstruction, the common practice is to do a normal reconstruction first, from which the ROI is identified and re-reconstructed.

Now we discuss how to extend the developed algorithm to targeted reconstruction of planar ROI on a planar object. But unlike conventional targeted reconstruction, the present method only needs one reconstruction process. Besides, it still possesses all advantages of the planar CT reconstruction technology such as the well-orientated reconstruction, flexible reconstruction resolution definition and easy visualization.

3.4.1 Simulation of scanning a planar object with a small planar ROI

To describe the concept of the proposed targeted reconstruction, as before, we first conduct a simulation to examine the projection property of the different parts of the components. As shown in Figure 32, a planar ROI (cross-sectional size: $w_{roi} \times t_{roi}$) is on top of a planar substrate with distances Δx and Δy to the centre-of-rotation respectively in x and y. By scanning this structure with a parallel-beam arrangement, we obtain a sinogram shown in Figure 33. Because only the shadow boundary information of the two parts is useful to us in determining the required parameters that are discussed later, the gradual variation in attenuation during the rotation is not considered in the simulation. Instead, we simply assume that the substrate and the ROI generate two different but constant shadow gray-levels during the scan.

Figure 34 shows the boundary curves of the two parts extracted from the sinogram in Figure 33, in which the dotted lines represent the projections of the substrate and the solid lines represent the ROI. As with the original method, the scan start angle can be determined by identifying the projection index that gives the narrowest shadow of the substrate on the detector (points A and B). Then the projected thickness (t_{roi}) of the ROI and its centre can be determined by identifying the two edge points of the ROI at this position.

Then we consider the determination of the other two parameters, i.e., w_{roi} and Δx in Figure 32, which are measured as the width and centre of the ROI shadow at a position 270 degree away for the narrowest position identified, as illustrated in Figure 34.

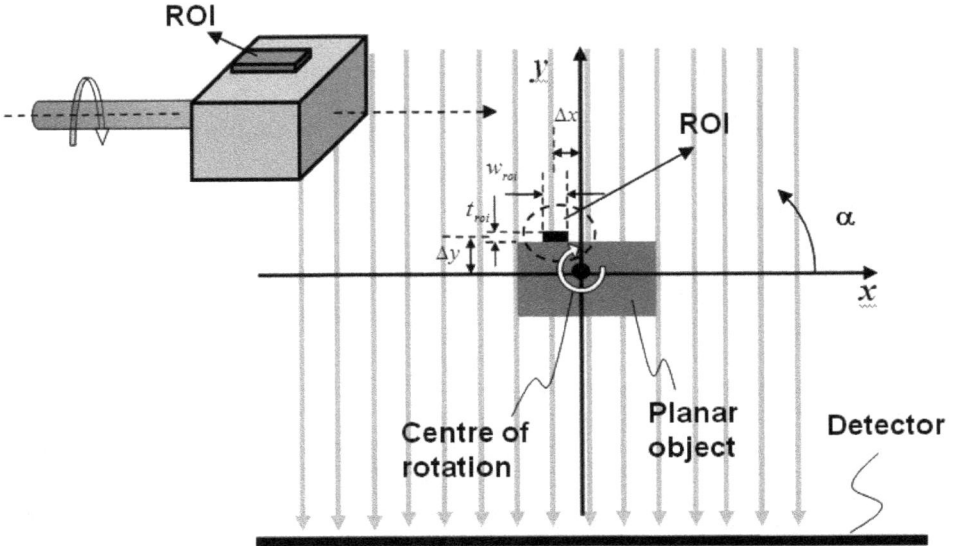

Fig. 32. Simulation of scanning a planar object with a small ROI

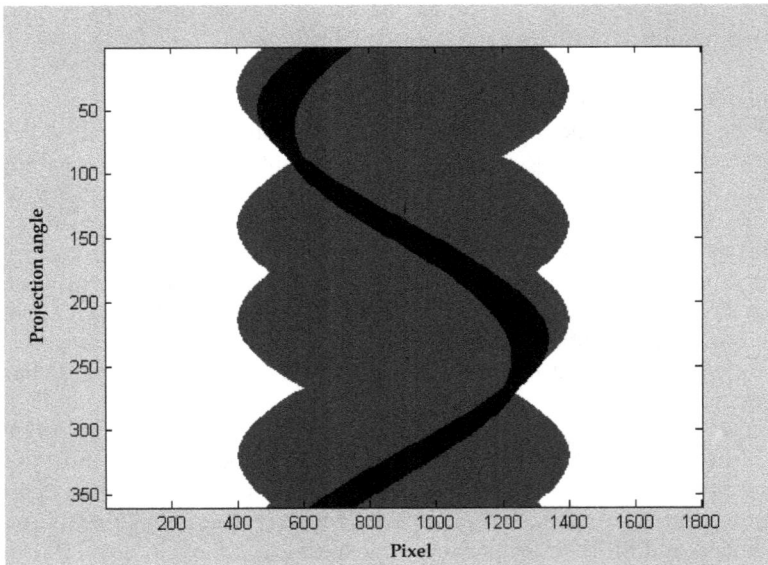

Fig. 33. Sinogram of simulated scanning with the arrangement shown in Figure 32.

The definition of the reconstruction with the obtained parameters of the ROI is exactly the same as the original reconstruction algorithm for planar object.

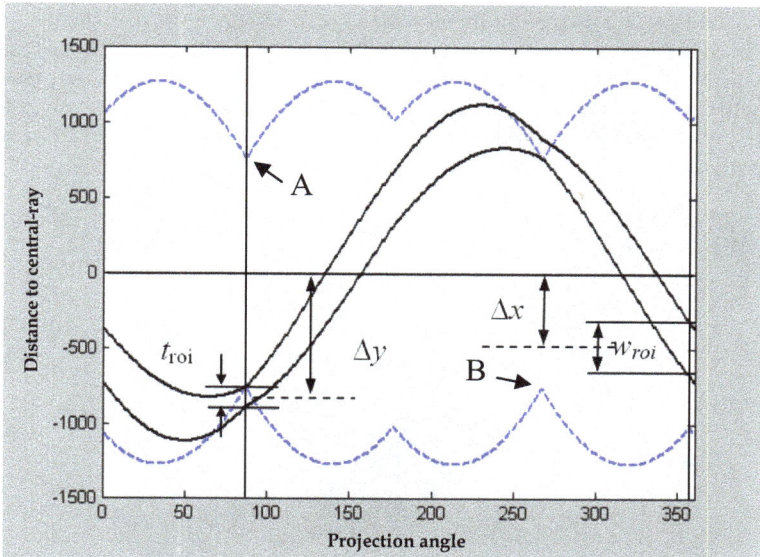

Fig. 34. The edge profiles of the two parts of the components

3.4.2 Implementation of the targeted reconstruction

A semiconductor packaging component used for demonstration is shown in Figure 35. It consists of three parts: the AIN substrate (l_a=3048µm, w_a=2032µm, t_a=1524µm), the aluminum solder interface layer (l_s=889µm, w_s=356µm, t_s=25µm) and the AuSn device layer (l_d=1400µm, w_d=400µm, t_s=100µm). In this CT inspection, we are particularly interested to the soldering quality of the solder layer, which has a direct impact on the interconnection function of the device. Obviously, the ideal CT result should be the individual aluminum solder layer with sufficient resolution and with good orientation for easy visualization.

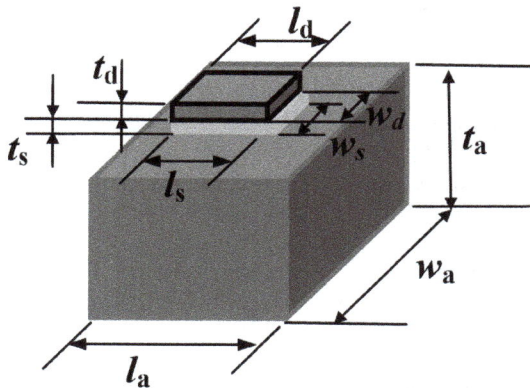

Fig. 35. The component to be inspected with X-ray CT

Figure 36 is one of the 2D projection images of the scan which clearly shows the geometrical relation among the three parts of the component. From which one actually can see that the device and the solder layer are very small compared to the substrate. The present scan is conducted with a tube voltage of 60KV and a tube current of 22μA. The source-to-detector distance (SID) and the source-to-object distance (SOD) are respectively 693mm and 22mm. Under this arrangement, the system's inspection resolution is about 4μm

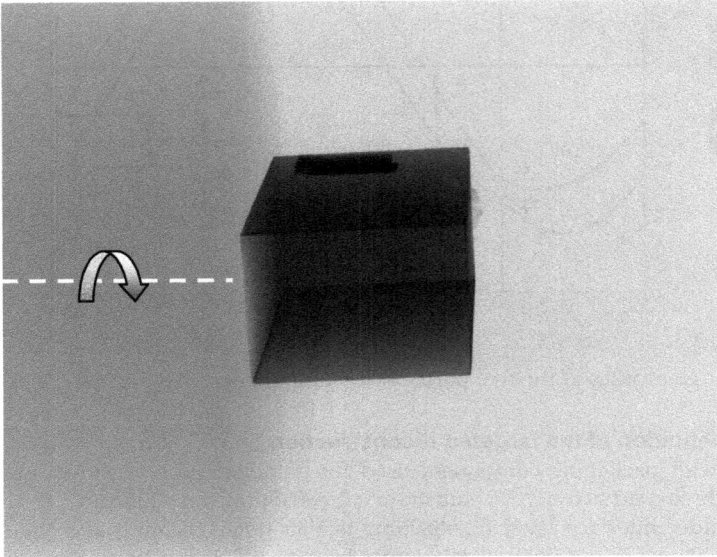

Fig. 36. A projection image of the component

Figure 37 shows a 3D CT image of the object reconstructed with traditional CT (Reconstruction studio V1.2, Comet GmBH 2006). Its volume is 512×512×512. The pixel size in each slice is $dx \times dy = 9.7\,\mu m \times 9.7\,\mu m$. One can immediately see that with this reconstruction the aluminum solder layer is less than 3 pixels on the image. This would make the subsequent de-layering process difficult. Also, on the CT image the device and the solder layer only occupy a small area. This means that the details of the features on the solder layer may not be properly reconstructed. Besides, due to the possibility of a tilted mounting of the sample with respect to the rotation axis, and a non-default start angle of the scan, the component will be reconstructed with a tilted orientation. This will make the subsequent layer-separation very time-consuming and tedious in the visualization process[18-19].

Figure 38 shows how to define the ROI and its offsets to the center-of-rotation (COR) with the real scan. First, with the central-slice singoram, the scan-start-angle is determined as 3.05°. Then, the thickness of the ROI, t_{roi}, and its offset Δy are determined directly at the position that corresponds to the narrowest shadow of the substrate (i.e., 87°). Then the width of the ROI, w_{roi}, and its offset to the COR in the x direction, Δx are determined at the position 270 degree away from above position (i.e., 357°).

Again, the axial-titlt-angle is determined with the projection that gives the the narrowest shadow, which is the 87th projection in this study. As shown in Figure 39, the edge points of the shadow are detected first, with which we can perform an line-fitting to identify the slope of the edge line, which is determined as -3.564°.

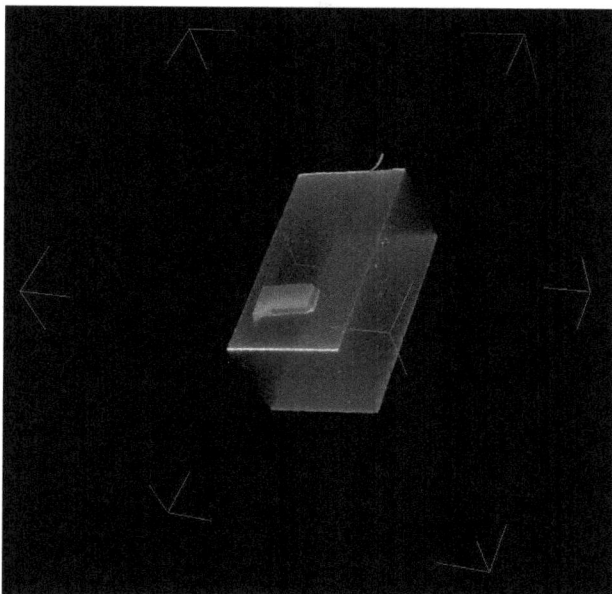

Fig. 37. The 3D CT image of the component reconstructed with traditional CT

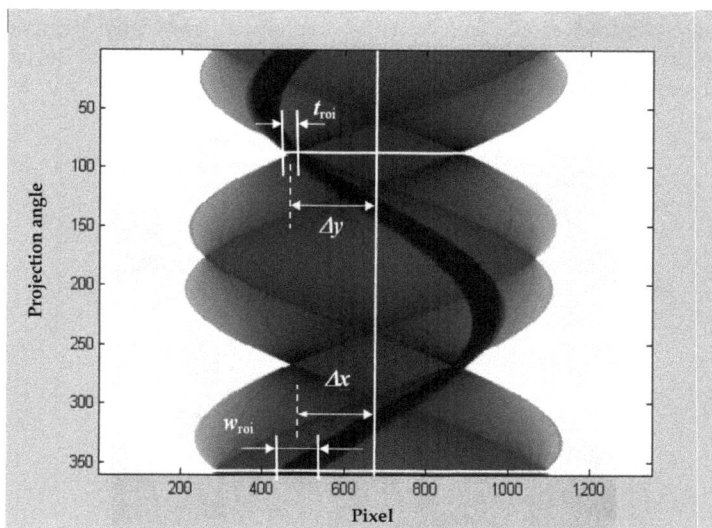

Fig. 38. Determination of the ROI dimensions and its offsets to the centre-of-rotation

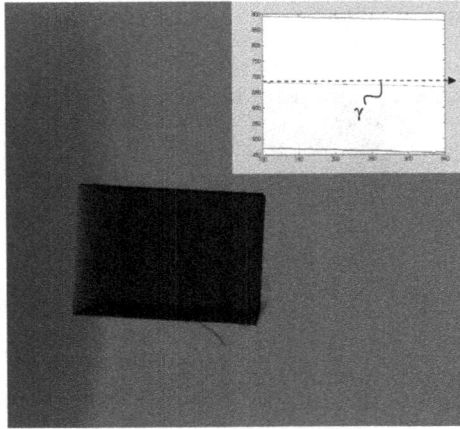

Fig. 39. Determination of the axial tilting angle

Figure 40 is the 3D CT image of the ROI (the solder layer and the device layer). Each slice is 512×100 and totally 380 slices are reconstructed with the differential CT reconstruction algorithm. The pixel size is defined as $dx \times dy = 1.2\mu m \times 3.4\mu m$. By comparison with Figure 37, one can find that although the present method has a much higher resolution in both the x and y directions. Its reconstruction volume size is still smaller than that with the traditional reconstruction.

The interface between the solder and the substrate and the interface between the solder and the device are shown in Figure 41. Because of the high reconstruction resolution in both the thickness and lateral directions, now it is available to see the voids on this solder layer. Most of these voids are through voids; however, they are smaller on the device side and become bigger on the substrate side. This can be explained from the perspective of the manufacturing process with which the solder paste is melted first On the device surface free of stress and then soldered on the substrate.

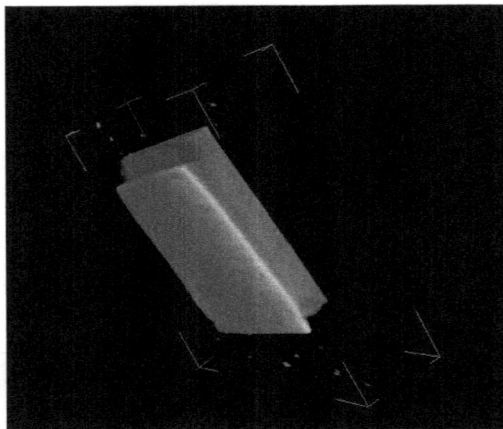

Fig. 40. 3D CT image of the ROI (solder layer plus the device layer)

Although in this targeted reconstruction the pixel size of dx =1.2µm is used, one must know that this is actually not meaningful. The reason is that with the system setting described above, the system's inspection resolution is only about 4µm. That means any reconstruction resolution more than 4um will not further improve the reconstruction resolution. In other words, we can make the present method more efficient by limiting dx =4µm and reducing the pixel number in the x direction to 154 ($\approx 512 \times (1.2 / 4)$).

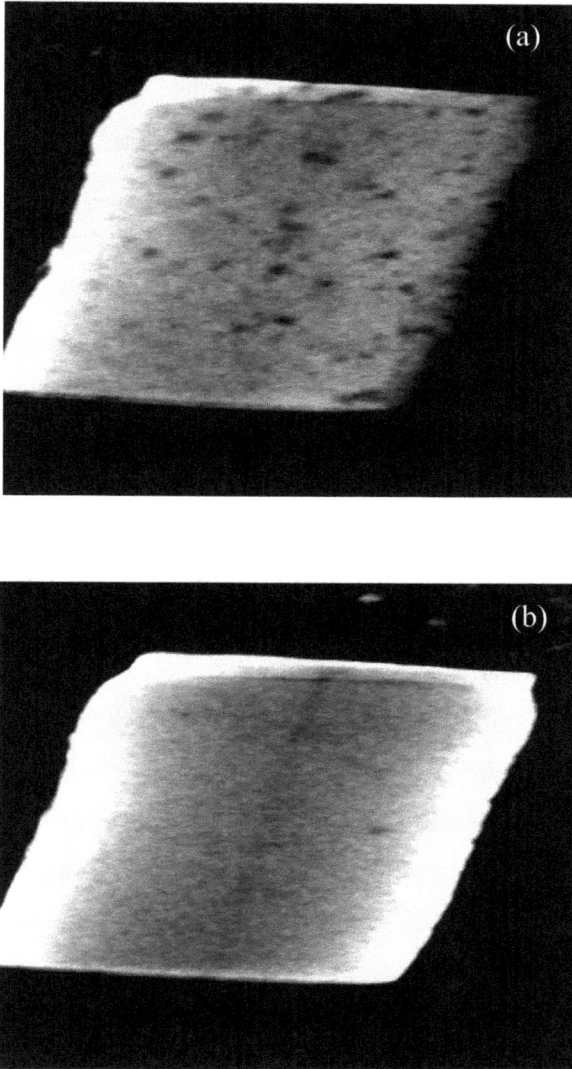

Fig. 41. The CT images of the solder layer surfaces: (a) on the substrate side; (b) on the device side.

3.5 CT inspection of a region-of-interest on a curved planar structure[20]

An interesting application of the targeted planar CT reconstruction algorithm is to conduct a orientation-preferred CT reconstruction for a tilted interesting part on an object. Figure 42 shows such an application: to inspect the impact damage that occurs at the curved region of a honeycomb composite sample. The objective of study is to evaluate the damage variation over the depth of the sample skin, therefore, it is preferred to reconstruct this particular region to be well-oriented with respect to the reconstruction volume. As a consequence the images of damage at different depths of skin can be obtained conveniently by displaying the reconstruction volume along one dimension of the volume.

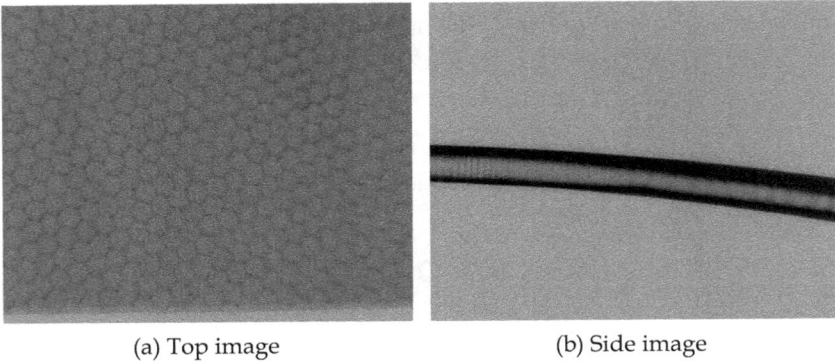

(a) Top image   (b) Side image

Fig. 42. Top view (a) and side view (B) of the object.

3.5.1 Methodology

Due to the curved-shape of the sample, when mounting the sample to the rotary system of the CT system, the ROI will form an angle β with the axis-of-rotation (Z) and the detector (represented as XZ plane) as shown in Figure 43. In this illustration, the shaded area is the region-of-interest, i.e. the location of the impact damage; and α is the scan-start-angle (when $\alpha = 0$, β becomes the axial-tilt-angle. To make these definitions clearer, we show them separately in Figure 44

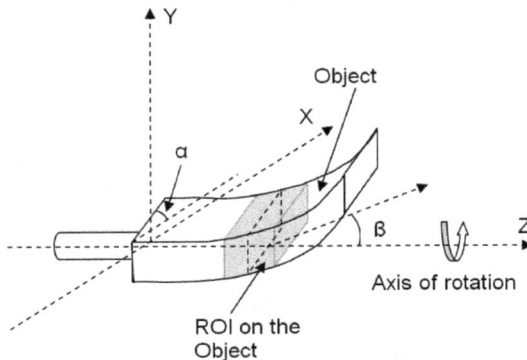

Fig. 43. Illustration of the scan start orientation of the object (shaded area is where the internal impact damage occurs)

Because α and β are generally not zero, with traditional CT reconstruction method, the ROI of the reconstructed object will be obliquely oriented with respect to the reconstruction volume, as illustrated in Figure 45(a). To obtain the impact damage pattern along the thickness dimension in this region, one has to use visualization software such as I-View or Volume Graphics. Both of them are powerful but expensive. However, even with these visualization software, in order to obtain the impact damage variation along the depth of the sample, one still needs a tedious and time-consuming process to carefully define a clipping plane which is parallel to the local plane of the ROI.

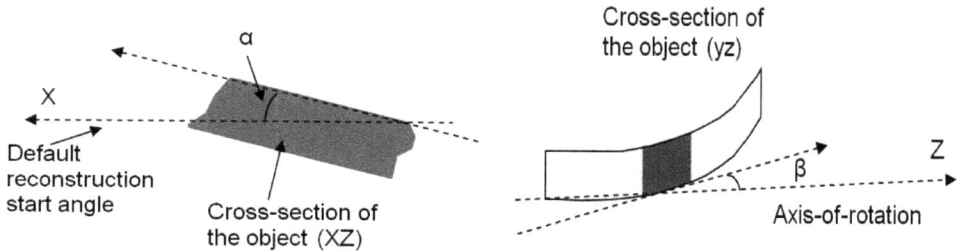

Fig. 44. Definition of angles α and β

If we can reconstruct the object with an orientation illustrated in Figure 45(b), that is, the local ROI is well-oriented with respect to the reconstruction volume, then we can directly see the impact damage pattern varying along the depth of the ROI by simply displaying the results slice-by-slice along the thickness (vertical) dimension of the reconstruction volume. This idea now becomes achievable with our developed planar CT reconstruction and the two following observations: Firstly the object is basically a planar object and secondly the local slope variation is relatively small and should not have meaningful inference to the inspection results and analysis if treated as a flat region.

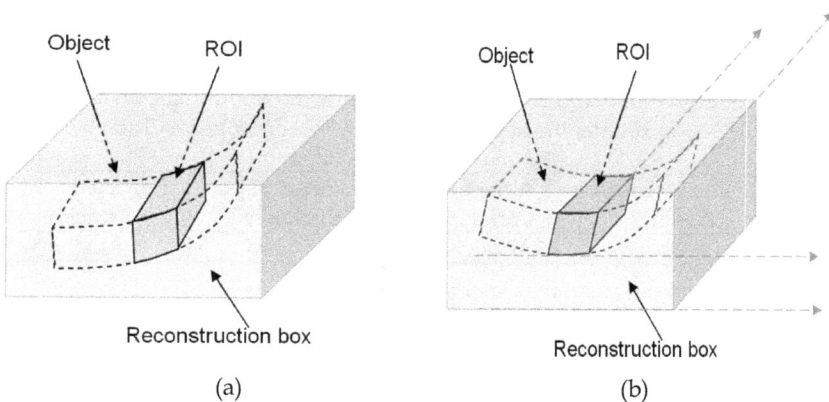

Fig. 45. Illustration of the reconstruction result of the scan: (a) with traditional method without considering object orientation; (b) the preferred orientation with planar CT reconstruction.

3.5.2 Determination of the parameters for the ROI region

The scan-start-angle is determined as usual, however, we need to explain in detail how to determine the axial-tilt-angle of the region-of-interest and other parameters so that the targeted region can be reconstructed as expected

The small image on the right side in figure 46 is the 2D projection that has the narrowest projected shadow of the sample. The left image to it is the interested region that is located at a curved part of the sample. In order to obtain a well-oriented reconstruction of this region, we should select this region for axial-tilt-angle determination. By detecting the edge points of the shadow, we can easily determine the axial-tilt angle, the projected thickness and its centre.

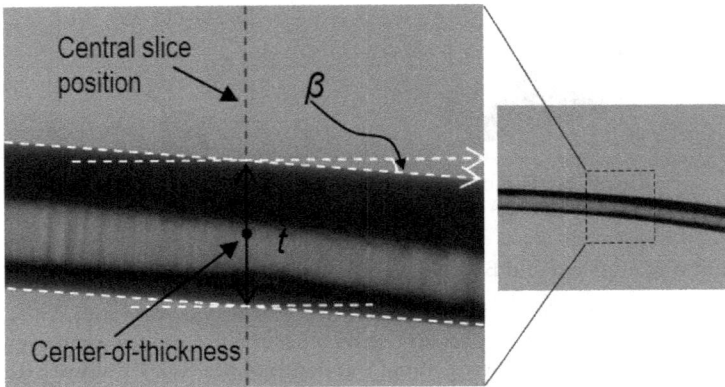

Fig. 46. Automatic determination of the axial tilting angle, the sample thickness under the set magnification, and centre position of the object thickness

Other processes will be similar to general CT reconstruction for planar objects

3.5.3 Results and discussion

This scan is conducted with a tube voltage of 110KV and a tube current of 12μA (according to the system specifications, the corresponding spot size is estimated to be 1 or 2 microns with this setting). The source-to-image distance (SID) and the source-to-object distance (SOD) are respectively 693mm and 286mm. A 360° scan was conducted with an angular step size of 1°. With the scanned data, the key parameters are summarized in Table 1.

Central ray	Scan-start-angle	Axial tilt angle	Projected object thickness	Projected centre-of-thickness
742.1 pixel	-1.96 degree	5.42 degree	193 pixel	823.5 pixel

Table 1. The determined orientation parameters of the ROI.

The reconstruction volume is (154 × 512) × 600, with the resolution in the thickness dimension being two times that in the lateral directions.

Figure 47 shows in one figure the three typical orthogonal views and the one 3D view as well. More details can be seen from one of the enlarged axial slice (Figure 48), in which the impact damage area is indicated in dotted box.

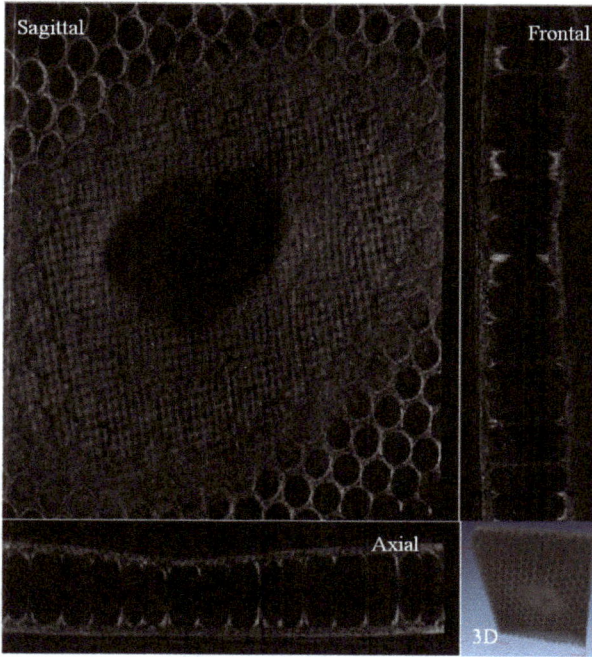

Fig. 47. 3D and the three orthogonal views

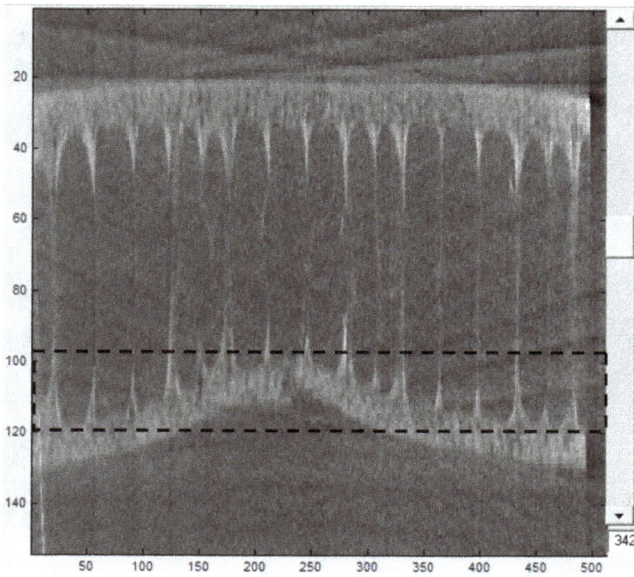

Fig. 48. An axial view with an the damaged region indicated

By analysing the frontal views slice by slice, one can observe the variation of the impact damage along the depth of the object. Limited by size of the paper, Figure 49 just shows 12 images with a 2-pixel step.

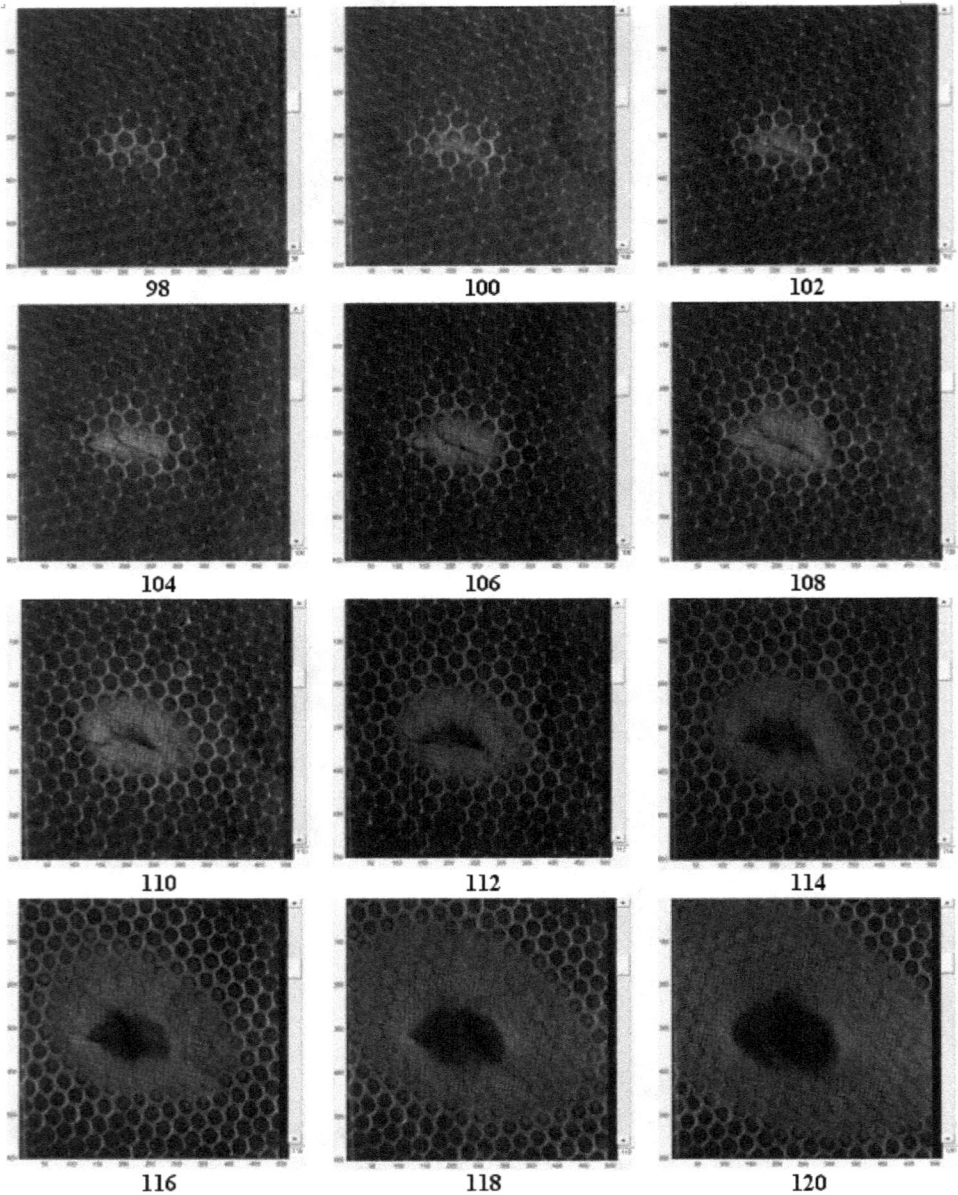

Fig. 49. Slices show the impact damage changing over the depth

4. References

[1] Sun, Y.; Hou, Y.; Zhao, F. & Hu, J. (2006).A calibration method for misaligned scanner geometry in cone-beam computed tomography. *NDT & E International* Vol. 39, pp.499–513

[2] Shepp, L. A.; Hilal, S. K. & Schulz, R. A. (1979). The tuning fork artifact in computerized tomography. *Computer Graphics Image Processiing*. Vol. 10, pp.246-255.

[3] Taylor, T.& . Lupton, L. R. (1986). Resolution, artifacts and the design of computed tomography system. In: computed Tomography Systems, Sect. VIII. New York: Elsevier, pp.603-609

[4] Azevedo, S. G.; Schneberk, D. J.; Fitch, J. P. & Martz, H. E. (1990). Calculation of the rotational centers in computed tomography sinograms. *IEEE Transaction on Nuclear Science*. Vol. 37(4) pp.1525-1540

[5] Olander, B. (1994). Center of rotation determination using projection data in X-ray micro computed tomography. *Report 77*. Linköping University, Sweden, *ISSN 1102-1799*

[6] Ramachandran, G. N. & Lakshminarayanna, A. V. (1971). Three-dimensional reconstruction from radiographs and electron micrographs: Application of convolutions instead of Fourier transforms. *Proceedings of the National Academy of Sciences of the USA*, 68, p.2236

[7] Hsieh, J. (2003). *Computed Tomography*, SPIE PRESS, ISBN 0-8194-4425-1, Bellingham, Washington

[8] Kak, A. C. & Malcolm, S. (1999). *Principle of Computerized Tomographic Imaging*, IEEE Press, ISBN 0-87942-198-3, New York

[9] Banhart, J. (2008). *Advanced Tomographic Methods in Materials Research and Engineering*. Oxford University Press, ISBN 978-0-19-921324-5, New York

[10] Feinfocus Fox 160.25 Operation Instruction. (2004), Version 1.0

[11] Liu, T. & Malcolm, A. A. (2006). Micro-CT for minute objects with central ray determined using the projection data of the objects. *9th European Conference on Non-Destructive Testing*. (2006), (September 2006), Berlin, Germany

[12] Liu, T. & Malcolm, A.A. (2006). Comparison between four methods for central ray determination with wire phantom in micro-CT system. *Optical Engineering*, Vol. 45(6), 066402 1-5

[13] Liu, T. (2009). Direct Central Ray Determination in Micro-CT. *Optical Engineering*, vol. 48(NA), pp. 46501-46501

[14] Liu, T. (2009). Differential Reconstruction for Planar Object in Computed Tomography. *Journal of X-ray Science and Technology*.Vol. 17(2), pp.101-114

[15] Liu, T.; Wong, B. S. & Chai, T. C. (2008). A CT Reconstruction with Good-Orientation and Layer Separation for Multilayer Objects. *17th WCNDT*, Shanghai, (October 2008)

[16] Liu, T (2011). Cone-beam reconstruction for planar objects. *NDT & E International*, under processing

[17] Liu, T.; Sim, L. M. & Xu, J. (2010). Targeted reconstruction with different planar computed tomography. *NDT & E International* Vol.43, pp.116-122

[18] User's Manual, VGStudio Max 2.1, (2011)

[19] Users Manual, i-View Workstation Version 1.0, (2003)

[20] Liu, T.; Malcolm, A. A. & Xu, J. (2010). High-resolution X-ray CT inspection of Honeycomb Composites Using Planar Computed Tomography Technology. *2nd*

International Symposium on DNT in Aerospace 2010 – We.4.B.4, (November 2010), Hamburg, Germany

[21] Kang, K.; Choi, M.; Kim, K.; Cha, Y.; Kang, Y.; Hong, D. & Yang, S. (2006). Inspection of impact damage in honeycomb composite plate by ESPI, Ultrasonic testing, and Thermography. *12th A-PCNDT– Asia-Pacific Conference on NDT*, Auckland, New Zealand

[22] Abou-Khousa, M.A.; Ryley,A.; Kharkovsky, S.; Zoughi, R.; Daniels, D.; Kreitinger, N. & Steffes, G. (2007). Comparison of x-ray, millimeter wave, shearography and through-transmission ultrasonic methods for inspection of honeycomb composites. *American Institute of Physics*

12

Cross-Sectional Imaging in Comparative Vertebrate Morphology - The Intracranial Joint of the Coelacanth *Latimeria chalumnae*

Peter Johnston
University of Auckland
New Zealand

1. Introduction

Vertebrate morphology, including developmental anatomy, has depended on dissection since anatomical study first began, and on microscopy since the 19th century, in particular since the invention of the microtome. These methods have limitations: dissection destroys tissues, and disturbs or destroys three-dimensional relationships. Microscopy is less destructive, in that sections can be preserved for periods of time, but cutting serial sections, as often used in developmental anatomy, is time-consuming, sections are easily lost in processing, and distortion can be a problem. Three-dimensional (3D) reconstruction for interpretation and demonstration of results was done with manual drawing techniques or physical reconstruction with sequential wax plates, but now can be done with image reconstruction software. Microscopy findings still need to be photographed, aligned and segmented — the tissues of interest identified and marked out on 2D slices — before a result can be obtained, all of which is still relatively labour-intensive.

Functional morphology became accessible with the invention of the motion-picture camera, and cinefluoroscopy with implanted radiological markers has provided many explanations. These traditional techniques have been supplemented in recent years by cross-sectional imaging and advanced techniques that depend on this imaging. CT (computed tomography) and MRI (magnetic resonance imaging) are best known as medical imaging technologies, but have a range of applications in morphology. Newer and more accurate techniques of imaging, real-time imaging for functional study and methods of image reconstruction are revolutionizing vertebrate morphology, bringing 3D information in a non-destructive manner. Rare museum specimens are often not made available for dissection, and these may be important taxa for biological and phylogenetic reasons; imaging techniques have an important application here.

This chapter will review a number of new imaging techniques used in comparative morphology, with examples of recent applications, and will present original research demonstrating a number of these techniques to investigate a morphological mystery, the intracranial joint of the coelacanth *Latimeria chalumnae*.

2. Imaging techniques in comparative morphology

2.1 MicroCT

MicroCT systems are now available at a size and cost suitable for laboratory equipment, with resolution to several microns. This is much more accessible than use of CT scanners at medical facilities, which are typically committed for medical use during office hours. The ability to produce 3D images of small structures replaces laborious and less accurate histological methods. Rieppel et al. (2009) used microCT to examine the skull of the anomalepidid (blindsnake) *Liotyphlops albirostris*, and were able to resolve a number of issues in the anatomy of the very small skulls of this snake. Preparation of skulls by the usual methods including digestion by enzymes and cleaning by insects may not give satisfactory results in small vertebrates, as the details are difficult to record, and the individual skull bones tend to disarticulate, making it impossible to study the relationships of the bones to the function of the whole skull. Rieppel et al (2009) have been able to make important functional deductions about adaptation to burrowing, and to compare these with another group of blindsnakes, typhlopids, which adapted the skull to a burrowing lifestyle with different morphological details but a similar result.

2.2 CT examination of fossils

Radiological examination is valuable for investigating internal cavities and structures in fossilized bones, and for preserving 3D relations and detail for both bones and soft tissues. Some fossils cannot be fully prepared from their rock matrix for fear of damage, and radiological examination can be the only way that details can be examined. Sutton (2008) gives an overview of methods available. CT examination depends mainly on differences in absorption of radiation by the fossil material and the enclosing matrix, although techniques using phase-contrast, which enhances detection of boundaries, are also showing promise.

Gardner et al. (2010) studied skull of the important Permian reptile *Youngina* with high-resolution CT scanning, enabling details of the braincase to emerge for the first time. This taxon is of great importance in the modern reptile evolutionary tree, being close to the stem leading to turtles, and the diapsid groups Archosauria (crocodiles, birds) and Lepidosauria (lizards, snakes, tuatara). The relationships among these modern groups remains uncertain: turtles were traditionally thought to retain their closed-in skull as a primitive feature, but recent evidence points to turtles as diapsid reptiles or even modified lepidosaurs. A number of hypotheses are current. Comparison of *Youngina* with these modern groups may help to give clearer answers.

2.3 MicroMRI

MicroMRI offers better soft tissue definition than microCT, and the output is based on the water content of the different tissues. Ruffins et al. (2007) set out the basis for an atlas of quail embryology with microMRI, achieving good images with resolution to 30 microns. These authors emphasize the ease of preparation of the sample tissue, absence of distortion from processing and ability to re-image the same embryo at a later stage as key advantages of this method. Real-time imaging of cardiac function in animals as small as mice has been achieved (Ross et al., 2002) and this offers considerable scope for investigation of reptiles with different cardiac morphologies. Disadvantages of microMRI are cost and access to suitable MR scanning facilities.

2.4 Synchrotron CT

Synchrotron CT imaging is a particularly exciting development, and a review of some of the applications of this technique is given by Westneat et al. (2008). Synchrotron radiation is produced from high-speed electrons constrained in a circular path, and the resulting X-ray beam is of high energy and narrow band-width ("monochromatic"). The latter feature enables the beam to be focussed, like a beam of light by an optical lens, and phase-contrast techniques are applied to enhance interfaces and edges. Resolution to 30nm has been achieved (see references in Westneat et al., 2008). The high photon flux used in this technique allows much faster acquisition times than with conventional radiation sources, and this enables real-time imaging of functions such as respiration and feeding in small invertebrates, which have previously not been amenable to observation. Imaging of soft tissues in 3D is also possible in fossils. Kleinteich et al. (2008) used synchrotron CT to define muscle fibre directions and thus the mechanical implications of muscle placement in caecilian amphibians. Much new data will emerge from this technology, but at present synchrotrons suitable for this purpose are only found in a few sites in the world, and access is thus limited.

2.5 Tissue contrast in preserved specimens

Another promising development for comparative morphology is the use of chemical agents for soft tissue contrast in preserved material. Metscher (2009) reviewed data on contrast agents for CT, and gave a variety of examples from original research. Iodine and phosphotungstic acid preparations can give good results, with much better soft tissue definition than microCT without these agents. Jeffery et al. (2011) investigated different protocols for iodine absorption contrast and showed muscle fibre definition in high-resolution microCT. Schmidt et al. (2010) used phosphotungstic acid contrast to demonstrate 3D muscle location in normal and genetically modified anuran larvae.

2.6 3D prototyping

The manufacture of physical models from 3D data derived from cross-sectional imaging is an example of 3D prototyping or 3D printing. Most of the systems available progressively build up a model in slices from image data, using thermoplastic materials. In morphology this method is particularly useful where possible movements between skeletal elements need to be defined. No doubt it will soon be possible to do this on computers with specific software, but for the present, this is a useful way to investigate the range of movement possible movement at joints. For example, Kleinteich et al. (2008) made a physical model of the jaw articulation in caecilian to help understand the movement of the jaw suspension (quadrate bone) on the skull and the musculature associated with this. The result of this was that the mandibular element of the joint enclosed the quadrate element to resist dislocation; this in turn permits a degree of mobility of the quadrate on the braincase. 3D prototyping has until now been an expensive technology, but desk-top systems are now available and the technique is likely to be applied more widely.

2.7 Movement analysis

3D data sets derived from cross-sectional imaging can be used in combination with animation software, which allows joints to be defined and their ranges of motions specified. Kargo and Rome (2002) used this method to define activity of hindlimb muscles involved in frog jumping, using the software SIMM (Musculographics Inc.), which allows muscle vectors to be applied to the skeleton and the results displayed. Gatesy et al. (2010) have used what they call "scientific rotoscoping" to build animations of skeletal motion modelled on movie sequences of real animals. In their study, skeletal data sets are acquired with CT or optical tomography, reconstructed into a 3D model, and animated with the 3D modelling software Maya (Autodesk) to correspond with live motion data. In a simpler system, Johnston (2010) used 3D coordinates of muscle origins and insertions to define vectors of muscle force acting on the basipterygoid joint in the tuatara *Sphenodon*. These studies are examples of new functional approaches that may yield important functional information on the skeleton, and may become useful in a phylogenetic context.

2.8 Methods of reconstruction
A number of softwares are available commercially and as freeware for reconstructing 3D surfaces and volumes from series of 2D slices. Images of the whole object scanned can be produced by volume rendering, but 3D reconstructions of individual structures or organs within the subject require identification ("segmentation") of these structures. This can be done in some cases with threshold methods, where a particular colour or grey-scale value can be selected and added to the slices, but often segmentation must be done manually, by drawing onto the 2D images. When this is complete, the software creates surfaces corresponding to the margins of the defined areas by adding a triangular mesh. Manual segmentation can be slow work and requires knowledge of what structures are to be expected in the subject. A useful guide to basic functions of three popular programs Amira (Visage Imaging), Osirix (Antione Rosset and Osman Ratib) and Voxx (Indiana University School of Medicine) is given by Corfield et al. (2008). Volumes can be calculated with these methods, and the surfaces generated can be used as a basis of 3D prototyping.

2.9 Image libraries
Libraries of cross-sectional images are maintained for access by researchers. The two largest such collections are Digimorph — the University of Texas Digital Morphology Group, http://digimorph.org, and the Digital Fish Library — University of California, San Diego, http://digitalfishlibrary.org. Digimorph offers a wide range of taxa in CT scan data, generally in sections in axial, horizontal and sagittal planes, cutaway movie sequences in the same planes, and roll movies of the whole subject. The Digital Fish Library comprises many fish from all groups in 3 planes of MRI. Both have full data on each specimen scanned. Images can be downloaded from the websites or provided on request for specific projects, both as movie animations and as the original voxel data. The voxel data is ideal for reconstruction work, but involves large files. The movie sequences are valuable for quick reference, and if needed for reconstruction can be turned into a series of aligned 2D images with software such as ImageJ (National Institutes of Health). With practice, the researcher can build up mental reconstructions by scrolling back and forth through 2D sequences. As 3D imaging progressively becomes a more important part of comparative morphology, these are essential resources for the vertebrate researcher. Smaller archives with specialist themes include those of Witmer (n.d.), Motani (n.d.), and the Computerized Scanning and Imaging Facility of Woods Hole Oceanographic Institute (n.d.). Access to and archiving of this increasing body of data is discussed by Ziegler et al. (2010) and Rowe and Frank (2011), who argue for a model such as the GenBank system for archiving of genetic sequence data.

3. The intracranial joint of *Latimeria chalumnae*

3.1 The living coelacanth, a relic of a flourishing lineage

Coelacanths were once a widespread group of sarcopterygian ("fleshy-finned") fishes, which were thought to have become extinct about 80 million years ago, until the finding in 1938 of an unusual fish in a trawler's catch in East London, South Africa, by Marjorie Courtenay-Latimer, a local museum curator. This was examined by the South African ichthyologist J. L. B. Smith and recognized as a coelacanth on the basis of its characteristic external shape, which has been conserved in coelacanths over 350 million years. The catch was said to have been trawled off the mouth of the Chalumna river, hence the name *Latimeria chalumnae*. Coelacanth means "hollow spines", referring to the hollow fin rays supporting the tail. In addition to their fleshy fins, which resemble short legs with terminal fins (as opposed to ray fins of teleost lineages), coelacanths present a number of other anatomical features: a double lower jaw articulation, the caudal of which is formed by hyoid arch elements articulating with the mandible; absence of vertebrae, with the notochord forming the axial structural element; ventral position of the kidney in *Latimeria*, a situation unknown in other vertebrates; a rostral sensory organ, presumed to be electroreceptive; a transverse joint across the middle of the skull, and a longitudinal muscle along the base of the skull, the basicranial muscle, in a position to ventrally flex the skull at this joint. The most important study of the anatomy of *Latimeria* has been the large general survey of Millot and Anthony and colleagues (Millot and Anthony, 1958; 1965; Millot et al., 1978) and colleagues. A variety of papers on specific anatomy have also been published, and are listed by Bruton et al. (1991). A comprehensive account of coelacanth osteology, together with general aspects of *Latimeria* biology, was given by Forey (1998).

Since the original discovery of *Latimeria chalumnae*, over 300 specimens have been taken from fishermen along the east coast of southern Africa, mostly in the Comores islands, which lie between Madagascar and Mozambique. *Latimeria* lives at depths not generally amenable to SCUBA diving, and observations in the wild have been few, and mainly conducted by submersible craft. Recently, detailed close-up photographs of *Latimeria* in natural habitat have been obtained at about 100 metres at Sodana Bay, South Africa (Butler and Ballesta, 2011). In 1997, living coelacanths were discovered in North Sulawesi, Indonesia, again being recognised by chance in a fisherman's catch by a biologist. Genetic testing suggests this is a different species, and it is now named *Latimeria menadoensis*.

3.2 The problem: The intracranial joint

The intracranial joint and its associated basicranial muscle are known in another group of sarcopterygian fossil fish, the rhipidistians, which are closer to the stem on the evolutionary tree that leads to tetrapods. A simplified tree after Yu et al. (2010) showing the relationships of gnathostomes (vertebrates with jaws) is given in Fig. 1. The function of the intracranial joint had never been convincingly explained despite its being a major feature of the sarcopterygian skull, and it was hoped that analysis of the *Latimeria* joint would lead to an understanding of its place in the predecessors of tetrapods (Forey, 1998). However, there has been debate about whether the joint is the same structure in coelacanths and rhipidistians; current opinion favours homology of this structure in these groups (Janvier, 1996). A variety of interpretations of the *Latimeria* intracranial joint have been advanced. The inability to sustain captive *Latimeria* has meant that direct observation has been very limited, and confined to manipulation of a few recently dead specimens. A number of notable

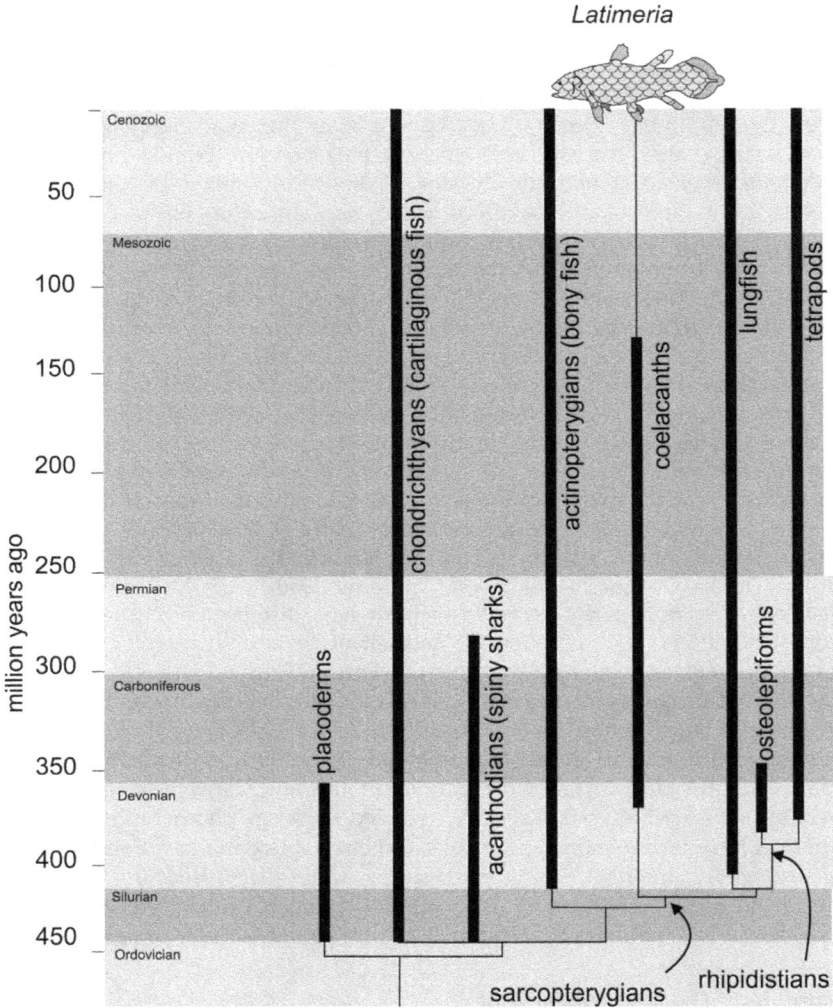

Fig. 1. Cladogram showing relationship of coelacanths to other gnathostomes.

ichthyologists and palaeontologists (and one distinguished ornithologist) have published on this structure. A summary of these studies is given below. The other important feature to be discussed in the sarcopterygian skull is the notochord. This was the primitive longitudinal support of the body before the evolution of the vertebral column, which is a series of ossifications around the notochord. The notochord is a prominent feature in developing vertebrates, and regresses to various extents in most taxa. The intracranial portion of the notochord regresses completely in all extant taxa except *Latimeria*. Fossil sarcopterygians also retained the intracranial notochord. In the embryo, the notochord has an important organizing function in development (Stemple, 2005). In the adult, where it is retained, it has a structural role as a hydraulic rod, having a viscous fluid-filled centre and a tough fibrous

Cross-Sectional Imaging in Comparative Vertebrate Morphology - The Intracranial Joint
of the Coelacanth Latimeria chalumnae

243

covering. The intracranial joint is situated between the ethmosphenoid and oto-occipital sections of the braincase; there is a dorsal articulation in the skull roof bones, and a ventral articulation at the base of the skull, immediately dorsal to the notochord. The location of the joint is shown in its location in the skull in Figs. 2a and 2b, and its components are labelled in Fig. 2c.

3.2.1 *Latimeria* cranial anatomy: Publications up to 1980

The work of Jacques Millot and Jacques Anthony (1958, 1965, 1978) and colleagues remain standard accounts of the morphology, based on dissection of a number of specimens. These authors considered that very little movement was possible at the joint in their first book, but by the time of the 1978 volume had been influenced by the mechanical theories of Keith Thomson (Thompson, 1966) and others. Thomson (1966; 1967) studied the intracranial joint in both rhipidistians and coelacanths. He reported that dorsal flexion at the joint in *Latimeria* to 20–30° is possible (Fig. 2d), around the fulcrum of the dorsal part of the joint in the skull roof, and related this to movements of the hyoid cartilages, jaw opening, and widening of the gape by dorsal flexion of the snout. These inferences were generalized to rhipidistians.

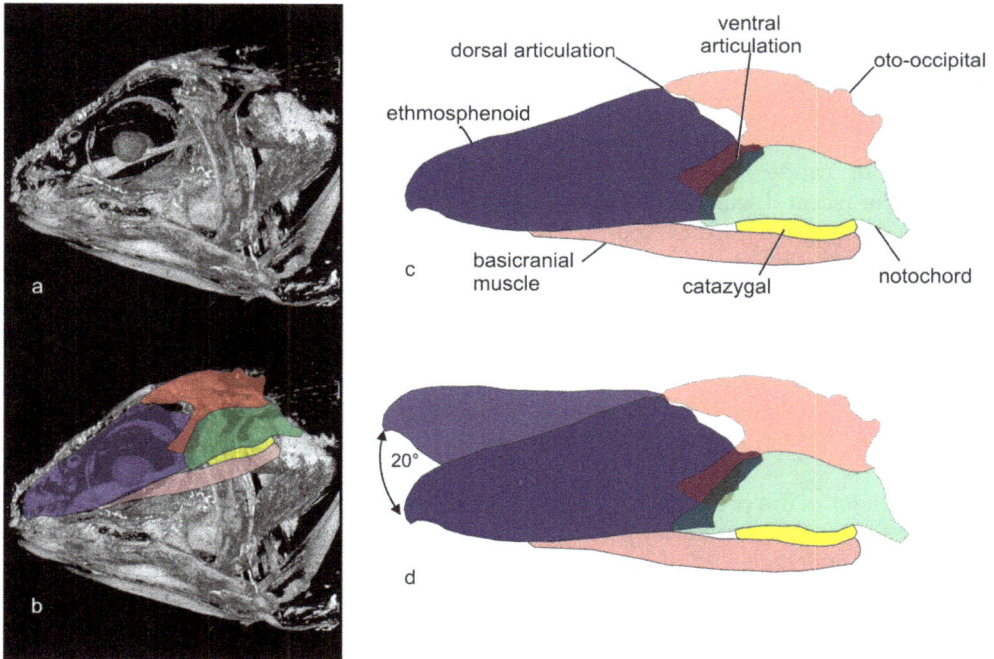

Fig. 2. a, b: *Latimeria* skull with braincase superimposed. c: median sagittal section of braincase with intracranial articulations and notochord. d: dorsal flexion of rostral braincase, as in previous hypotheses.

R. McNeil Alexander (1973) presented a rather similar analysis in *Latimeria*, having examined an unfixed specimen, and concluded that dorsal flexion to perhaps 15° is possible.

Other interpretations also included dorsal flexion at the dorsal articulation, to widen the gape (Adamicka and Ahnelt, 1976; Cracraft, 1968)

3.2.3 *Latimeria* cranial anatomy: After 1980

George Lauder (1980) also accepted dorsal flexion, and proposed a more detailed model involving initiation of jaw opening by dorsal flexion of the occiput on the body by the epaxial muscles and retraction of the hyoid apparatus by the sternohyoideus muscle, causing rostral displacement of the main jaw articulation, such that the axis of dorsal force on the palatoquadrate lay rostral to the intracranial joint, with consequent dorsal flexion. This dorsal flexion is an integral part of the jaw-opening mechanism in Lauder's plan. Erik Jarvik (1980) summarized many years' experience with rhipidistians and considered that little translatory or angular movement was possible in any coelacanth or rhipidistian. Edward Hitchcock (1995) accepted dorsal flexion in both coelacanths and rhipidistians.

Philippe Janvier's (1996) book offers a detailed survey of early vertebrates and discusses the existence or possibility of an intracranial joint in all lineages. He considered the *Latimeria* skull to permit very limited movement on morphological grounds. Peter Bernstein (2002) examined the morphology of the intracranial joint in a serially sectioned juvenile *Latimeria* head. His principal finding was that in the ventral part of the joint, the ethmosphenoid component articulates closely as longitudinal rails within grooves in the oto-occipital part of the joint. He concluded that this arrangement allows longitudinal, plunger-type mobility but not dorso-ventral flexion.

Kanyukin (2009) advanced a more complex proposal for movement of the hyoid apparatus than that of Lauder (1980), again requiring dorsal flexion of the ethmosphenoid. The inference of recent discussions (Bernstein, 2002; Forey, 1998; Janvier, 1996) is similar to that of Jarvik (1980): even if *Latimeria* does have dorsal flexion of the joint, this is not relevant to rhipidistians or even to other coelacanths, in which the morphology would not permit this. *Latimeria* is a derived (end of an evolutionary branch) rather than plesiomorphic (showing generalized features) coelacanth.

The basicranial muscle has given rise to interesting discussion about its innervation and homologies; the conclusion of Bemis and Northcutt (1991) that the muscle is supplied by the sixth cranial nerve is the most robust, and the homology of this muscle with the m. retractor bulbi of tetrapods has thus been considered.

3.3 Statement of the problem

The function of the intracranial joint in *Latimeria* remains unclear, and it is also uncertain whether an understanding of the coelacanth joint can be generalized to rhipidistians. A major feature of the skull in the forerunners of tetrapods is still a mystery.

4. Original research

4.1 Aims

The aims of the current study are to reconstruct the ethmosphenoid and oto-occipital sections of the braincase from CT and MRI scan images, build physical models with 3D prototyping to establish what mobility is possible at the intracranial joint, and discuss this mobility in the context of sarcopterygian evolution.

4.2 Methods

Most of the braincase in *Latimeria* is cartilaginous, and not visible on the CT scans available, thus MRI scans are needed in addition. The dermal skull roof bones are, however, well shown with CT, as is the palatal bone assembly, which is not reconstructed here. These bony structures are not well seen on MRI, and a variable degree of signal loss is present in and around the bones; the combination of CT and MRI is thus necessary. The identification of individual structures is still a complex process, and requires correlation with published anatomical resources on *Latimeria*.

4.2.1 Image sources

CT scan images were provided by the University of Texas Digital Morphology Group, from the Digimorph archive; specimen: American Museum of Natural History AMNH 32949, an embryo. MRI scan images were provided by the Digital Fish Library, University of California, San Diego; specimen: Marine Vertebrate Collection, Scripps Oceanological Institute, SIO 75-347, a 950mm long adult. Cross-sectional images drawn from macroscopic slices by Millot and Anthony (1958) and from microscopic sections by Bernstein (2002) were used to help identify structures in the scans.

4.2.2 Segmentation and reconstruction

DICOM image series were viewed with ImageJ (NIH). QuickTime (Apple Inc.) movie animations were converted to serial images with ImageJ. Segmentation and reconstruction were done with Amira 5.2.1 (Visage Imaging), tracing structures onto the MR images with frequent reference to CT data. Although Amira has a facility for registering two sets of data, this was not possibly here as the scans were of different specimens. The ethmosphenoid and oto-occipital blocks were outlined, and also the cranial part of the notochord. The anazygal, which bridges between the oto-occipital blocks dorsal to the notochord, has been included with the oto-occipital for the purposes of 3D prototyping. Other cranial structures including the hyoid arch elements and palatoquadrate were also segmented but not included in the present analysis. Fig. 3 shows equivalent CT and MRI slices, and the segmentation window in Amira 5.2.1.

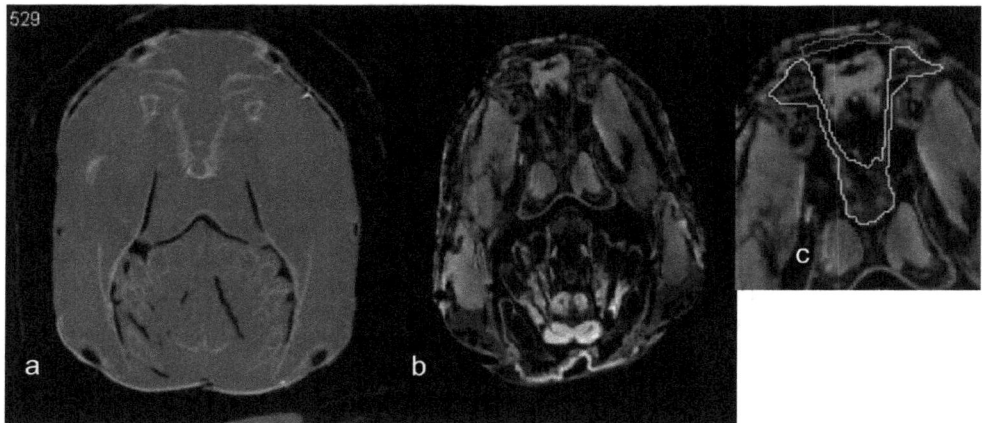

Fig. 3. a: CT axial (coronal) slice; b: equivalent MRI slice; c: segmentation window in Amira 5.2.1, ethmosphenoid in blue, oto-occipital in red.

4.2.3 3D prototyping

The ethmosphenoid and oto-occipital blocks were generated as surfaces in Amira, and saved as .stl files for 3D prototyping, which was done with a fused deposition modelling (FDM) system, using ABS (acrylonitrile butadiene styrene) plastic.

4.3 Results

The reconstructed ethmosphenoid and oto-occipital blocks are shown in Fig. 4a. The dorsal part of the intracranial joint is a simple butt joint, as described by all previous authors. The ventral joint has the rails-within-grooves morphology described by Bernstein (2002), with an angle of 40° to the horizontal. The ethmosphenoid "rails" are the condyles of Millot and Anthony (1958) (Fig. 4c), and diverge laterally within the oto-occipital components to form a locking mechanism resisting longitudinal displacement (Fig. 3e). When the two sections are articulated, they lock neatly together, and only a 5° angulation ventrally is possible from the "neutral" position in which both specimens were scanned (Fig. 4b). This small rotation takes place around an axis between the dorsal and ventral intracranial joints. No dorsal flexion of the ethmosphenoid component is possible at all.

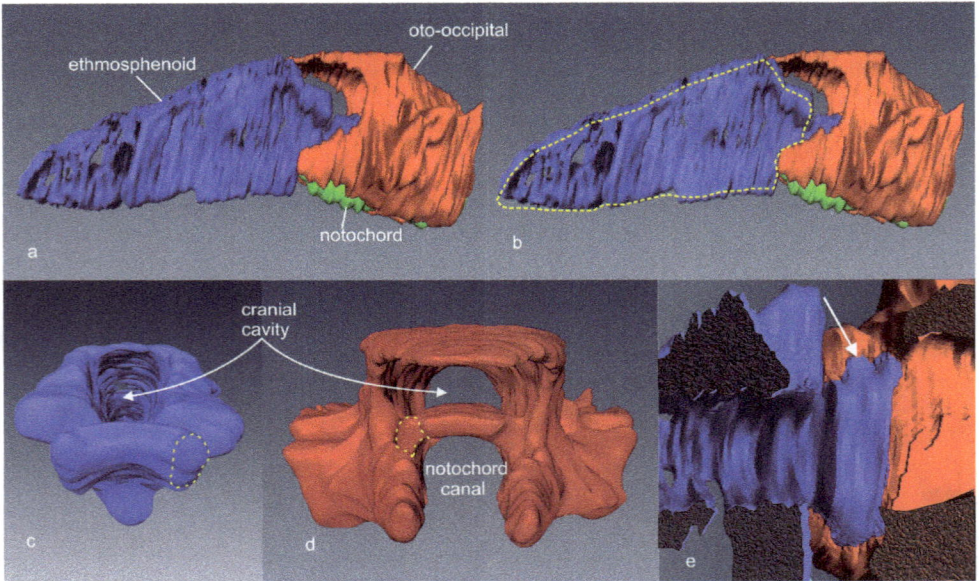

Fig. 4. Reconstructions of braincase and notochord, left lateral view; b: the limit of mobility at the intracranial joint is indicated by the dotted line; c: caudal view of ethmosphenoid, the articular condyle is outlined on the right side; d: rostral view of oto-occipital, socket for the condyle outlined; e: dorsal view of intracranial joint after removal of the roof of the braincase, the arrow points to the locking of the components.

4.4 Interpretation

These findings accord with those of Millot and Anthony (1958) and with the interpretation of Jarvik (1980). The analyses involving dorsal flexion at the intracranial joint (sections 3.2.2

and 3.2.3) are not compatible with the morphology revealed here. The jaw-opening mechanism suggested by Lauder (1980) is otherwise convincing however, and remains the best explanation of the hyoid apparatus and double jaw articulation of the coelacanth. The minor amount of movement allowed by this result provides no easy explanation for the basicranial muscle, which is relatively large in *Latimeria*. The studies involving manipulation of a recently dead or thawed specimen (Thomson, 1966 and Alexander, 1973) have not used radiological confirmation of movement at the joint, and the dorsal flexion observed must have been movement of the whole skull on the notochord at the occiput.

5. Discussion

5.1 The intracranial joint of sarcopterygians

The intracranial joint of adult sarcopterygians, excluding lungfish, represents a major difference from the fused sphenoid and otic regions of modern chondrichthyans (cartilaginous fish), actinopterygians (ray-finned bony fish) and tetrapods. The putative ancestors of lungfish also had such a joint: the taxa *Youngolepis* and *Powichthys* are Dipnomorpha, on the branches leading to lungfish. These taxa have an intracranial joint that is identifiable but either very narrow or closed, and retain an incomplete intracranial notochord. In the actinopterygian lineage, in quite a similar morphology, the taxa *Mimia* and *Kansasiella* had the notochord still present within the base of the skull but regressed caudally from the intracranial joint, which was narrow or closed (Janvier, 1996). The incompletely closed ventral part of the joint appears to be represented in later actinopterygians by the ventral cranial fissure; there has been some debate about this, but this interpretation offers the best explanation (Janvier, 1996).

In the absence of an obvious function in jaw action of this joint in *Latimeria*, it is appropriate to consider possible functions of the joint applicable to all sarcopterygians. The presence of the intracranial notochord is closely linked with the existence of an intracranial joint (Janvier, 1996), and the explanation which has been assumed, and not examined in detail, is that the notochord is needed to provide flexibility to the base of the skull so that the joint can operate. The basicranial muscle in this model is the ventral flexor of the joint.

5.2 The primary role of the intracranial notochord

I would like to turn this association around, and suggest that the retention of the intracranial notochord is the primary evolutionary event, and that the intracranial joint exists to deal with pressure and length changes in the notochord. No research on the physical properties of the *Latimeria* notochord has been published. The closest similarity to the *Latimeria* notochord in a living animal is the sturgeon, which has an unconstricted extracranial notochord as its axial support. Studies on the sturgeon notochord (Long, 1995) have examined its flexibility and contribution to an undulating swimming motion, but not the effects of movement on the notochord itself. Koehl et al. (2000) have investigated the physical properties of the *Xenopus* tadpole notochord with models of a fibre-wound hydraulic skeleton. It was found that bending and straightening of the model resulted in lengthening or shortening, depending on the angle at which the fibres (collagen in life) are wound onto the viscous core. A model of the *Latimeria* notochord with an appropriate viscous core and fibrous coating would be needed to advance this suggestion, but from present knowledge it is reasonable to conclude that the notochord in *Latimeria* may be subject to changes in length and pressure with swimming motion.

The intracranial joint and basicranial muscle could thus be seen as a shock-absorbing mechanism, to deal with these changes in the intracranial notochord. The skull elements, notochord and basicranial muscle are thus in a dynamic balance. The mechanical opposition of the notochord and the basicranial muscle has been recognised by Millot and Anthony (1958) and subsequent authors, but in the context of the intracranial joint being the primary functional element, rather than the notochord.

Key taxa for evaluating this hypothesis further in sarcopterygian evolution are those in which the intracranial joint is closed (or very narrow) and the intracranial notochord has not regressed to the back of the skull. Such taxa are the dipnomorph *Youngolepis* (Chang, 2004), as mentioned above, and the tetrapodomorphs *Acanthostega gunnari* (Clack, 1998) and *Mandageria fairfaxi* (Johanson et al., 2003). Correlation with the morphology of the postcranial axial skeleton will also be important, both in these transitional forms and in sarcopterygians as a group.

6. Conclusions

6.1 Imaging techniques

The various recent advances based on cross-sectional imaging set out in section 2 above are new tools for the morphologist, and depend on the ability of computer systems to record, calculate and display 3D data. With the availability of high resolution CT and MRI, and real-time display with synchrotron imaging, these tools are now applicable to invertebrate as well as vertebrate study. Hopefully costs of some these relatively expensive techniques will come down in time, and access to synchrotron imaging or a similar high-energy radiation source will become wider.

6.2 The intracranial joint of *Latimeria*

The original research on the intracranial joint presented here demonstrates the use of some the tools described in section 2: CT and MRI scanning, 3D reconstruction and 3D prototyping. These methods have enabled new functional anatomical data to be applied to the unresolved problem of the sarcopterygian intracranial joint. It is very unlikely that museum specimen of *Latimeria* would be made available for such a study, emphasizing the value of these non-destructive techniques.

6.2.1 Future research

Further work can be done with the data described here, adding the segmentation of the hyoid elements, palatoquadrate and mandible to the reconstruction, and then adding mobile joints in an animation software, probably with the help of more 3D prototyping. Lauder's (1980) scheme for the function of the hyoid apparatus, mandible and skull can then be revised in light of the data on intracranial joint mobility described above. Building a physical model of the *Latimeria* notochord, with an accurately copied fibre-wound external sheath and viscous interior, would also elucidate the issues raised here.

6.2.2 The problem - reframing the question

In an evolutionary context, the hypothesis offered here, that the sarcopterygian intracranial joint exists to deal with mechanical effects of notochord bending, can be developed by close examination of taxa with transitional states of reduction of the joint. If this hypothesis is upheld, the major question then changes from "what is the function of the intracranial joint?" to "why does the intracranial notochord persist in sarcopterygian lineages?". The regression of the notochord from the base of the skull in the rhipidistian-tetrapod transition is not difficult to understand: the development of the occipito-vertebral joint, separation of the dorsal skull form the shoulder girdle and regression of the notochord all increase mobility of the head on the body as an adaptation to life on land. On the other hand, the retention of the notochord in the adult sarcopterygian skull contrasts with its loss or reduction in all other cartilaginous and bony fish, and no developmental or functional explanation has yet been suggested.

7. Acknowledgements

For the CT scan images I am grateful to Timothy Rowe and Jessie Maisano, University of Texas Digital Morphology Group, and for the MRI scans, Larry Frank and Rachel Berquist of the Digital Fish Library, University of California, San Diego. The Digital Fish Library project is funded by NSF grant number: DBI-0446389. I thank Brett Cowan for technical discussion on MRI, and Andrew Kersley for information on 3D prototyping. I am grateful to Casey Holliday for pointing out literature on contrast use for CT.

8. References

Adamicka, P. & Ahnelt, H. (1976). Beiträge zur funktionellen Analys und zur Morphologie des Kopfes von *Latimeria chalumnae* Smith. *Annal des (KK) Naturhistorischen (Hof) Museums, Wien* 80:251-271.

Alexander, R.M. (1973). Jaw mechanisms of the coelacanth *Latimeria*. *Copeia* 1973:156–158. ISSN 0045-8511

Bemis, W.E. & Northcutt, R.G. (1991). Innervation of the basicranial muscle in *Latimeria chalumnae*. *Environmental Biology of Fishes* 32:147–157. ISSN 0378-1909

Bernstein, P. (2002). *Die evolutive Transformation der Oticalregion der Sarcopterygii beim Übergang vom Wasser- zum Landleben.* Thesis: Tübingen, Eberhard-Karls-Universität. 179 p.

Bruton, M.N., Coutouvidis, S.E. & Pote, J. (1991). Bibliography of the living coelacanth *Latimeria chalumnae* with comments on publication trends. *Environmental Biology of Fishes* 32:403–433. ISSN 0378-1909

Butler, C. & Ballesta, L. (2011). Ancient swimmers. *National Geographic* 219(3):86–93.

Chang, M-M. (2004). Synapomorphies and scenarios – more characters of *Youngolepis* betraying its affinity to the Dipnoi. In: Arratia G, Wilson MVH, Cloutier R, editors. *Recent advances in the origin and early radiation of vertebrates*. München: Verlag Dr Freidrich Pfeil. p 665–686. ISBN 3899372052X

Clack, J.A. (1998). The neurocranium of *Acanthostega gunnari* Jarvik and and the evolution of the otic region in tetrapods. *Zoological Journal of the Linnean Society* 122:61-97. ISSN 0024-4082

Corfield, J.R., Wild, J.M., Cowan, B.R., Parsons, S. & Kubke, M.F. (2008). MRI of postmortem specimens of endangered species for comparative brain anatomy. *Nature Protocols* 3:597-605. ISSN 1750-2799

Cracraft, J. (1968). Functional morphology and adaptive significance of cranial kinesis in *Latimeria chalumnae* (Coelacanthini). *American Zoologist* 8:354. ISSN 0003-1569

Forey, P.L. (1998). *History of the Coelacanth Fishes*. London: Chapman and Hall. 419 p. ISBN 0412784807

Gardner, N.M., Holliday, C.M. & O'Keefe, F.R. (2010). The braincase of *Youngina capensis* (Reptilia: Diapsida): new insights from high-resolution CT scanning of the holotype. *Palaeontologia Electronica*. p 16. ISSN 1094-8074

Gatesy, S.M., Baier, D.B., Jenkins, F.A. & Dial, K.P. (2010). Scientific rotoscoping: a morphology-based method of 3-D motion analysis and visualization. *Journal of Experimental Zoology* 313A:244-261. ISSN 1548-8969

Hitchcock, E.C. (1995). A functional interpretation of the anteriormost vertebrae and skull of *Eusthenopteron*. *Bulletin du Muséum national d'Histoire naturelle, 4ieme séries, section C* 17:269–285.

Computerized Scanning and Imaging Facility of the Woods Hole Oceanographic Institute. (n.d.). Accessed April 2011. Available at: http://www.whoi.edu/csi.

Janvier, P. (1996). *Early Vertebrates*. Oxford: Clarendon Press. 393 p. ISBN 0198540477

Jarvik, E. (1980). *Basic structure and evolution of vertebrates*. London: Academic Press. 575 p. ISBN 0123808014

Jeffery, N.S., Stephenson, R.S., Gallagher, J.A., Jarvis, J.C. & Cox, P.G. (2011). Micro-computed tomography with iodine staining resolves the arrangement of muscle fibres. *Journal of Biomechanics* 44:189-192. ISSN 0021-9290

Johanson, Z., Ahlberg, P. & Ritchie, A. (2003). The braincase and palate of the tetrapodomorph sarcopterygian *Mandageria fairfaxi*: morphological variability near the fish-tetrapod transition. *Palaeontology* 46:271-293. ISSN 0031-0239

Johnston, P. (2010). The constrictor dorsalis musculature and basipterygoid articulation in *Sphenodon*. *Journal of Morphology* 271:280-292. ISSN 0362-2525

Kanyukin, A.A. (2009). The role of hyobranchial skeletal elements in the Rhipidistian intracranial kinetic mechanism. *Doklady Biological Sciences* 428:278-281.

Kargo, W.J. & Rome, L.C. (2002). Functional morphology of proximal hindlimb muscles in the frog *Rana pipiens*. *Journal of Experimental Biology* 205:1987-2004. ISSN 0022-0949

Kleinteich, T., Haas, A. & Summers, A.P. (2008). Caecilian jaw-closing mechanics: integrating two muscle systems. *Journal of the Royal Society Interface* 5:1491-1504. ISSN 1742-5662

Koehl, M.A.R., Quillin, K.J. & Pell, C.A. (2000). Mechanical design of fiber-wound hydraulic skeletons: the stiffening and straightening of embryonic notochords. *American Zoologist* 40(28–41). ISSN 0003-1569

Lauder, G.V. (1980). The role of the hyoid apparatus in the feeding mechanism of the coelacanth *Latimeria chalumnae*. *Copeia* 1980:1-9. ISSN 0045-8511

Long, J.H. (1995). Morphology, mechanics and locomotion: the relation between the notochord and swimming motions in the sturgeon. *Environmental Biology of Fishes* 44:199–211. ISSN 0378-1909

Cross-Sectional Imaging in Comparative Vertebrate Morphology - The Intracranial Joint
of the Coelacanth Latimeria chalumnae

251

Metscher, B.D. (2009). MicroCT for comparative morphology: simple staining methods allow high-contrast 3D imaging of diverse non-mineralised animal tissues. *BMC Physiology* 9:11. ISSN 1472-6713

Millot, J. & Anthony, J. (1958). *Anatomie de Latimeria chalumnae*. Paris: CNRS. 122 p.

Millot, J., & Anthony, J. (1965). *Anatomie de Latimeria chalumnae. II Système nerveux et organes des sens.* Paris: C.N.R.S. 131 p.

Millot, J., Anthony, J. & Robineau D. (1978). *Anatomie de Latimeria chalumnae.* Paris: CNRS. 198 p.

Motani, R. (n.d.) Accessed April 2011. Available at: http://3dmuseum.org.

Rieppel, O., Kley, N.J. & Maisano J.A. (2009). Morphology of the skull of the white-nosed blindsnake, *Liotyphlops albirostris* (Soclecophidia: Anomalepididae). *Journal of Morphology* 270:536-557. ISSN 0362-2525

Ross, A.J., Yang, Z., Berr, S.S., Gilson, W.D., Peterson, W.C., Oshinski, J.N. & French, B.A. (2002). Serial MRI evaluation of cardiac structure and function in mice after reperfused myocardial infarction. *Magnetic Resonance in Medicine* 47:1158–1168. ISSN 0740-3194

Rowe, T. & Frank, L.R. (2011). The disappearing third dimension. *Science* 331:712–714. ISSN 0036-8075

Ruffins, S.W., Martin, M., Keough, L., Truong, S., Fraser, S.E., Jacobs, R.E. & Lansford, R. (2007). Digital three-dimensional atlas of quail development using high-resolution MRI. *TSW Development and Embryology* 2:47–53.

Schmidt, J., Schuff, M. & Olsson, L. (2011). A role for FoxN3 in the development of cranial cartilages and muscles in *Xenopus laevis* (Amphibia: Anura: Pipidae) with special emphasis on the novel rostral cartilages. *Journal of Anatomy* : 218: 226-242. ISSN 0021-8782

Stemple, D.L. (2005). Structure and function of the notochord: an essential organ for chordate development. *Development* 132:2503-2512. ISSN 0950-1991

Sutton, M.D. (2008). Tomographic techniques for the study of exceptionally preserved fossils. *Proceedings of the Royal Society B* 275:1587-1593. ISSN 0950-1193

Thomson, K.S. (1966). Intracranial mobility in the coelacanth. *Science* 153:999–1000. ISSN 0036-8075

Thomson, K.S. (1967). Mechanisms of intracranial kinetics in fossil rhipidistian fishes (Crossopterygii) and their relatives. *Zoological Journal of the Linnean Society* 46:223-253. ISSN 0024-4082

Westneat, M.W., Socha, J.J. & Lee, W-K. (2008). Advances in biological structure, function and physiology using synchrotron X-ray imaging. *Annual Review of Physiology* 70:119-142. ISSN 0066-4278

Witmer, L. (n.d.) Accessed April 2011. Available at:
http://www.oucom.ohiou.edu/dbms-witmer/3D-visualization.htm.

Yu, X., Zhu, M. & Zhao, W. (2010). The origin and diversification of osteichthyans and sarcopterygians: new Chinese fossil findings advance research in key areas of evolution. *Bulletin of the Chinese Academy of Sciences* 24(2):71–75.

Ziegler, A., Ogurreck, M., Steinke, T., Beckmann, F., Prohaska, S. & Ziegler, A. (2010). Opportunities and challenges for digital morphology. *Biology Direct.* 5:45. ISSN 1745-6150

13

Conventional - and Cone Beam – CT - Derived Stereolithographic Surgical Guides in the Planning and Placement of Dental Implants

Volkan Arısan

Department of Oral Implantology, Faculty of Dentistry
Istanbul University
Turkey

1. Introduction

The prevalence of tooth loss and edentulism is still posing a serious health problem especially for the elderly population. A removable denture was the only option in the treatment of total edentulism. However, serious complaints related to poor retention, mastication and perception of the prosthesis are common among edentulous patients (Raghoebar et al., 2000).

The discovery of osseointegration, -the direct bone contact to the load bearing titanium implant surface under 100X light microscopy- has led to a radical change in the rehabilitation of the edentulous patients. Especially upon the loss of posterior teeth, removable prosthesis was the only available option for patients suffering from severe decay, periodontal or root fracture problems (Lekholm, 1985). Anchorage of such removable prosthesis to the existing dentition yielded additional stress on the remaining teeth and increased the risk of decay in case of insufficient patient hygiene. Osseointegrated dental implants were especially vital for totally edentulous mandible which in other case will likely to result with an unsatisfactory denture due to various muscle attachments and tongue activity. With the help of orthopantomogram (known as panoramic x-rays) the vertical available bone height in mandibular symphisis was evaluated and the longest possible implant fixture (the only available implant diameter was the 3.75mm) was inserted after a surgical flap exposure. The implants were left to undisturbed healing for an approximate of 4 to 6 months. Following the osseointegration period a second surgery was performed for uncovering the implants and restorative phase (George et al., 1985).

Since then many technological advances have been accomplished from the titanium surface enhancements to the prosthetic aspect of the implant dentistry allowing better satisfaction of the patients' needs. Unlike early implant-supported hybrid prosthesis, the acceptable standard of care in implant dentistry requires not only the restoration of the lost function but also the appearance of the natural anatomy. This has become a criterion of success in the maxilla where the facial expression is conveyed through a pleasant aesthetic smile. Accurate positioning of the implant fixture has therefore become extremely critical to ensure a "natural" look (Belser et al., 1996).

Various attempts were undertaken to improve the relation of the implant positions and the prosthetic plan (Akca et al., 2002). In order to incorporate prosthetic information in the planning stage, the so known basic conventional implant placement approach was revised and called as "backwards planning" (Gotfredsen and Karlsson, 2001). With the use of radiopaque markers (Basten and Kois, 1996), the ideal position of the final prosthesis could be visualized on the x-rays which and they were transferred to the patients' mouth by a custom surgical template (Basten, 1995). The use of these templates provided help to some degree in partially edentulous cases. Furthermore, the inclusion of three dimensional (3D) tomographic data also assisted in deciding the implant diameter and axial inclination (Blanchet et al., 2004). From a prosthetic point of view, the parallelism of the implants would provide significant ease of clinical handling during the restoration phase. However due to trajectory of the jaws the parallel placement of multiple implants is extremely difficult. Also there is a risk of lethal haemorrhages or neural injuries as a result of the collision of the drills and/or implant apex were reported (Kalpidis and Setayesh, 2004).

2. Recent radiographic examination methods in oral implantology

Similar to many of those minor surgical interventions in dentistry ,the planning is generally based on the two-dimensional images of the radiographic techniques such as, peri-apical, orthopantomogram (panoramic x-ray), sephalometric and occlusal. Among these four techniques the two mentioned former are the most commonly used (Amet and Ganz, 1997). All these methods, however, are subject to distortion, blurring and also do not provide any information regarding the z-dimension; the "bone thickness". Consequently, clinical implant dentistry quickly recognised the importance of tomographic imaging (Klein et al., 1993) and its interactive implementation in the computer environment via a dedicated "implant planning" software (Rosenfeld et al., 2006). The technologic advances led emerging of newer and more specific imaging instruments such as cone-beam computed tomography (CBCT). The lack of sufficient comparative studies coupled with the rapidly evolving technologies (Reddy et al., 1994), however, has revealed many doubtful aspects of the recently marketed tomographic scanners which are briefly discussed below.

2.1 Multi-slice computed tomography (CT)

Conventional multi-slice CT was primarily developed for medical imaging of the body such as abdominal pathologies and investigation of the extremities. The sophisticated tube-detector assembly rotates 360° along the axis of the scan area which is positioned by the table the patient is lying on. Each increment of the patient induces the rotation of the tube-detector assembly and consequent radiation exposure. The resulting transversal images are then transferred to a computer with dedicated software. Thanks to the advanced tube-detector assembly, the released ionizing energy of the ray of x-ray photons can be calculated to construct various diagnostic parameters with robust accuracy. Amongst these parameters, the Hounsfield unit is the most widely utilized parameter which is used for the assessment of the bone density on the basis of the gray-density values. By the attenuation of the x-ray energy to the air (-1000 HU) and water (0 HU) local bone density can be objectively measured on a quantitative basis (Shapurian et al., 2006). The measured gray density values may help predicting the local density of the implant recipient bone (Turkyilmaz et al., 2007). Due to complex structure and space needs, multi-slice CT scanners are operable in hospitals and/or radiology canters.

Conventional - and Cone Beam – CT - Derived Stereolithographic Surgical Guides
in the Planning and Placement of Dental Implants

255

2.2 Cone-beam computed tomography (CBCT)

Advancements in the computer processing and the reconstruction process as well as the mathematical conversion algorithms used for the CT led emerging of a new approach that is based on rendering "volumes" instead of "slices" (Araki et al., 2004). As opposed to the CT where a full-360° turn of the tube-detector assembly is required for each slice, in the CBCT the whole image of the object to be screened is "radiated" with an array of conic-rays (Arai et al., 1999). The resulting data is then transferred to the computer and the axial, sagittal or frontal views are re-formatted by the computer according to the user demand. As a result of single-turn of the x-ray source the emitted dose (and relevant scanning time) is significantly lower than the CT (Carrafiello et al., 2010). This was a result of the re-designed tube assembly which emits remarkably lower doses of radiation as compared to the multi-slice CT.

As opposed to the multi-slice CT, the cone-beam CT scanners are quite small and have become available in size of an orthopantomogram (panoramic) device. This technology was primarily developed for cardiovascular purposes and promising outcomes led extension to different disciplines such as dentistry. The first generation of CBCT machines was equipped by an "image-intensifier" detector; a CMOS or CCD based technology used mainly in the digital camera industry. The resulting images were rather sufficient for visual examination purposes. However, in certain circumstances the images were subjected to severe distortion in terms of dimensional accuracy. Moreover, areas with high density caused heavy halation and beam hardening effects (Katsumata et al., 2006). Later use of flat-panel amorphous-silicone detectors improved the accuracy of the images but also led a slight increase in the emitted radiation dose (Baba et al., 2002). The efficacy of the CBCT-based grey-density values as compared to the CT-based Hounsfield unit (HU) is, however, unclear.

3. Stereolithography and biomodelling in implant dentistry

The need of a rapid 3D model of the computer-aided-designed (CAD) components in particular industries (i.e. automotive, space craft jewellery) leaded emerging complex technologic advances. The term "streolithography" (abbreviated as SLA or SL) first introduced in 1986 by Charles W. Hull, defines the method and apparatus for making solid objects by successive printing of light-curable material one on top of the other (Asberg et al., 1997). The procedure is entirely computer-controlled and named by various tags such as "3D printing", "additive manufacturing", "rapid manufacturing/prototyping" etc. This process was termed as "biomodelling" in the medicine and initially used to obtain 3D models of the particular bones. Thanks to the realistic dimensions of the models the clinicians were able to explore the future surgical site and decide particular plans specific to the local bone geometry of the patient. Biomodelling is widely used especially in cranial and spinal surgery.

3.1 Virtual dental implant planning on reformatted CT images

The need of a thorough planning of the dental implants prior to the surgical placement yielded emerging of many implant planning software on the market. The ability of working on true-sized 3D models is however, featured in only few of them. With the help of the advanced capabilities of some software, the clinician may outline critical anatomy (i.e. *n.alveolaris, sinus maxillaris*), prosthetic priorities and special circumstances which can never be assessed without exploring the actual surgical site. This may not only prevent the occurrence of adverse outcomes but can also diminish the stress on the surgeon in the surgical theatre (Rosenfeld et al., 2006); (Fig. 1).

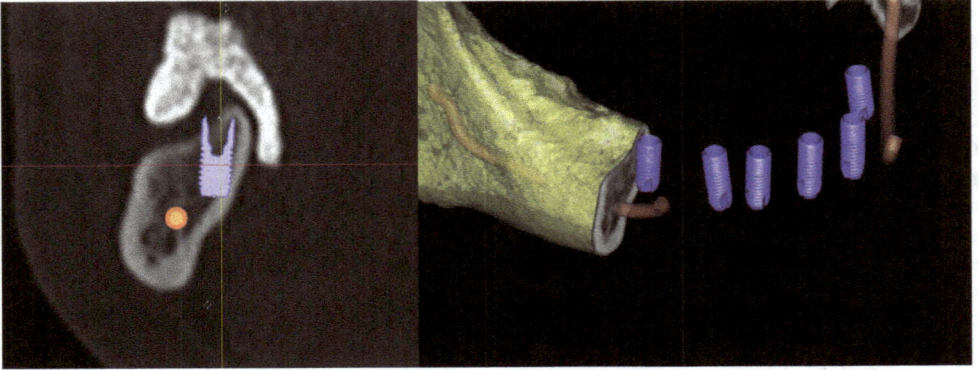

Fig. 1. Depiction of the mandibular nerve (orange point and line) and the implant body (blue cylinders) on cross sectional images and 3D reconstruction. Enhanced viewing capabilities of some software allow 3D depiction of critical anatomic structures in relation with the true-sized implants. The interactive features of the planning software allow 360° rotation of the planning either collectively or individually.

3.2 SLA surgical guide manufacture

Utilization of the virtual implant planning in conjunction with the CT-based surface modelling on the basis of the gray-density values (known as the Hounsfield unit) allows rapid manufacturing of biomodels according to the aforementioned SLA technology (Ganz, 2003). In this respect, the spatial position of the virtually planned implants can be outlined by a surgical guide since implants are basically cylindrical objects inserted after the use of cylindrical drills. Therefore, the "SLA guide" can simply locate the point of drilling by outlying the implants entry point on the virtual planning.

Most often this is done by placing "guide tubes" in the central axis of the planned virtual implant which will guide the direction of the drilling during surgery. Accurate positioning of the drills is maintained by the supporting surrounding material: the CT- or CBCT-derived stereolithographic model. Since all modelling manufacturing process is based on a mathematical process, the process is virtually error-free (fig. 2).

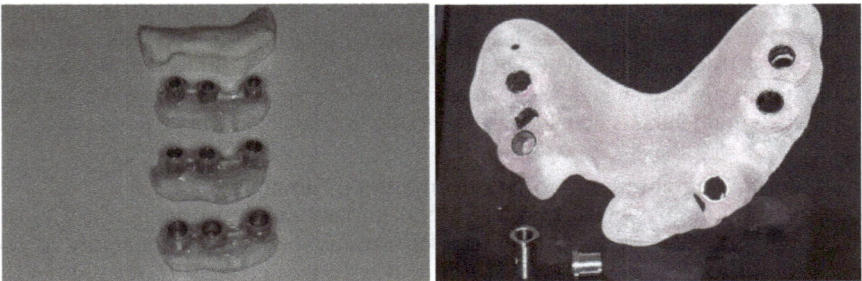

Fig. 2. SLA model (white block) and the multiple-type drill guides with guiding metal sleeves prepared according to the consecutive drill diameters. The guides are replaced after the use of each drill (left). A single-type tooth- and mucosa-suported SLA guide. The drilling is completed via the special metal sleeves (the two-metal tubes located infront of the guide) placed into the guide tubes in the SLA guide (right).

Since the planning and the production of the SLA guides are realised on the basis of the tomographic data, the reliability and the safety of the whole procedure is mainly dependent on the proper execution of the clinical and radiographic steps revised below.

Most often the placement and restoration of the implants are accomplished by different clinicians usually consisting of a surgeon and a restorative dentist. The surgeon places the implant where the alveolar bone is abundant whereas restorative dentist would prefer proper alignment of the implants according to the emergence profile and root eminence of the prosthesis. In fact, the disregard of the prosthetic conformity in the placement of dental implants usually compromise aesthetic, phonetic, prosthetic and periodontal outcome. For instance, interproximal emergence of the implant between the two teeth implants is one of the most frequently encountered positioning error in implant dentistry. This incidence not only causes an unpleasant aesthetic appearance (especially in cases with high smile line) but also seriously complicates the ability of patients' access to peri-implant area for daily hygiene procedures (Fig. 3).

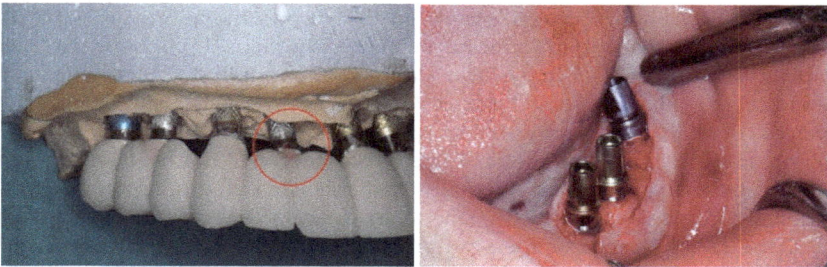

Fig. 3. The emergence point of the implant invades the inter-proximal area of two neighbouring teeth (left). The posterior implant has been placed with an excessively labial inclination and this will complicate the restorative phase (right).

Among such positioning errors, improper parallelism or excessive angulation of multiple implants can also be regarded highly challenging for the restorative dentist.

4. Potential pitfalls and sources of error in computer-aided implant planning and surgery using stereolithographic guides

Although its medical utilization was initiated by the late 1980's, comprehensive use of CT technology incorporating prosthetic data in relation with the implant treatment has been recently   introduced by a scanning technique employing a radio-opaque scan prosthesis. The process was, however, not uneventful since the CT technicians were mostly trained for medical purposes. Due to their unfamiliarity with dento-maxillofacial scanning procedure and the dental scan prosthesis, the proper execution of the process was prone to error risk in the imaging stage of the "guided implant treatment" sequence. Furthermore the clinician, patient, radiology technician and the auxiliary personnel (if present) -responsible for the segmentation and preparation of the raw CT or CBCT data for the implant planning- may cause errors which may unfortunately become apparent in later stages of the treatment sequence. Proper execution of each step in the computer-aided implant planning sequence is therefore mandatory to avoid undesired circumstances. It should also be noted that in case of adverse events or outcomes, the primary responsible and legitimate respondent will solely be the clinician and therefore a thorough understanding and control of the possible error sources is of utmost importance for the practising dentist. The errors could be due various reasons; resulting from human error(s) and/or technical flaw(s) of the employed equipment.

4.1 Possible errors and relevant sources

The cascade of computer aided implant treatment sequence incorporating the "backwards planning" should start with a tooth setup that will be the representation of the final prosthetic goal. In this manner, the clinician should initially create an articulated diagnostic model to evaluate the maxillo-mandibular relationship as well as with the prosthetic allowance and prosthodontics options. This is usually done with plasters models and a consequent wax setup for the bite registration. The clinical try-ins is similar to that of performed for a total prosthesis consisting of registering the vertical dimension and centric occlusion as well as overjet, overbite and smile line. Then the wax-setup of the final tooth positions should be tried intra-orally for ensuring to achieve an accurate prosthesis in terms of aesthetic, functional and phonetic aspects. In this respect the approval of the patient is also an important and motivating factor for the rest of the steps throughout the "computer-aided implant treatment". This step is also a unique opportunity to determine and discuss patient expectations which in some instances may carry unrealistic aspects and non-dental issues such as overall correction of the facial appearance (Fig. 4).

It is also important to notice that the final fixed restoration will not have labial flanges and consequently the labial support. Usually patients expect important relief of the circumferential wrinkles around the lip due to an "inflation effect" from the prosthesis. In such cases, the labial flanges of the scan-prosthesis can be removed in order to better simulate the final facial appearance after completion of the treatment.

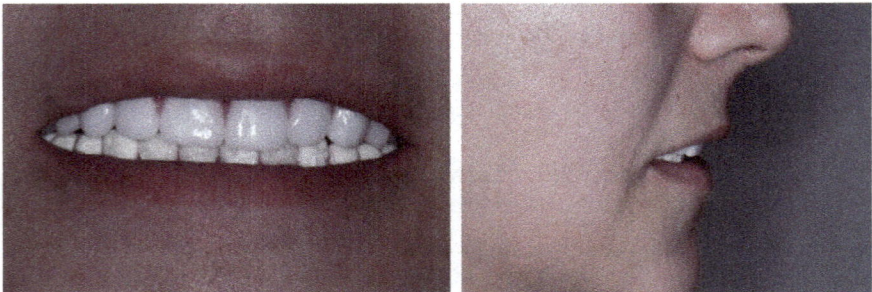

Fig. 4. Try-in of the wax-up dentures representing the final prosthetic goal. Different radio-opaque objects were used to prevent interference of upper and lower jaws in the tomographic image. $BaSo_4$-based radio-opaque teeth were used in lower jaw and upper jaw only included a $BaSo_4$-based base (left). The patient should be informed that the final prosthesis will not have the lip-support of the labial flanges (right).

The patient should be able to evaluate and discuss the limitations and consequences of the treatment at this stage. Minor correction of the incisal line and tooth eminence could be performed by the clinician. The resulting phonetics should also be evaluated. A retention medium (i.e, tissue conditioner or prosthesis fixation powder) can be used to hold the prosthesis in the proper position especially if the patient is using the total denture for the first time. For such patients it is also important to consider the interference of the scan prosthesis with the healing extraction sockets (if present) and creation of sufficient relief in the impression surface is mandatory to ensure a comfortable fit during the tomographic scan. Usually due to periodontal and/or endodontic disease, the remaining teeth of the patient in the designated jaw have to be extracted prior to the implant surgery. This situation combined with the unfamiliarity of the use of a total prosthesis may lead to serious loss of control regarding the patient holding the prosthesis. Such an incidence is potentially dangerous for the sake of the procedure because the patient is likely to alter the accurate position of the scan prosthesis during tomographic imaging. It should also be noted that an estimated minimum of 2 to 3 weeks which are necessary for the completion of the pre-operative stages, will also yield minor soft and hard tissue changes due to extraction-related remodelling.

The clinician should be precautious and should allow prolonged healing periods before the tomographic imaging to ensure that the scan prosthesis is correctly positioned within the patients' mouth. Pain and discomfort during the try-in of the prepared scan prosthesis should be taken as a precaution and the implications of this situation should be explained to the patient. Improper positioning or dislocation of the scan prosthesis during the tomographic scan could be induced by the clinician, patient, radiology technician and the auxiliary post-imaging processor. Some of the most often occurred instances are in table 1.

Errors could be related due to clinician, patient, radiology technician, post-image processing auxiliary personnel. After the tomographic imaging, the preparation and insertion of the implants should be realised without any prolonged time before an additional remodelling occurs in the seating surface of the scan-prosthesis (Table 2).

Besides the errors affecting the scan prosthesis, a number of image artefacts and/or errors can also compromise the quality of the tomographic data (Table 3). Metal scattering is one of the most frequent image artefact in tomography. Ideally, the clinician should remove the metal objects from the mouth prior to the scan as they will introduce serious effects on the resulting image. As a result of the reduced radiation dose the severity of metal scatter (or so known starbust effect) may be less prominent in CBCT. The removal of all possible metallic objects is recommended either in CT or CBCT.

Most likely due to typical daily routines, the CT imaging technician and auxiliary personnel may simply disregard performing key actions for the patient under the computer-aided dental implant treatment sequence. Misalignment of the imaging plane (gantry tilt) is one of the most frequent mistakes made by the CT technicians. In order to facilitate the planning on the cross sectional images, the scan plane should be parallel to the occlusal table identified on the scan prosthesis. Nevertheless the CT technician should be acknowledged regarding the occlusal table – a dentistry related issue-. Arbitrary alignment of the scanning plane may inevitably lead misleading reconstruction and consequent planning as the ideal positioning of the implants is expected to be vertical to the occlusal table. Some planning software incorporate special tools to correct the gantry tilt according to the clinicians' desire. However, such tools may introduce additional errors in CBCT.

4.2 Segmentation and threshold-processing of CT- and CBCT data

The aim of this process is to prepare an optimal view of the imaging data including mandible or maxilla, scan prosthesis and existing teeth, if present. Although the tools and processes may differ amongst different software, the basic methodological approach is standard.

Respondent	potential sources of error
Clinician	-The clinician may have not sufficiently instructed the patient regarding the procedure and the role of the scan prosthesis. - Insufficient healing-time allowed following tooth extraction(s). - Failure to provide a proper fit of the scan prosthesis to the underlying mucosa. - Direct use of existing removable denture without improvements for the double-scan procedure. - Insufficient number and/or positioning of the guta markers on the existing denture in the double-scan procedure. - Poor result in the duplication of the existing prosthesis. - Absence of a bite-index
Patient	- Patient is unaware of the importance of sustaining the proper position of the scan prosthesis. - Gag reflex. - First time use of a removable denture - Pain due to irritation of the scan prosthesis to the recent extraction sockets.
Radiology Technician	- Technician is unaware of the "guided implant surgery" procedure and the role of the scan prosthesis, failed to provide the appropriate bite-position index prior to scan
Post-tomographic image processing auxiliary personnel	- Auxiliary personnel is not trained in "jaw and scan prosthesis matching" procedure.

Table 1. Potential error sources and relevant respondents in case of improperly placed scan-prosthesis observed in the tomographic images.

Respondent	Potential source of error
Clinician	- The clinician may have not sufficiently instructed the patient regarding the procedure and the role of the scan prosthesis. - Auxilary personnel (or radiology technician) is unaware of the need of a scan prosthesis for the procedure.
Patient	- Patient forgot or refrained wearing the scan prosthesis. -Patient assumed to achieve a better result by complying the "well-known" tomographic principle: "removal of possible objects during scan".
Radiology Technician	-Technician intentionally removed the scan prosthesis and unaware of the "guided implant surgery" procedure and the role of the scan prosthesis.
Post-tomographic image processing auxiliary personnel	-Auxiliary is unaware of the double-scan procedure and omitted "scan-prosthesis" data. -Gray-density thresholds were not properly adjusted. -Variant nature of the gray-density values in CBCT was not emphasized by the auxiliary.

Table 2. Potential error sources and relevant respondents when the scan prosthesis was found unpresent in the planning data.

Usually, an auxiliary personnel who is trained in this step performs this time-consuming process. Initially the gray-density values are adjusted according to relevant density levels of the bone, scan prosthesis and remaining teeth if present. This is rather tricky in CBCT since the gray-density values are not absolute and may need precise manual adjustment to fully visualize intact 3D structures in the software. Due to standard distribution of the HU in the CT, segmentation according to the pre-determined HU values usually reveals satisfactory results. As compared to the CT, the CBCT images also include higher radiographic "noise" which requires manual removal prior to the planning. The use of CBCT however is advantageous in the presence of the metallic objects in the mouth. The intensity of the metal-scattering (or starbust) effect is significantly reduced with the lower exposure of CBCT. The quality of the segmentation procedure will ease the planning of implants by providing clear visibility in the constructed 3D model.

5. Dental implant planning on cross-sectional images

The modification of the recently available medical 3D examination and planning software has led to the introduction of various "dental implant planning" software in the market. The majority of these software simply make use of well-known re-formatting algorithms to

Image artefact/ error	Clinician-related	Patient-related	Radiology technician-related	Post-scan processing auxiliary technician-related	Effects
Heavy scattering (Starbust effect).	-Failed to remove metal-containing restorations prior to the scan	-Forgot removing opposing denture including metallic components.	-Failed to adjust exposure parameters to reduce scattering.	-Failed manual removal of scattering objects from the 3D rendering	Mostly CT Also CBCT
Blurred image	none	-Patient moved during scanning -Gag reflex -Failure to keep still due to anxiety.	-Technician failed to notify patient to hold still during scan. -Technician did not checked the resulting images or unaware of the dento-facial imaging.	none	Mostly CT Also CBCT
Improper gantry tilt	- Failure to provide sufficient information to the radiology technician	None	Technician is unaware of the guided-surgery imaging procedure.	-Auxilary did not corrected the tilt of the images during post-tomography processing	CT and CBCT
Impartial structures in the 3D model	None	None	CBCT technician may have not provided sufficient current (radiation dose or duration) for the procedure	-Threshold values were improperly adjusted. -Segmentation process was poor. - Auxiliary is unaware of the variant gray-density values in CBCT.	Mostly CBCT Also CT

Table 3. Possible artifacts/errors on CT and CBCT images and relevant sources.

provide cross-section views of any desired area. Also a 3D reconstruction accompanies the planning steps by providing better visualisation and thorough understanding of the complete intervention including implant-prosthesis relationship. The implants are generally constructed and modelled by basic cylinders of varying length and diameter. Some software additionally incorporates realistic implant shapes and abutments of commercially available dental implants as well. The panning and zooming of the reconstructed 3D model significantly enhances the quality of the planning and assures the accuracy of the final outcome. The clinician should practice and emphasize the use of these features of the implant planning software before starting to treat patients with this method.

5.1 Determinaiton of the "panoramic line" relevant cross-sections

Initially, a guide line (called as panoramic line), along the body of the alveolar crest has to be marked by the clinician. Connected by a group of points marked by the clinician, the software calculates re-formatted images along the route of this line and displays axial, sagittal and frontal views in relevant windows. On these views, the clinician is able to see critical anatomy, the inferior and superior borders of the jaw and the scan prosthesis. By using the navigation options on the software, the clinician may "explore" the best possible location for the implant regarding the scan-prosthesis and the patients' jaw anatomy. All cross-sectional views as well as the 3D construction simultaneously interact with the response of the planning clinician (Fig. 5).

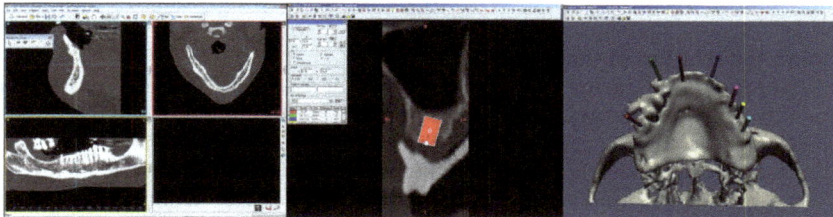

Fig. 5. Marking of the panoramic line should center the available alveolar bone width (left). The virtual implant (red rectangle) planned in relation with the scan prosthesis on the reformatted cross-sectional image (middle) simultaneously interacts with the 3D model (right).

5.2 Depiction of important anatomic structures

Proper identification of the critical anatomy relevant to the implant insertion surgery is one of the most beneficial advantages of SLA-guided surgery. By means of dedicated tools in the software, the clinician may outline mandibular nerve (*n. alveolaris inferior*), the foramens (*foramen mentalis*) as well as the maxillary structures such as sinuses (*sinus maxillaris*) and nasal base (*vomer*). Using the navigation feature on the cross-sectional images the clinician can mark these important anatomies as bright-coloured 3D structures which are also displayed on the 3D view window. The automated collision detectors of the software will warn the clinician in case of an approximation and/or collision with any of the marked structures.

5.3 Planning a virtual implant

After ensuring the best possible location of an implant the clinician may select from a variety of available virtual implants and place on any of the axial, sagittal or frontal views.

Then the length and the diameter of the implant can be adjusted according to the available bone volume. The use of the reconstructed 3D model is especially useful in the alignment of the proper implant angulation in accordance with the scan prosthesis. This procedure is rather easy if guide holes have been previously drilled on the scan prosthesis. Also, enhanced viewing capabilities of some software which allows "toggling" the view of implant, bone and the scan prosthesis either collectively or individually, may significantly improve the accuracy of virtual planning (Fig. 6).

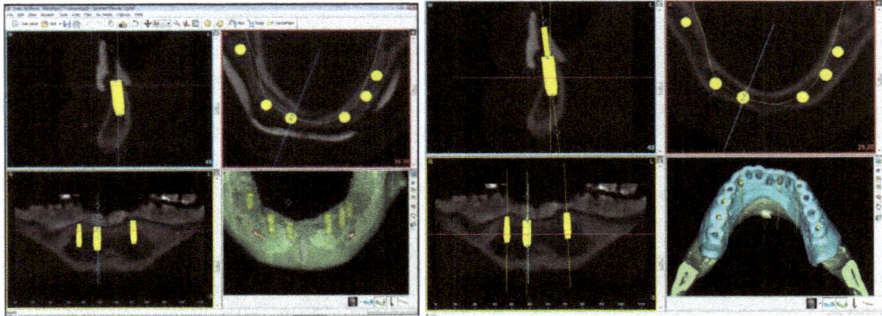

Fig. 6. The view of jaw bone, implants and the scan prosthesis can be visualized collectively (right) or individually (left).

5.4 Planning the fixation of the guide
The rigidity of the guide during osteotomy is essential for ensuring the accurate transfer of the virtual implant positions into the patients' mouth. Especially in totally edentulous cases, the guide is likely to tilt and move during the procedure. Patients'' movement, clinicians' posture and frictional resistance between the tubes and the drills can be regarded as potentially intruding during the surgery. In a previous study it was demonstrated that the use of 3 or more fixation screws decrease the transfer-error of implants placed by SLA guides (Arisan et al., 2010b).

If a solely mucosa-supported guide is planned for the case, incorporation of rigid fixation by means of osteosynthesis screws, pins etc. is essential. In tooth- and bone- supported guides this is not mandatory and depends on the clinicians' decision. Author suggests incorporation of fixation screws for all guides at the stage of virtual planning. By doing so, the manufacturer will incorporate dedicated guide holes with the exact dimensions of the fixation element. To prevent tilting and dislocation of the SLA guide during screwing (or insertion), fixation elements should be planned with a 45° angle to the horizontal plane. Manual access to the planned fixation elements should be predetermined carefully, since screws planned too apical or distal may not be managed within the patients' mouth (Fig. 7).

5.5 Deciding the type and the support type of the SLA guide
The basic role of the SLA guides is to control the direction of the implants during the osteotomy. To do so, a guide cylinder in comply with the drill diameter, is embedded into the guide. Initial use of this method was involved with multiple guides (Fig 2). Formerly, SLA guides usually consisted of multiple guides which were replaced after each use. This is of course clinically impractical and was shown to be increasing the deviations of the placed implants in comparison to the planned implants (Arisan et al., 2010b).

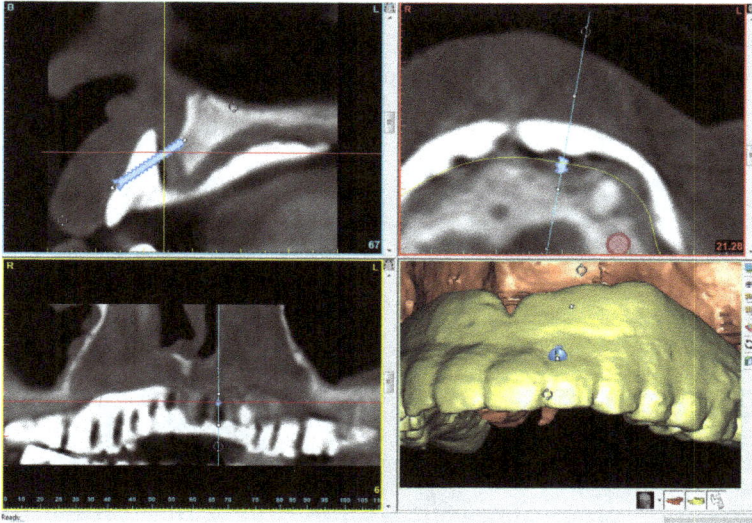

Fig. 7. To avoid shifting of the SLA guide, the fixation screws should be planned with a 45° angle to the horizontal plane.

At the stage of computer-planning, the clinician should also decide the type of support for the SLA guide. Thorough evaluation of the patients jaw characteristics is crucial when deciding the support type. It should be noted that jaws exhibiting insufficient alveolar bone thickness to accommodate the designated implant diameter have to be operated by additional augmentative procedures following a flap exposure. Basically the SLA guides can be seated on the alveolar bone, existing tooth and the mucosa. The production of bone and tooth supported SLA guides are independent of a scan prosthesis. For a mucosa-supported SLA guide, CT/CBCT imaging of the patient with perfectly fitting scan-prosthesis (the impression surface) is essential since the seating surface of the SLA guide will be an modified replicate of the involved scan prosthesis.

5.5.1 Mucosa support

Using a mucosa-supported guide the clinician may execute a flapless surgery by just removing the circular tissue over the implants by a special guided mucotome and a drill-kit with depth controlling physical stoppers. By doing so, the surgical duration as well as with the post-operative complications may significantly diminish (Arisan et al., 2010a). For performing a "flapless surgery", the alveolar bone receiving the implant body should be wide enough to accommodate a narrow-diameter (usually between 3.00 to 3.50 mm) implant. It is known that, a minimum of 1mm bone thickness should cover the implant for ensuring long-term survival. Therefore the clinician should seek for sufficient bone thickness when considering a flapless implant surgery for the patient. If any of the planned implant sites reveals a bone thickness below 1-mm in the lingual or buccal aspect of the virtual implant, clinician should consider the need of flap exposure for augmentation procedures.

In such cases, the support type can be bone or teeth (if present) or even mucosa which requires an incision for bone exposure. Alternatively, a bone calliper can be used to measure the local bone thickness under infiltrative anaesthesia. By doing so, patients exhibiting severe bone atrophy can be determined and if a fixed metal-ceramic prosthesis is not an option, the patient could be sent straight to tomographic imaging without a scan prosthesis. Because the prosthetic conformity of the implants would not be that critical in cases where gross amount of bone is missing.

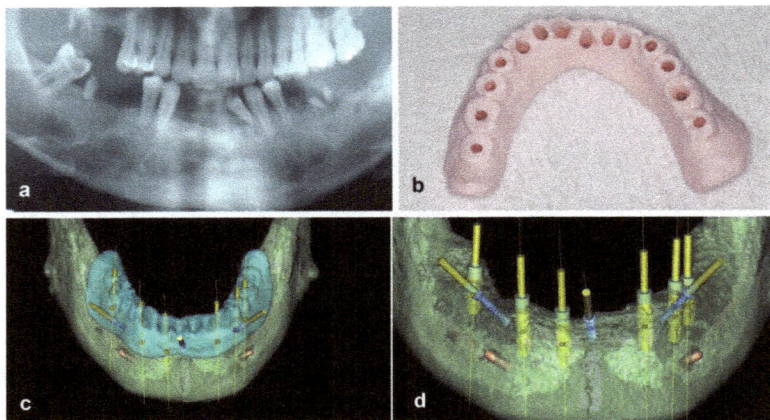

Fig. 8. a) Panoramic x-ray of the patient exhibit progressed decay and periodontal disease, b) a radiopaque scan prosthesis is prepared with guide holes to facilitate planning, c) implants were planned in relation with the scan prosthesis, d) planned implants are fully embedded into the alveolar bone and there is no need of bone augmentation.

If all of the planned implants are surrounded by a minimum of 1-mm bone, the clinician may consider executing the implant surgery without raising a flap. Delicate oral mucosa may wrap around the mucotome and drills during osteotomy and the patient may get injured. This is an additional point of concern in deciding "flapless implant surgery" using the support of mucosa. A minimum of 5 mm attached mucosa should therefore be sought on the designated implant site for ensuring the safety of the procedure. Though not generalizable, it can be claimed that the percentage of patients suitable for a mucosa-supported flapless implant surgery would be relatively small compared to bone- or tooth support. However, due to lack of incision and suturing (flapless implant surgery), the comfort of the patient can significantly be enhanced during surgery and in the post-operative period (Fig. 8); (Arisan et al., 2010a).

5.5.2 Tooth support

Healthy tooth can be used to support the SLA guide during surgery. By matching the stereolithographic implant planning data and the laser scan model of the patients' mouth (by a plaster model) a very precise fit can be assured. In the majority of the available dental literature, the tooth supported SLA guides were shown to be superior to other types of SLA guides in terms of minimizing the transfer error from the planning due to the stiff support of the teeth. This is, however, mainly dependent on the number and the rigidity of the existing teeth. It is of no doubt that the rigidity of the tooth-supported SLA guide will dramatically differ if the SLA guide is supported by a couple of periodontally compromised

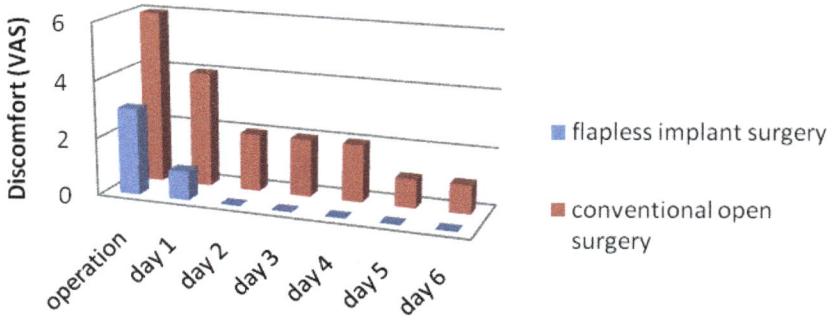

Fig. 9. Discomfort scores of patients in the week after treated by conventional implant and flapless implant surgery techniques (Visual analog scale: 0:no discomfort, 10: extremely high discomfort.).

teeth in a uni-lateral position. Heavily rotated or super-erupted teeth should also be avoided due to the presence of undercuts. The use of teeth support for the SLA guide seems feasible especially in the presence neighbouring teeth in the distal and mesial aspect of the designated implant area.

5.5.3 Bone support

Bone-support is the basic type of support in SLA-guided implant surgery and can be used in any cases irrespective of the aforementioned criteria regarding mucosa and tooth support. Simply by placing the SLA guide on the alveolar bone tissue, the osteotomy can be completed. Some clinicians prefer to use this type of support for just marking the beginning point of drilling and then continue the osteotomy and additional procedures (i.e. augmentation, bone splitting, sinus lifting) if required. Bone-supported SLA guides require additional extension of the flap borders than normal because the edges of the SLA guide may interfere with the soft tissue and hamper proper fit. This is of particular importance if multiple guides are used during the surgery as the edge of the flap may relapse under the SLA guide while switching to another guide. Amongst other type of SLA guides, bone-supported guides have the highest number of available scientific documentation.

The following diagram can be used in the consideration of support type. Nevertheless, special circumstances of each individual case should always be respected.

The final data could be sent to the production facility and usually the SLA guide can be retrieved within 2 weeks.

6. Surgical phase

The retrieved SLA guide should be checked for possible errors. The seating (or impression) surface may contain minor porous particles and may cause discomfort of the patient. Such sharp edges and irregularities should be carefully removed by proper tools. Also it is important to check the operability of the surgical hand piece on the SLA guide as some hand piece instruments may have large connections or rotational parts interfering with the SLA guide. In such cases, an alternative handpiece should be considered. Following these steps the patient must be re-examined to check the proper fit of the SLA guide when mucosa

Attached mucosa width
<5mm; possible soft tissue problems & use of mucotomes are <u>not</u> indicated : Bone -or teeth- supported SLA guides
>5mm; the use of mucotomes are possible : Flapless implant surgery via mucosa-supported SLA guides

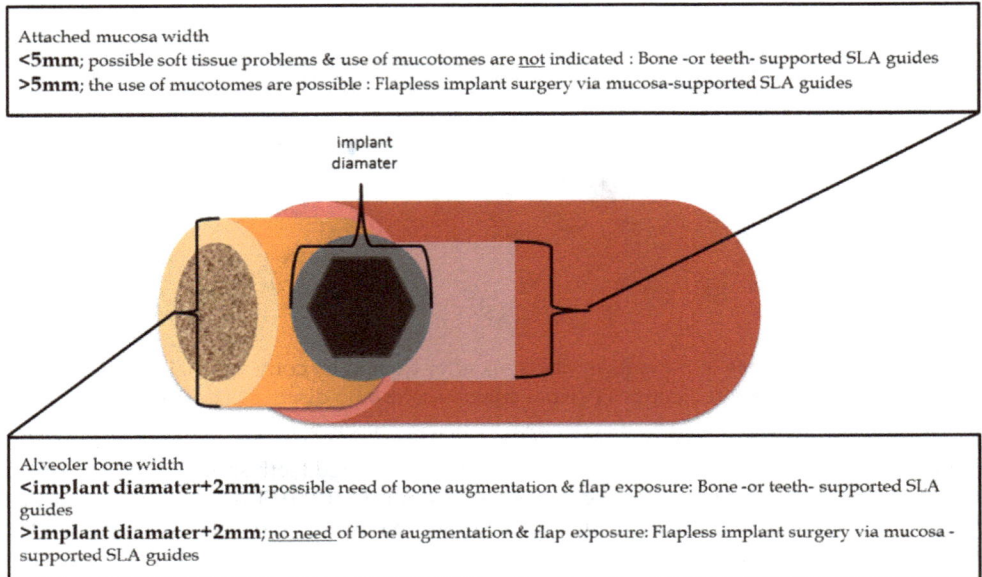

Alveoler bone width
<implant diamater+2mm; possible need of bone augmentation & flap exposure: Bone -or teeth- supported SLA guides
>implant diamater+2mm; <u>no need</u> of bone augmentation & flap exposure: Flapless implant surgery via mucosa - supported SLA guides

Fig. 10. Schematic representation of the criteria that should be considered in deciding the SLA guides' support type. The clinician should use transversal, sagittal and frontal cross-sections in relation with the intra-oral records (intra-oral photographs, bone-thickness measurements via bone-calliper and plaster models) of the patient. The need of possible bone augmentation should be evaluated for each planned implant.

and/or tooth support is used. Care should be given to ensure the accurate fit of the guide and a bite-index should be obtained to repeat the accurate SLA guide position in surgery. Additional steps can also be undertaken in this step if an immediate loading protocol is planned for the patient. By using any of the available technologies such as CAD/CAM design& manufacture or SLA-based laboratory modelling, an interim prosthesis can be fabricated prior to the surgery.

6.1 Implant surgery via CT- or CBCT-derived SLA guides

The surgical tray and related *armamentarium* should be made available in the surgical theatre. Alternatively, the equipment for the conventional surgical sequence should be ready in case of an adverse event involving the SLA guide and relevant instruments. The drilling sequence and the implants to be inserted (planned on the software) should also be prepared in a concise manner to prevent unnecessary confusion during the surgery. Some manufacturers provide a printed list of drills and implants with exact length and diameter information whereas others expect this to be listed by the clinician particularly. If a special osteotomy kit is to be used in the surgery, the relevant components and handles (or so called "spoons") should be examined before the surgery. The insertion of implants is also guided via the guided-fixture-mounts in some systems. To facilitate the surgery, guided-fixture-mounts could be connected on top of implants and could be laid-out in the proper order on the special surgical tray. With such setup, the clinician would not get confused in sustaining the right order of the implants during insertion (Fig 11).

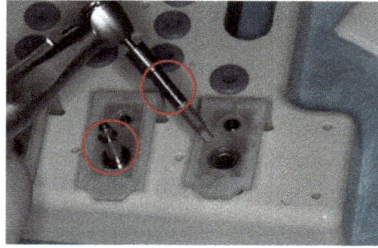

Fig. 11. Guided implant mounts (encircled by red) connected to the implants which were
laid onto the special surgical tray in the right order.

The exact replication of the accurate positioning of the SLA guide as it was during the
tomographic scan is of utmost importance for ensuring the accuracy of the implants placed
by mucosa-supported guides. To do so, the bite-index obtained in the previous examination
is extremely convenient. Using this index, the clinician should position the guide properly.
Swelling of the mucosa after infiltrative anaesthesia may slightly alter the position of the
mucosa-supported SLA guide. Therefore, anaesthetic administration through the holes of
the SLA guide while the guide is in occlusion with the antagonist jaw may be beneficial in
terms of preventing the shifting of the SLA guide. The diffusion of the anaesthetic liquid
will be slower than normal and the clinician should allocate an extended amount of time for
the anaesthesia. In tooth-supported guides, the process can be accomplished as usual if there
is no interaction of the guide with the mucosa.
Care should be given to ensure that the bone-supported guide seats properly on the alveolar
bone surface. When multiple-type SLA guides are used, the clinician must ensure proper fit
of all consecutive guides throughout the osteotomy.
If fixation screws were planned (on single-type guides only), they should be screwed while
the guide is in occlusion with the antagonist jaw. When fixing the SLA guide to the
underlying bone, all screws should be initially screwed to the end, but the final tightening of
each screw should be realised simultaneously as possible. Because tightening just one screw
to the end at once may provoke shifting of the guide towards the direction of the screw.
Also the tightness of these screws should be checked frequently during the osteotomy
because the drilling forces may loosen these screws and may induce deviations.

6.1.1 Risk of over-heating
A non-traumatic surgery is essential for ensuring the osseointegration process of dental
implants. Since the osteotomy is performed in a closed manner through the guide sleeve
holes on the SLA guide, abundant irrigation of the osteotomy area is critical to prevent
overheating. The surgeon must be aware of this risk and control the osteotomy procedure
with precaution. The operational rpm of the surgical motor should be reduced. An
auxillary irrigation source can also be utilized. Another option is to chill the irrigation
solution before the surgery. Prolonged periods of drilling should be avoided while the
drill is fully inserted into the tube. Frictional resistance will reveal itself by a metallic
sound during drilling and must be regarded as an incator of heat generation. To prevent
this, the surgeon must check and initiate the drilling in parallel to the axis of each guide
cylinder. If the SLA guide provides depth-control of the osteotomy, the surgeon can

realize the process by a simple in-and -out motion. This is particularly useful in flapless surgeries. If no depth control is provided, then the surgeon must check the exact osteotomy depth visually. This may constitute an important amount of time in cases where multiple numbers of implants are simultaneously placed. Copious irrigation of the osteotomy hole may help removal of debris prior to the insertion of implants. The clinician may insert the implants manually (following the removal of the SLA guide) if the SLA guide provides no guided-implant-insertion (Fig. 12).

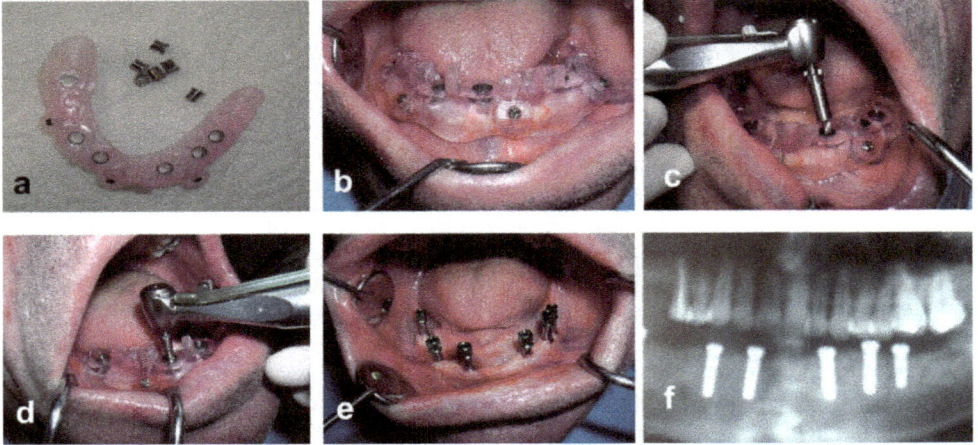

Fig. 12. a) Single-type mucosa-supported SLA guide and corresponding guiding sleeves, b) the guide is firmly fixed via three osteosythesis screws, c) a special guided-mucotome was used to remove the mucosa over the implant recipient areas, d) the guiding seleeves were mounted on the tubes of the SLA guide and osteotomy was completed with the special drill which controlled the depth of the osteotomy, e) clinical view after the insertion of 6 implants, f) post-operative radiographic view exhibits uneventful placement of 6 implants.

6.2 Guided implant insertion

Some SLA-guide systems provide guided implant insertion via the guided implant mounts provided in the special surgical kit. The length and the diameter of these implant mounts differ according to the planned implants' length and placement level and therefore the clinician must assure the correct choice of implant mounts. Guided-implant-mounts with a mismatching diameter may simply not fit into the guide tube (or will stay loose in the tube) during insertion. Similarly, an incorrect guided-implant-mount length either will not let full insertion of the mount into the tube or will leave implants partially inserted into the alveolar bone.

For the insertion of implants, the surgeon may use a torque-controlled surgical motor or may manually screw the implants using the hand-ratchet provided in the surgical tray. If the insertion of implants is to be realised through the SLA guide, the surgeon may utilize the "tripodial" placement approach to prevent the tilting of the guide. Placement of posterior implants followed by an implant in the anterior aspect will provide the "tripodial" position and prevent tilting of the SLA guide. As long as a minimum of three tripodial implants support the SLA guide, one of the implants in these positions could be removed after the insertion of neighbouring implants. Consecutive insertion of all implants without removal of any mounts may cause undesired tightening of the implant mounts and complicate the removal of mounts.

After insertion of all implants, the mounts are unscrewed and carefully removed. Following the removal of the SLA guide the implants can be checked for primary stability- a critical perquisite for assuring osseointegration (Abdel-Haq et al., 2011). Implants posing a risk of insufficient primary stability can be predetermined on the planning stage according to the gray-density values. Usually, implants placed in a bone with a gray-density value of below 250HU may yield insufficient stability upon insertion (Shapurian et al., 2006). Nevertheless, primary stability also depends on the macroscopic design of the implant body.

The clinician may decide to leave implants to "submerged" or "non-submerged" healing according to the specific conditions of the case. Additionally procedures such as bone augmentation could be performed followed by the flap repositioning and suturing. If the surgery is completed without a flap exposure, the healing caps could be screwed and the additional second stage surgery (for exposing the implants) can be eliminated.

7. Conclusion

The field of Implant Dentistry, Oral and Maxillofacial Surgery and relevant oral surgery disciplines have been recently adapted 3D imaging and virtual planning which can be regarded as performing a virtual surgery in advance of the actual intervention. Up until now, the use of 3D tomographic imaging was more common in the medical community. However, the emerging of more affordable and maintainable cone-beam tomographic scanners enabled dental professionals to provide treatment-specific planning especially for cases requiring implant insertion. Implementation of dedicated implant software the guesswork of where, which implant fixture and how to firmly place an implant is potentially eliminated.

Since implant dentistry is a matter of life quality rather than life necessity, alleviation of the discomfort throughout the treatment sequence may significantly improve the acceptance and the appreciation of the candidate patient. It is of no doubt that the technology will continue its rapid evolution delivering more efficient tools to the professionals aiming to provide better standard of care for the edentulous patient.

8. Acknowledgments

Author would like to thank Prof.Dr. Cüneyt Karabuda, Prof.Dr. Tayfun Özdemir, Assoc.Prof.Dr. Selim Ersanlı and Prof. Dr. Serdar Yalçın from the Department of Oral Implantology, Faculty of Dentistry, Istanbul University for their support. The charity and help of collaborating colleagues in the same department and assistance of Ms. Ayca Kabaoglu is also gratefully acknowledged. Last but not least author thanks Istanbul University Research Fund for the generous support.

9. References

Abdel-Haq, J., Karabuda, C., Arisan, V., Mutlu, Z. & Kurkcu, M. (2011) Osseointegration and Stability of a Modified Sand-Blasted Acid-Etched Implant: an Experimental Pilot

Study in Sheep. *Clinical Oral Implants Research,* Vol.22, No.3 (March 2011), pp.265-274, ISSN 0905-7161.

Akca, K., Iplikcioglu, H. & Cehreli, M. C. (2002) A surgical guide for accurate mesiodistal paralleling of implants in the posterior edentulous mandible. *Journal of Prosthetic Dentistry,* Vol.87, No.2, (Febryaury 2000), pp.233-235, ISSN 0022-3913.

Amet, E. M. & Ganz, S. D. (1997) Implant treatment planning using a patient acceptance prosthesis, radiographic record base, and surgical template. Part 1: Presurgical phase. *Implant Dentistry,* Vol.6, No.3, (Fall 1996), pp.193-197, ISSN 10566163.

Arai, Y., Tammisalo, E., Iwai, K., Hashimoto, K. & Shinoda, K. (1999) Development of a compact computed tomographic apparatus for dental use. *Dento-Maxillo-Facial Radiology,* Vol.28, No.4, (July 1998), pp.245-248, ISSN 0250-832X.

Araki, K., Maki, K., Seki, K., Sakamaki, K., Harata, Y., Sakaino, R., Okano, T. & Seo, K. (2004) Characteristics of a newly developed dentomaxillofacial X-ray cone beam CT scanner (CB MercuRay): system configuration and physical properties. *Dento-Maxillo-Facial Radiology,* Vol.33, No.1, (January 2002), pp.51-59, ISSN 0250-832X.

Arisan, V., Karabuda, C. Z. & Ozdemir, T. (2010a) Implant surgery using bone- and mucosa-supported stereolithographic guides in totally edentulous jaws: surgical and post-operative outcomes of computer-aided vs. standard techniques. *Clinical Oral Implants Research,* Vol.21, No.9, (September 2010), pp.980-988, ISSN 0905-7161.

Arisan, V., Karabuda, Z. C. & Ozdemir, T. (2010b) Accuracy of two stereolithographic guide systems for computer-aided implant placement: a computed tomography-based clinical comparative study. *Journal of Periodontology,* Vol.81, No.1, (January 2010), pp.43-51, ISSN 1600-0765.

Asberg, B., Blanco, B., Bose, J., Garcia-Lopez, M., Overmars, G., Toussaint, G. & Wilfong, B. (1997) Feasibility of design in stereolithography. *Algorithmica,* Vol.19 (Special Issue on Computational Geometry in Manufacturing), No.1/2, (January 1997), pp.61-83, ISSN 0302-9743.

Baba, R., Konno, Y., Ueda, K. & Ikeda, S. (2002) Comparison of flat-panel detector and image-intensifier detector for cone-beam CT. *Computerized Medical Imaging and Graphics,* Vol.26, No.3, (May-June 2002), pp.153-158, ISSN 0895-6111.

Basten, C. H. (1995) The use of radiopaque templates for predictable implant placement. *Quintessence International,* Vol.26, No.9, (September 1995), pp.609-612, ISSN 0033-6572.

Basten, C. H. & Kois, J. C. (1996) The use of barium sulfate for implant templates. *Journal of Prosthetic Dentistry,* Vol.76, No.4, (October 1996), pp.451-454, ISSN 0022-3913.

Belser, U. C., Bernard, J. P. & Buser, D. (1996) Implant-supported restorations in the anterior region: prosthetic considerations. *Practical Periodontics and Aesthetic Dentistry,* Vol.8, No.9, (November-December 1996), pp.875-883; quiz 884, ISSN 1042-2722.

Blanchet, E., Lucchini, J. P., Jenny, R. & Fortin, T. (2004) An image-guided system based on custom templates: case reports. *Clinical Implant Dentistry and Related Research,* Vol.6, No.1, (January 2004), pp.40-47, ISSN 1708-8208.

Carrafiello, G., Dizonno, M., Colli, V., Strocchi, S., Pozzi Taubert, S., Leonardi, A., Giorgianni, A., Barresi, M., Macchi, A., Bracchi, E., Conte, L. & Fugazzola, C. (2010)

Comparative study of jaws with multislice computed tomography and cone-beam computed tomography. *Radiological Medicine,* Vol.115, No.4, (June 2010), pp.600-611, ISSN 0033-8362.

Ganz, S. D. (2003) Use of stereolithographic models as diagnostic and restorative aids for predictable immediate loading of implants. *Practical Periodontics and Aesthetic Dentistry Dentistry,* Vol.15, No.10, (November-December 2003), pp.763-771; quiz 772, ISSN 1042-2722.

George, A., Zarb, G. & Tomas, J. (1985) Tissue- Integrated Prosthesis: Osseointegration in Clinical Dentistry. In: *Tissue- Integrated Prosthesis: Osseointegration in Clinical Dentistry,* (ed.) P. I. Branemark, Zarb, G, Albrektsson T., pp. 241-282. Quintessence, ISBN 0-86715-129-3, Chicago, USA.

Gotfredsen, K. & Karlsson, U. (2001) A prospective 5-year study of fixed partial prostheses supported by implants with machined and TiO2-blasted surface. *Journal of Prosthodontics,* Vol.10, No.1, (March 2001), pp.2-7, ISSN 0893-2174.

Kalpidis, C. D. & Setayesh, R. M. (2004) Hemorrhaging associated with endosseous implant placement in the anterior mandible: a review of the literature. *Journal of Periodontology,* Vol.75, No.5, (May 2004), pp.631-645, ISSN 1600-0765.

Katsumata, A., Hirukawa, A., Noujeim, M., Okumura, S., Naitoh, M., Fujishita, M., Ariji, E. & Langlais, R. P. (2006) Image artifact in dental cone-beam CT. *Oral Surgery, Oral Medicine, Oral Pathology, Oral Radiology, and Endodontics,* Vol.101, No.5, (May 2006), pp.652-657, ISSN 1079-2104.

Klein, M., Cranin, A. N. & Sirakian, A. (1993) A computerized tomography (CT) scan appliance for optimal presurgical and preprosthetic planning of the implant patient. *Practical Periodontics and Aesthetic Dentistry,* Vol.5, No.6, (August 1993), pp.33-39; quiz 39, ISSN 1042-2722.

Lekholm, U., & Zarb GA. (1985) Patient selection and preperation. In: *Tissue-integrated prosthesis,* (ed.) P. Branemark, Zarb G, Albrektsson T., pp. 199-209. Quintessence, ISBN 0-86715-129-3, Chicago, USA.

Raghoebar, G. M., Meijer, H. J., Stegenga, B., van't Hof, M. A., van Oort, R. P. & Vissink, A. (2000) Effectiveness of three treatment modalities for the edentulous mandible. A five-year randomized clinical trial. *Clinical Oral Implants Research,* Vol.11, No.3, (June 2000), pp.195-201, ISSN 0905-7161.

Reddy, M. S., Mayfield-Donahoo, T., Vanderven, F. J. & Jeffcoat, M. K. (1994) A comparison of the diagnostic advantages of panoramic radiography and computed tomography scanning for placement of root form dental implants. *Clinical Oral Implants Research,* Vol.5, No.4, (December 1994), pp.229-238, ISSN 0905-7161.

Rosenfeld, A. L., Mandelaris, G. A. & Tardieu, P. B. (2006a) Prosthetically directed implant placement using computer software to ensure precise placement and predictable prosthetic outcomes. Part 1: diagnostics, imaging, and collaborative accountability. *International Journal of Periodontics and Restorative Dentistry,* Vol.26, No.3, (June 2006), pp.215-221, ISSN 0198-7569.

Shapurian, T., Damoulis, P. D., Reiser, G. M., Griffin, T. J. & Rand, W. M. (2006) Quantitative evaluation of bone density using the Hounsfield index. *International Journal of Oral and Maxillofacial Implants,* Vol.21, No.2, (March-April 2006), pp.290-297, ISSN 0882-2786.

Turkyilmaz, I., Tumer, C., Ozbek, E. N. & Tozum, T. F. (2007) Relations between the bone density values from computerized tomography, and implant stability parameters: a clinical study of 230 regular platform implants. *Journal of Clinical Periodontology,* Vol.34, No.8, (August 2007), pp.716-722, ISSN 0303-6979.

14

Gamma-Ray Computed Tomography in Soil Science: Some Applications

Luiz Fernando Pires[1], Fábio Augusto Meira Cássaro[1],
Osny Oliveira Santos Bacchi[2] and Klaus Reichardt[2]
[1]*State University of Ponta Grossa, Department of Physics*
[2]*Center for Nuclear Energy in Agriculture, Laboratory of Soil Physics*
Brazil

1. Introduction

The first computed tomography (CT) apparatus was developed by Godfrey Hounsfield, at the beginning of the seventies of the last century (Hounsfield, 1973). For its development Hounsfield and Allan M. Cormack (Cormack, 1963), who developed the mathematical basis of image reconstruction, were rewarded by the Nobel Prize in medicine in 1979. Cormack's developments were basically focused in the reconstruction of bodies with geometries with no medical interest, like for instance, the human head.

After these first developments, some CT scanners were developed and gradually introduced into other areas of knowledge like engineering, agronomy, biology, physics, chemistry, etc. Most of the modern scanners make use of gamma and X-ray sources. However some instruments make use of neutron and positron ray sources.

Recent developments describe the use of synchrotron X-ray beams to investigate fluid transport at the pore scale (Coles et al., 1998). Some other applications of CT involve: investigation on morphological changes in small animals (Stenstrom et al., 1998); determination of soil macroporosity by chemical mapping (Brandsma et al., 1999); and dental analysis of the anatomy and some restorative materials through X-ray microtomography (Braz et al., 2001). More recently, Vontobel et al. (2006) and Winkler et al. (2006) presented the use of neutron tomography to investigate the morphology or structure of rocks and metal melts. CT allowed demonstrating the behaviour of metal melts with different densities. Voronov et al. (2010) used the micro CT (with micrometric resolution) to analyze the distribution of flow-induced stresses in highly porous media of interest for bioengineering. Flow-induced stresses have been found to stimulate the growth of cells.

Reports describing the use of the CT in soil science were published few years later of the invention of the first tomography scanner system by Hounsfield. Petrovic et al. (1982) followed by Hainsworth and Aylmore (1983) and Crestana et al. (1985) successfully reported the use of CT scanners for soil bulk density studies, soil water content and water movement measurements.

CT is a non destructive and non invasive investigation technique used to assess some attributes in the interior of an object of interest. It is essentially based on the principle of the attenuation of an electromagnetic radiation beam by the object. CT technique has been well accepted in agricultural research, due to its non invasive and non destructive characteristics, which allow repeated measurements on the same sample that does not need any pre treatment. Another important fact is that modern scanners allow investigating a sample with increasingly better resolutions. It is also important to mention that conventional image analysis techniques commonly used in soil physics (Horgan, 1998; Li et al., 2004; Pires et al., 2008) inevitably destroy the inner structure of the soil or do not allow a second measurement at the same position.

In soil science, Phogat et al. (1991) showed the potential of the use of dual-gamma energy CT for non destructive studies of the structural status and stability of soils. Rasiah and Aylmore (1998) used CT to analyze the influence of wetting and differences in structural stability on the spatial continuity of soil parameters. Perret et al. (1999) using the CT determined the geometry and topology of macropore networks. Gantzer and Anderson (2002) measured the macroporosity of soils affected by different tillage managements. Langmaack et al. (2002) and Jégou et al. (2002) studied soil rehabilitation after earthworm activities. Appoloni et al. (2002) applied X-ray microtomography to investigate thin layers of soil clod particulate systems and porous microstructures. Baveye et al. (2002) showed the importance of soil sampling volume in the determination of macroscopic parameters, like volumetric water content, volumetric air content, gravimetric water content, and bulk density. Wildenschild et al. (2002) have compared three different X-ray CTs to characterize hydrological soil properties. Elliot and Heck (2007) proposed the CT as a complementary methodology of the optical method for void space determination. In Taina et al. (2008) an interesting and vast literature review is presented for the application of X-ray CT to soil science.

In Brazil, soil science studies were firstly carried out using CT medical scanners. However, their high costs and difficulties involved in their calibrations for soil investigations make them practically unavailable for this kind of studies. This problem was solved by developing cheaper dedicated 1st generation CT scanners, designed for specific use in agronomy research (Cesareo and Giannini, 1980; Cesareo et al., 1994; Crestana et al., 1986; Cruvinel et al., 1990; Naime, 1994; Naime, 2001). Nowadays, some research groups in Brazil have been conducting studies using scanners of 1st and 3rd generation, which use gamma or X-ray radiation sources; most of their studies are in the millimetric or micrometric resolution level.

The use of CT for measurements of soil water retention and movement was introduced in Brazil by Crestana et al. (1985). Afterwards, Vaz et al. (1989), using a gamma-ray tomograph with millimetric resolution evaluated soil bulk density modifications due to conventional management practices. Cruvinel et al. (1990) presented the development of a 1st generation CT scanner which makes use of X-ray (60 kVp, 60 mA) or gamma-ray (^{241}Am, 60 keV, 300 mCi) sources, exclusively for soil physics research in Brazil. Biassusi et al. (1999) presented an investigation of soil bulk density changes in a swelling soil submitted to several hydration levels. Lopes et al. (1999) showed that the neutron tomography is able to detect small differences in soil moisture and that the methodology using neutrons provides more representative results of soil moisture variations in comparison to CT using gamma-rays. Fante Júnior et al. (2002) compared the methods of the paraffin sealed clod and CT for soil bulk density evaluations and found a good correlation between these two methods. Nonetheless, CT has the additional advantage of being a non-destructive measurement method that allows the measurement of soil density with a spatial resolution of millimeters. Pedrotti et al. (2003) described aspects of the choice of sample size for measurements of soil density by CT. Balogun and Cruvinel (2003) employed Compton scattering CT to study the soil density distribution inside samples with different degrees of compaction. Pires et al. (2004) applied CT in studies of soil structure disturbance produced by traditional sampling methods. Pires et al. (2007) used the CT technique to evaluate the radius of influence of tensiometer and soil solution extractors in field measurements. Modolo et al. (2008) used a 3rd generation microtomograph scanner to analyze changes produced by soybean seeding procedures in a non-tillage management field. In Pires et al. (2011a), the use of CT is presented to investigate the modifications that might occur in soil samples submitted to several wetting and drying cycles. A better picture of the use of CT technique applied to soil science investigation, in the past 25 years, in Brazil can be found in Pires et al. (2010).

This chapter presents some possible uses of single energy gamma-ray computed tomography (GCT) applied to soil science studies, such as: 1) soil bulk density (ρ_s) and soil porosity (ϕ) detailed determinations, 2) soil crust characterization, and 3) soil structure changes.

2. Theoretical background

2.1 Interaction of radiation with matter

Alpha and beta particles and gamma and X-radiation interact with matter in completely different ways. Due to their charges and masses alpha and beta particles interact with matter producing excitations and ionizations, what makes them lose rapidly their energy during the interaction. In the case of X and gamma-radiation, which is composed by photons, the interaction with matter is basically via: the photoelectric effect, Compton scattering, and pair production (for photons with energies higher than 1.02 MeV). These interactions make the attenuation of the radiation by matter to follow an exponential behaviour (Kaplan, 1963). The energy of the gamma-photons of interest in soil science falls in the range between 50 and 700 keV. The characteristic of an absorbing material to scatter or absorb a photon is called the attenuation coefficient. The linear attenuation coefficient (κ, cm^{-1}) represents the probability of absorption of a photon beam per unit path length (Chase and Rabinowitz, 1968). It is dependent of the density of the absorbing material (ρ, g cm^{-3}). For example, even being composed by the same material ice, water, and steam have different linear attenuation coefficients (Ferraz and Mansell, 1979). Nevertheless the mass attenuation coefficient μ (κ/ρ, cm^2 g^{-1}) of these materials are the same and are frequently tabulated as the probability of an individual element to attenuate a determined type of gamma or X-ray radiation (Jenkins et al., 1981).

For a given composit material, κ corresponds to the sum of all its chemical components (Kaplan, 1963):

$$\kappa = \sum \kappa_i w_i \tag{1}$$

where w_i represents the weight fraction of component i in the absorbing material.

The change in intensity "ΔI" of a gamma or X-ray beam interacting with an absorber of thickness, Δx (cm) is given by:

$$\Delta I = -\kappa I \Delta x \tag{2}$$

When integrated this relation provides the Beer-Lambert equation, which relates I_0 and I, the intensities of the beam before and after passing through the absorber, respectively (Colgate, 1952; Wang et al., 1975):

$$I = I_0 \exp(-\kappa\, x) \tag{3}$$

For heterogeneous systems x is considered as the sum of the length x_i of the path corresponding to each component i. For the case of soils, this summation is made over soil solid component (soil particles), soil liquid component (soil solution), and soil gaseous component (soil air). As the attenuation of the air is negligible in comparison with the other components equation (3) can be rewritten as follows (Ferraz and Mansell, 1979):

$$I = I_0 \exp-(\kappa_w\, x_w + \kappa_s\, x_s) = I_0 \exp-(\mu_w\, \rho_w\, \theta + \mu_s\, \rho_s)\, x \tag{4}$$

where the subscripts s and w stand for soil and water, respectively, and θ is the volumetric soil water content (cm^3 cm^{-3}). The density of water ρ_w (g cm^{-3}) is generally considered as unity. From equation (4) it follows that (Cesareo et al., 1994):

$$\kappa = \mu_s\, \rho_s + \mu_w\, \theta \rho_w \tag{5}$$

and it becomes clear that measurements of κ provide information about soil bulk density and soil water content. Therefore, it is possible to evaluate these soil properties using X or gamma-ray attenuation techniques (Elzeftawy et al., 1976; Ferraz, 1974).

2.2 Basic principles of computed tomography

When n regions with different thicknesses and different linear attenuation coefficients are placed along a radiation beam, the Beer-Lambert law (Equation 3) can be written as (Herman, 1980):

$$I = I_0 . \exp\left(-\sum_{j=1}^{n} \kappa_j x_j\right) \tag{6}$$

Having a set of simple transmission measurements, obtained in different orientations across a plane of an object makes it possible to map the attenuation coefficients of the material in this selected plane.

The method used for image reconstruction uses mathematical manipulation to generate a unit called TU (tomographic unit) that is assigned to each position of the plane (Vaz et al., 1989). Different colours or gray intensity values are assigned to these units, what permits to visualize or investigate the image or tomography of the plane. For instance, the tone of one point of the image can vary from white (no attenuation of the beam) to black (maximum attenuation of the beam), passing through different gray tonalities depending on intermediate degrees of interaction of the object with the beam (Brooks et al., 1981).

When a tomographic image is obtained for a heterogeneous material, the beam will cross different directions in a chosen plane of the sample and travel through regions of distinct physical properties with different thicknesses l. For the reconstruction of the image with a heterogeneous distribution of densities it is necessary to use a coordinate system (x, y) on the chosen plane to locate the measured points. In the tomographic analysis the intensity of the emerging beam is proportional to the integral of all $\mu(x, y)$ of a given path L, which is represented by the straight line for a particular source-detector pair arrangement (Kak and Slaney, 1988):

$$\ln\left(\frac{I_0}{I}\right) = \int_{r,\varphi} \kappa(x, y)\, dl \tag{7}$$

where dl denotes the integration along the beam path, the subscript r represents the measurements made in different parallel paths separated by a constant distance Δr and φ is the rotation angle of the sample, made in regular steps $\Delta\varphi$ around the line formed by source and detector.

Mathematically it is possible to define a function f(x, y), called density function M, which represents the distribution of a given physical property M along a cross section of the sample. The main objective of CT is to reproduce as precisely as possible the function f(x, y), which represents the attenuation coefficient κ of the slice of the material, that in turn is related to M. The line integral of this function in relation to (r, φ) is called ray sum or projection ray P(r, φ), given by (Herman, 1980):

$$P(r,\varphi) = \int_{r,\varphi} f(x,y)\,dl \tag{8}$$

When f(x, y) represents κ(x, y) it is possible to obtain a set of ray sums using equations (7) and (8), for a defined angle φ, called projection. Acquiring a large number of projections for different values of φ it is possible to construct the function f(x, y), which will provide a 2D image (composed of squares called pixels with a gray level that is related to its density) of the slice (Martz et al., 1990).

2.3 Computed tomography calibration

The evaluation of soil physical properties like bulk density and water content using CT depends on the calibration of the system, that basically consists in finding a relation between TU and κ for some 'homogeneous' materials.

The tomographic unit, which is related to κ of the soil in each crossing position, takes the air as the medium with the minimum possible κ value. In the case of heterogeneous materials like soils, TU is a result of the contributions from solid mineral and organic components, water, and air crossed by the radiation beam, which makes κ different for each path through the sample. Attenuation of the beam by the air is insignificant as compared to soil particles and water, and it can therefore be neglected. For a dry soil sample the relation between TU and κ is given by:

$$TU = \alpha\kappa = \alpha\ (\mu_s\ \rho_s) \tag{9}$$

For example, if the value of TU obtained by CT scanning is known for a given portion of a soil, the value μs is determined by gamma-ray attenuation measurements and the value of α is also known, it is possible to determine ρs using equation (9).

The choice of materials for the calibration determines the goodness of fitting between TU and κ. In general, homogeneous materials produce better calibration fittings than heterogeneous materials like soils (Figure 1).

During the CT calibration κ of each material is determined using the Beer-Lambert law, and in general represents an average of several measurements taken in different positions of this material. Values of TU are extracted from the tomographic images (Vaz et al., 1989; Crestana et al., 1992; Pires et al., 2011b).

3. Gamma-ray CT scanner

The results presented in this work were obtained with a first generation CT scanner with a fixed source-detector arrangement and translation/rotational movements of the samples (Figure 2).

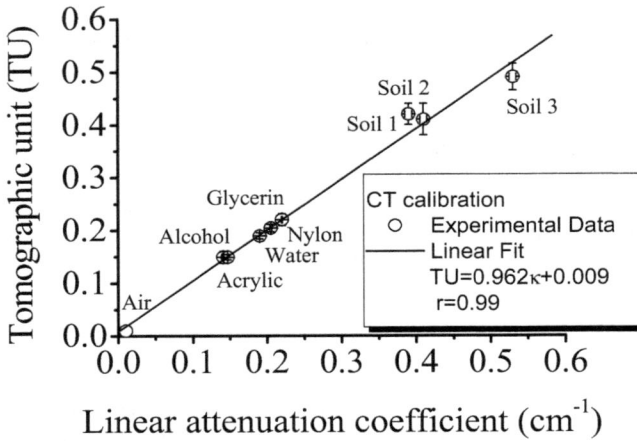

Fig. 1. Computed tomography (CT) calibration curve for [241]Am gamma-ray radiation. Error bars represent the standard deviation of the measurements. Soil 1, 2 and 3 are sand, clay loam and clay sieved soils.

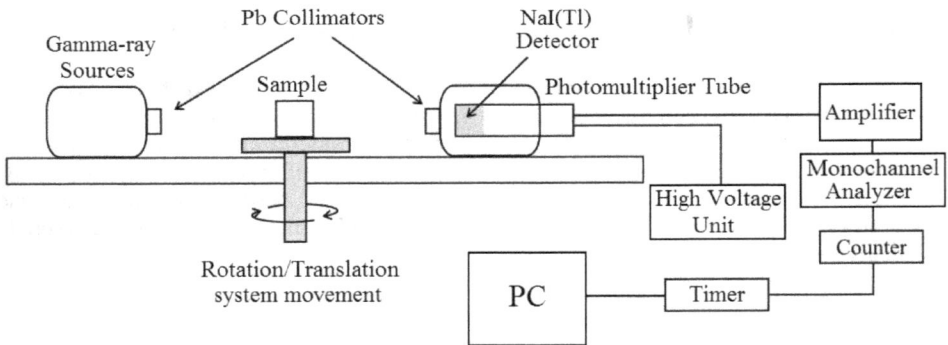

Fig. 2. Schematic diagram of a first generation CT scanner. Adapted from Pires et al. (2011c).

The radioactive sources used in the study were [241]Am (59.54 keV) and [137]Cs (661.6 keV), protected by a lead block. A NaI(Tl) scintillation crystal (7.62 x 7.62 cm) coupled to a photomultiplier tube was used to detect the monoenergetic photons passing through cylindrical lead collimators placed either in front of the source as the detector (Figure 3). The gamma detector is also protected by a lead block to minimize background radiation detection. The acquired data were stored in a PC and CT images were obtained using the reconstruction algorithm Microvis (2000).

The angular and linear steps were chosen as: 2.25° and 0.11 to 0.15 cm, respectively.

4. Soil science applications

This section presents some applications of the gamma-ray computed tomography (GCT) in soil science. The analyses were accomplished with the first generation scanner shown at the last section, which has millimetric resolution. Qualitative and quantitative results were obtained by examining 2D images of soil sample sections. The following applications will be presented to give a general notion of the power of GCT as a tool for soil science studies.

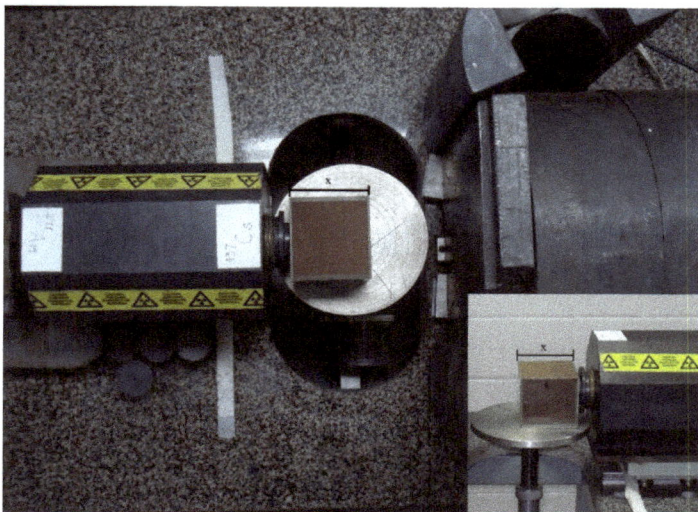

Fig. 3. Picture of the gamma-ray CT scanner located at the Laboratory of Soil Physics (Center for Nuclear Energy in Agriculture, Piracicaba, Brazil). At the left side there is the gamma-ray source, at the center the sample and at the right side the lead block covering the gamma detector and photomultiplier tube. Courtesy of Costa (2011).

4.1 Application of GCT to study soil bulk density and porosity

In this item the use of GCT is presented as a tool to obtain detailed information of soil bulk density and porosity distributions.

The soil bulk density is represented by the ratio of the mass of the solid phase of the soil for its total volume, and is determined using dried samples, i.e. samples of which the liquid phase was eliminated of its total volume using an oven at 105 °C until constant weight.

The soil porosity represents the portion of the total soil volume not occupied by soil solids. Sample features such as structure, texture and organic matter content largely influence soil porosity. Same values of soil porosity can be related to completely different soil structures and pore distributions.

By soil bulk density or porosity characterization it is possible to obtain important information about soil quality. For example, compacted soils have a much lower porosity. Soil compaction causes modifications on soil porosity and structure that are related to soil water and gas movement inside them. Soil porosity modification has as consequence the decrease of water infiltration rate, which in turn can increase the water runoff volume on soil surface which is related, for example, to furrow irrigation erosion.

Tomographic images of two soil clod samples are shown in figure 4, collected from the soil surface (0-10 cm).

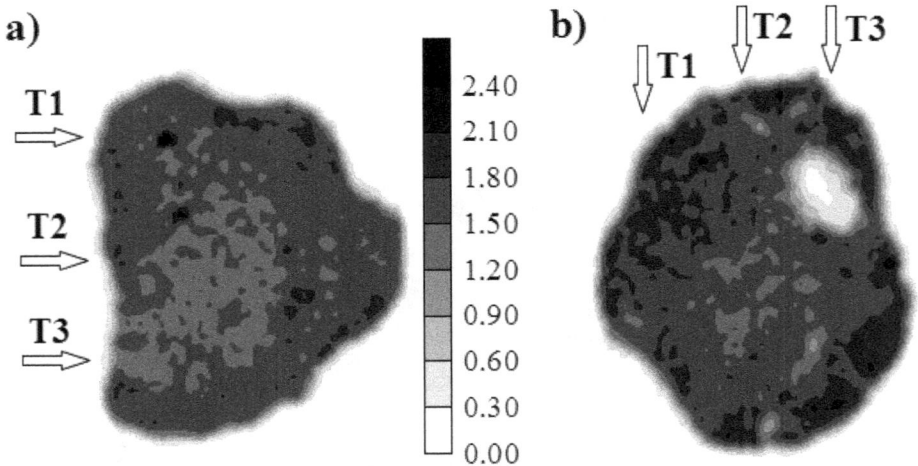

Fig. 4. (a,b) Tomographic images of soil clods collected from soil surface. T1, T2, and T3 represent transects used for quantitative soil bulk density (ρ_s) analysis. The gray scale represents the distribution of ρ_s, where white refers to the lowest ρ_s value and black to the highest.

As it can be seen in figure 4 tomographic images permit firstly a qualitative analysis of soil structure. For example, it is possible to observe dense regions (dark gray spots) and great holes (light gray or white spots) (Figures 4a and 4b) inside the soil samples. Denser regions inside the sample are probably related to stones inside the soil while the less dense regions are in general related to macropores (*e.g.* biopores caused by worms or roots).

From the images it is possible to obtain a 2D arrangement of tomographic units and consequently the global density distribution inside the investigated sample. Another advantage of the technique is that modifications inside the sample can be followed by redoing the image after any treatment imposed on it, something that is not possible by the traditional techniques such as the paraffin clod method for bulk density determination.

Using tomographic images it is possible to investigate the soil bulk density distribution and variability inside a sample. Figures 5a and 5b present ρ_s values inside samples, at each 0.115 cm (Figure 5a) and at each 0.104 cm (Figure 5b), along the linear transects T1, T2, and T3 presented in figures 4a and 4b.

From these figures some very distinct values of bulk density can be observed inside the sample. Generally these values are related to the presence of stones and holes. Along T1 of figure 5a, a global density of 2.57 g cm^{-3} can be noticed, a value close to the average stone density of 2.65 g cm^{-3} , which represent the very dark point in figure 4a. On the other hand, low bulk density values are related to holes in the sample. An example of this is observed in T3 of the second investigated clod (Figures 4b and 5b). Using information extracted from the images and the transects it is also possible to calculate an approximation of the area occupied by the hole, 1.17 cm^2, which can be related to the presence of a dead root or a wormhole.

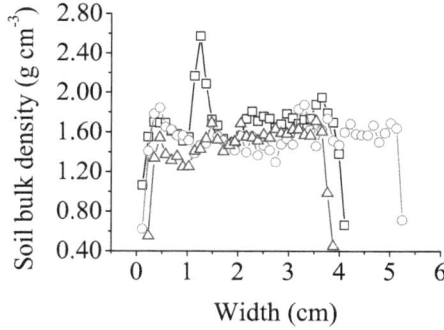

(a)

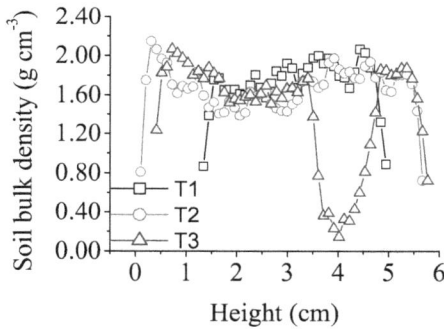

(b)

Fig. 5. Soil bulk density (ρ_s) values along linear transects (T) inside the soil clods. (a) Analysis along soil width and (b) analysis along soil height.

The average bulk density values resulted from the GCT analysis were 1.57±0.06 and 1.62±0.10 g cm^{-3} for clods A and B, respectively. Comparable values of ρ_s were obtained by the paraffin sealed clod method, average of 1.56 g cm^{-3} for these clods. The GCT technique was also used for determining the porosity (ϕ) of the samples. By the traditional method this determination is made by using soil bulk density and soil particle density (ρ_p) values, using the following expression (Flint and Flint, 2002):

$$\phi = \left(1 - \rho_s / \rho_p\right) 100 \qquad (10)$$

One artificially packed soil sample in a cylindric container of 5.0 cm in diameter was produced to show the potential of the GCT for ϕ analysis (Figure 6). To prepare the sample, 2.0 mm sieved air-dry soil was homogeneously packed in the cylinder. The tomographic image represents a cross section taken at the middle of the sample.

By the analysis of the sample (Figure 6a) it is possible to observe its heterogeneity, although such samples are in general considered as homogeneous. The analysis of the ϕ distribution shows that the soil porosity is (55±5)% (for 1880 points in the investigated plane). The large number of investigated points shows the ability of the GCT as a tool for detailed analysis of this physical property inside soil samples.

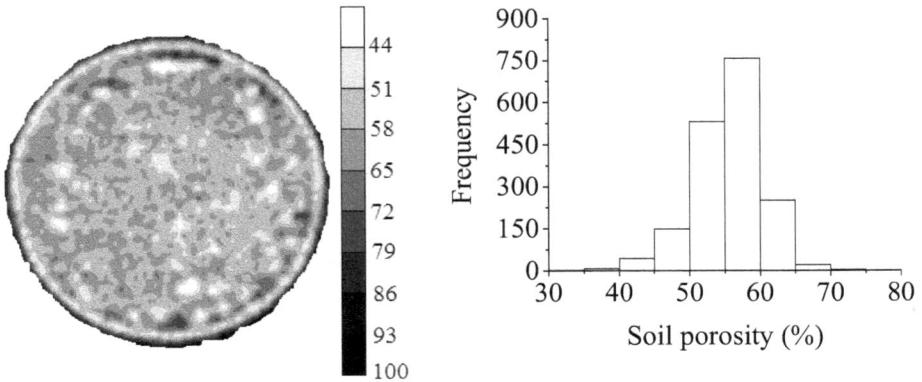

Fig. 6. (a) Tomographic image of an artificial soil sample packed inside a cylinder and (b) distribution of soil porosity (ϕ). The gray scale represents the distribution of ϕ, where white refers to the lowest ϕ value and black to the largest.

For the case of the soil clods presented earlier (Figure 4), the average values of ϕ (n=18) obtained by GCT and the traditional paraffin sealed methods were 36.2±2.6% and 36.6±2.4%, respectively, showing a very good agreement between methods.

Having in mind the potential of tomography to give detailed analysis of soil bulk density and porosity the next two items explore the use of GCT in studies of soil porosity and structure changes due to natural and/or artificial processes.

4.2 Application of GCT to study soil crust

Soil surface sealing or crusting is an important phenomenon that may occur on soil surface as a result of clay migration/orientation processes and pore plugging. The impact of raindrops promotes the disintegration of soil aggregates and the dispersion of the clay particles in soil suspension. The finest particles in suspension migrate into soil pores along with water, plugging these pores. During the drying process, deposition, migration and orientation lead to the formation of a fine hard surface layer or soil crust (Baver et al., 1973). This layer produces soil surface flooding, increasing run-off volume, which can promote laminar and furrow erosions (Pagliai and Vignozzi, 1998; Pla, 1985).

In this sub-section the GCT was utilized to investigate soil surface crusting caused by application of sewage sludge as a fertilizer. The CT technique was employed as a tool to 1) identify differences in soil density due to the sewage sludge application and 2) determine the soil crust density and thickness in the compacted layers.

Soil samples for GCT analysis (Figure 7) come from an experimental field consisted of 3 treatments [2 sludge rates (SR) + 1 control (0SR)]. The sludge rates were calculated on the basis of dry weight of sludge, that correspond to: 10 and 80 t ha^{-1} (1SR and 8SR). Soil samples were collected in steel rings of 3 and 5 cm (height and diameter) at the soil surface.

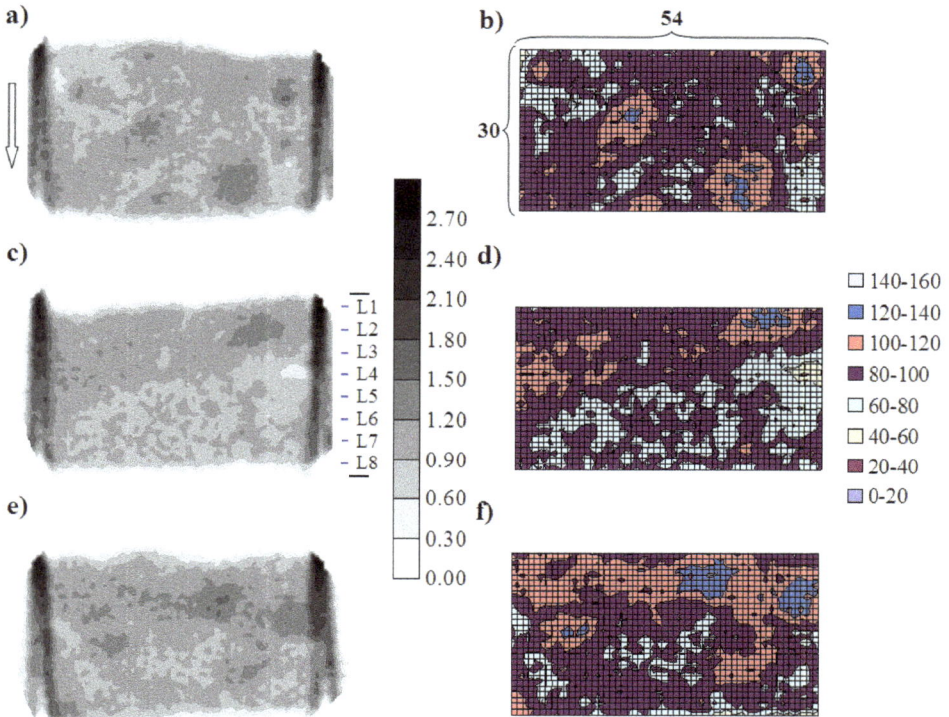

Fig. 7. (a) Absolute control sample (0SR), (b) Tomographic unit (TU) distribution (matrix of 54x30) map of the control sample; (c) Sample submitted to 10 t ha^{-1} (1SR) of sewage sludge application; (d) TU distribution map of the sample 1SR; (e) Sample submitted to 80 t ha^{-1} (8SR) of sewage sludge application and (f) TU distribution map of the sample 8SR. The gray scale represents the distribution of soil bulk density (ρ_s), where white refers to the lowest ρ_s value and black to the largest. The color scale represents the TU distribution for a matrix of data selected inside the soil image. The arrow indicates the direction of sampling at the soil surface and L represents soil layers of 3 mm each.

Soil images were obtained using a ^{137}Cs as radiation source due to the stainless steel rings. The tomographic images of soil samples were taken for vertical planes crossing the center of the sample.

GCT images (Figure 7) allowed a qualitative observation on the upper soil sample surface of the influence of the sewage sludge application. This result is more evident by the analysis of TU distribution maps (Figures 7b, d and f). For example, the comparison of the control sample (Figure 7b) and the sample with an application of 80 t ha^{-1} of sewage sludge (Figure 7f) indicates a region with higher densities in the surface. This kind of crust was induced or incremented by the application of sewage sludge at the soil surface. Nonetheless, due to sampling variability, the sample submitted to the sewage application of 10 t ha^{-1} did not present great changes in soil density at the surface in comparison to the control sample. This result is important as the appearance of a crust at the soil surface due to the sewage sludge application as fertilizer, as already said, can affect water infiltration and favor laminar and furrow erosion.

To quantify the impact of sewage sludge application on soil bulk density, linear transects were constructed (Figure 8). Each transect presents the ρ_s distribution along soil depth.

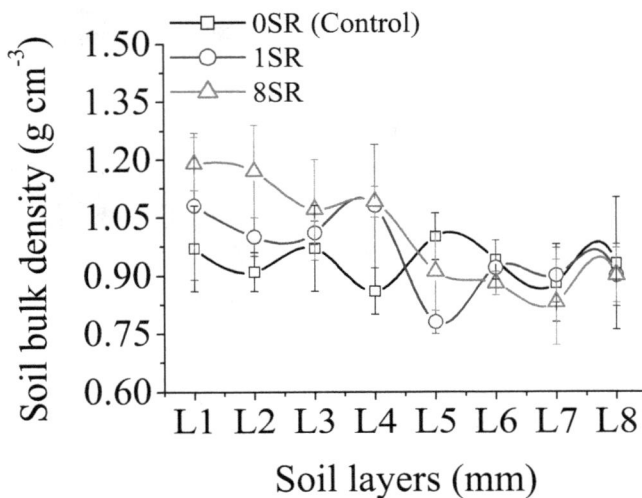

Fig. 8. Linear transects indicating soil bulk density (ρ_s) variation. Soil layers (L1 to L8) represent average values of three consecutive ρ_s determinations for layers of 1 mm. Error bars represent the standard deviation of the mean (n=3).

The analysis of the selected linear transects (Figure 8) show that the application of 80 t ha[-1] of sewage sludge induces the appearance of a crust in the upper soil surface in comparison to the control samples. Also the samples submitted to 10 t ha[-1] of this fertilizer present higher values of ρ_s at the soil surface. As expected, for the control samples (0SR) it is not possible to observe this more compacted region at the soil surface. For these samples the soil bulk density oscillates around a mean (0.93 ± 0.05 g cm[-3]). This low average value of ρ_s is influenced by the amount of organic matter content in the samples collected at the soil surface.

After the layer L5 (13-15 mm) all soil samples practically present similar values of ρ_s (0.92 ± 0.03 g cm[-3] for 0SR, 0.91 ± 0.01 g cm[-3] for 1SR, and 0.87 ± 0.04 g cm[-3] for 8SR). This result shows the impact of sewage sludge application in the upper soil surface. However, it is important to mention that if another column of the soil matrix is selected for the analysis of ρ_s variation, distinct results of those presented can be obtained due to sample variability. On the other hand, when average values of ρ_s are evaluated considering all columns a similar behavior of that reported here would be obtained.

In order to avoid the influence of artifacts of the GCT images in the quantitative results the linear transects were selected about 3 mm below and above of the superior and inferior soil sample parts. To conclude the GCT analysis allowed determining that the thickness of the soil crust induced by the sewage sludge application varied from 2 to 4 mm.

4.3 Application of GCT to study soil structure changes

In this item two applications of the GCT technique to verify changes in soil structure will be presented. The first is related to the procedure of soil sampling and the second one to the application of wetting and drying cycles in samples used to evaluate soil water retention curves.

4.3.1 Soil sampling procedure effect on soil structure

Many soil scientists have investigated the influence of the sampling volume on the evaluation of soil physical properties such as, soil bulk density, air volume, water volume, and porosity (Rogasik et al., 1999). VandenBygaart and Protz (1999) tried to define a representative elementary area (REA) in the study of pedofeatures for quantitative analysis. They showed that there is a minimum area to represent pedofeatures and that it is not possible to make quantitative analyses for smaller areas. Baveye et al. (2002) showed the importance of the soil sampling volume in the determination of macroscopic parameters, and that small sampling volumes exhibit significant and seemingly erratic fluctuations.

Instruments used for soil sampling may also affect measurements. Camponez do Brasil (2000) showed that for four different soil sampling devices, certain soil physical properties could be strongly affected by the sampling process. The equipment could cause compaction of the samples, resulting in modifications of the porous system and consequently in soil structure.

Soil compaction and changes in soil structure can cause serious alterations of soil physical properties such as bulk density. Soil bulk density as said earlier is represented by the ratio between soil mass and soil volume. So, this property gives an idea of the percentage of voids that define soil structure. Low porosity represents a more compact region of the soil sample. These compacted regions can cause modifications in the soil water storage capacity and matric soil water potential, which are parameters used in irrigation and drainage management, and therefore have economic significance in agriculture.

Soil core samples were taken from a soil profile of a Geric Ferralsol according to FAO classification (FAO, 1998), from an experimental field located in Piracicaba, SP, Brazil (22°40′S; 47°38′W; 580 m above sea level). Two different soil sampling devices were used and correspond to inox cylinders of different sizes: (1) Sampler A (4.2 cm high, 2.7 cm i.d., 25 cm^3 volume) and (2) Sampler B (5.3 cm high, 4.9 cm i.d., 100 cm^3 volume).

All samplers permit the introduction of the steel cylinders in their inner space and soil samples are collected in these cylinders by a procedure that starts with a rubber mass falling from different heights to introduce the sampler containing the steel cylinder into the soil, down to the desired depth.

After complete introduction of the set into the soil, the surrounding soil is removed with a spade. The excavation is made carefully allowing the extraction of the cylinder containing the sample for density evaluation. Caution is needed during this process to minimize vibration, scissoring and compaction effects on the structure of the soil sample.

CT analysis was performed on 10 soil samples (5 from each soil sampler) carefully collected close to the soil surface. The pixel sizes were 1.0 x 1.0 mm for sampler A and 1.4 x 1.4 mm for sampler B. The pixel size was calculated by the ratio between the inner diameter of the soil sample and number of data of the reconstruction matrix (80x80). A [241]Am (59.54 keV) was used with an activity of 3.7 GBq.

For image analysis different concentric rectangular areas (from 0.4 to 6.7 cm^2 – sampler A and from 0.8 to 24.7 cm^2 – sampler B) were selected inside soil sample images (Figures 9 and

10), where the arithmetic means of TU were calculated and converted into ρ_s, giving a general idea of the spatial variability of this parameter, in depth as well as laterally, within the sample.

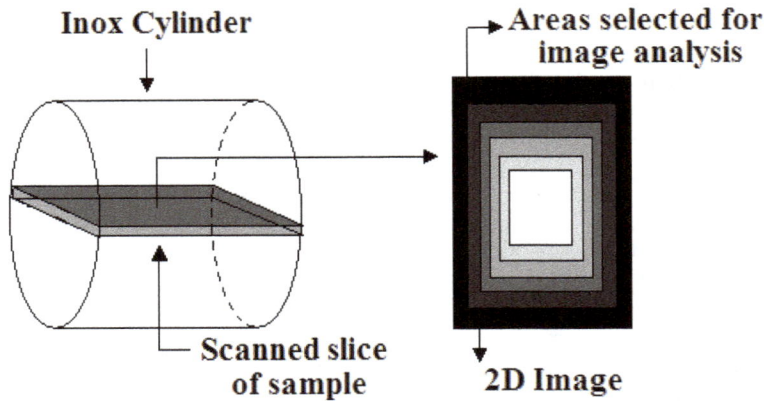

Fig. 9. Schematic diagram of the region selected for GCT image analysis and concentric rectangular areas utilized for soil sample quantitative analysis.

The mass attenuation coefficients for soil and water were 0.244±0.003 and 0.199±0.001 cm^2 g^{-1}, respectively. The obtained parameter calibration (α) used to calculate ρ_s (Equation 9) was 0.955 cm. The planes of image acquisition were vertical and the available data permitted a continuous 2-D analysis of the density distribution along the soil sample. The soil samples were air dried for several weeks before scanning.

Soil images (Figure 10) show a clear heterogeneity of ρ_s and the occurrence of larger values next to the edges of the samples. There is a density gradient for samples obtained by both soil sampler devices. However this ρ_s gradient seems to be more prominent for sampler A. For this sampler it is possible to observe a compaction at the bottom and at the top of the sample, due to the smaller internal diameter of the cylinder. Pires et al. (2004) have shown through of the analyses of transects of CT images that small soil-sampling volumes may induce compaction at the top and at the bottom of the soil sample.

The graph of ρ_s (Figure 11) confirms the existence of a density gradient from the center to the edge of samples. These results indicate that there is a compaction near the edge of sample and consequently a decrease in soil porosity. Decreases in soil porosity indicate variations in soil structure, which can affect soil hydraulic properties. Modifications in hydraulic properties can lead to important practical problems of water management of irrigated crops as said earlier.

In order to quantify the effect of sampler size in soil structure mathematical linear adjustments were constructed between ρ_s and A (ρ_s=0.09A+1.16, r=0.99 for sampler A and ρ_s=0.02A+0.84, r=0.98 for sampler B). Soil samples collected by sampler A presented the largest slope value, which indicates the great impact of this soil sampler device on sample structure in comparison to sampler B.

In order to avoid the effects of possible artifacts or fluctuations in images, as observed by other authors (Herman 1980; Paulus et al. 1999), in the evaluation of soil density, the quantitative analyses should be made selecting areas smaller than the real soil sample size inside the cylinder. With this procedure we excluded the sample strip borders very close to the cylinder walls where the abrupt density changes (inox/soil) may cause the known image distortions.

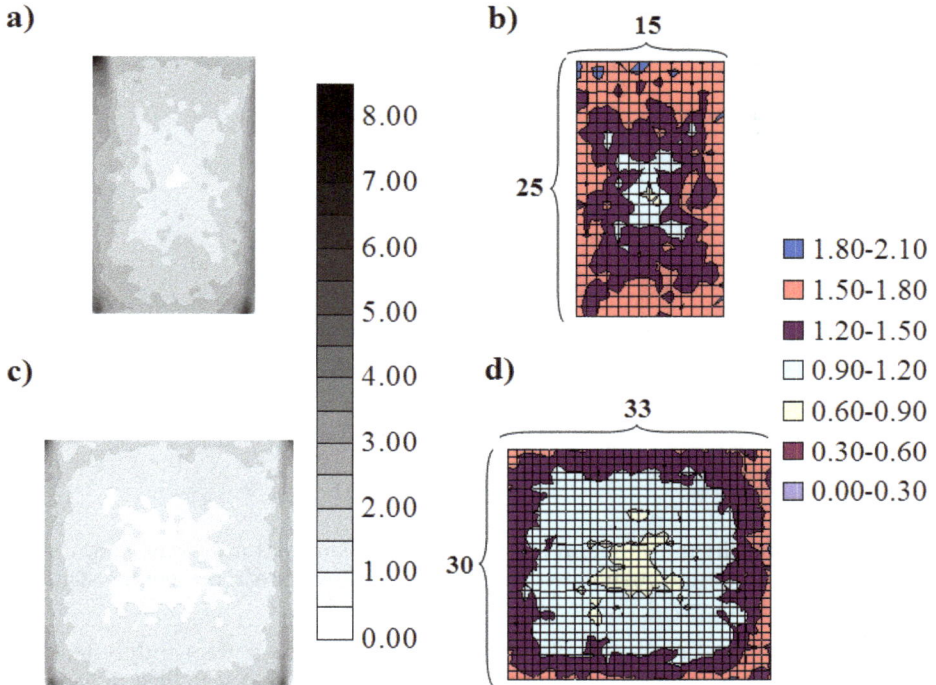

Fig. 10. (a) Soil image of the sample collected with the sampler A (4.2 cm high, 2.7 cm *i.d.*, 25 cm³ volume), (b) Tomographic unit (TU) distribution (matrix of 25x15) map of an area selected inside the sample presented in (a), (c) Soil image of the sample collected with the sampler B (5.3 cm high, 4.9 cm *i.d.*, 100 cm³ volume), (d) TU distribution (matrix of 30x33) map of an area selected inside the sample presented in (c). The gray scale represents the distribution of soil bulk density (ρ_s), where white refers to the lowest ρ_s value and black to the largest (in this specific case represent the attenuation by the inox cylinder wall). The color scale represents the ρ_s distribution for a matrix of data selected inside the soil image.

4.3.2 Soil structure changes due to wetting and drying cycles

Soil structure is influenced by several phenomena such as organic matter dynamics, soil genesis, human action, wetting/drying (W-D) cycles, and other (Kutílek and Nielsen, 1994). An important aspect of soil structure is the porosity, which consists of a continuous branching of pores of sizes classified in different categories like macro, meso and micropores (Oliveira et al., 1998). Adequate soil porosity is very important for soil aeration, water infiltration, and root distribution, allowing a better crop development. W-D cycles can cause great modifications of the structure of a soil, especially in pore distribution, which reflects the temporal and spatial distribution of soil water and, consequently, these processes can affect soil water and nutrient retention and movement. These alterations have important practical consequences when calculating soil water storages and matric potentials, widely used in irrigation management.

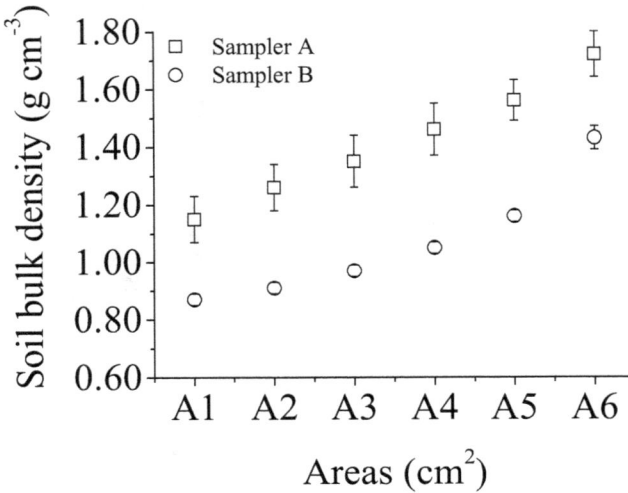

Fig. 11. Soil bulk density (ρ_s) variation with the cylinder diameter for the schematic areas (A) presented in figure 9 for the quantitative image analysis. Error bars represent the standard deviation of the mean (n=5).

The effect of W-D cycles on soil physical properties has been frequently cited in the literature (Sartori et al., 1985; Pagliai et al., 1987; Hussein and Adey, 1998; Rajaram and Erbach, 1999; Bresson and Moran, 2003; Pires et al., 2005). Soil structure, as a dynamic property, can be influenced by W-D cycles, pores being filled by water during wetting, with soil particles being rearranged irreversibly during drying. Thus, W-D cycles can affect soil resistance measured by cone penetration, particle cohesion, internal friction, aggregate size and their mechanical stability (Rajaram and Erbach, 1999). These cycles can also result in aggregate formation in non-aggregated soils restoring the damaged structure of some soils (Telfair et al., 1957; Newman and Thomasson, 1979).

According to Dexter (1988), W-D cycles affect directly soil aggregation due to the action of forces among soil particles and soil aggregates. Consequently, the soil porous system is strongly influenced by the sequences of wetting and drying cycles (Baumgartl, 1998). Wetting and drying processes produce small changes in the soil core sample volume, caused by stresses due to water/air interfaces originated from capillary forces. Therefore, after each new wetting step, the soil structure will undergo to a new state of energy, which most of the time promotes definitive changes in soil structure (Viana et al., 2004).

For this study a radioactive gamma-ray source of [241]Am was used. Circular lead collimators were adjusted and aligned between source and detector. Angular sample rotation steps $\Delta\phi$ were 2.25° until completing a scan of 180°, with linear steps Δr of 0.14 cm. The pixel size was 1.14 x 1.14 mm, calculated by the ratio between the inner diameter of the soil sample and number of pixels of the reconstruction matrix.

In order to avoid effects of possible artifacts or fluctuations in the images the quantitative analyses to determine the soil porosity was made selecting areas inside the cylinder smaller than the real soil sample size.

Core samples were taken from profiles of an Eutric Nitosol from an experimental field in Piracicaba, SP, Brazil. Six samples (3.0 cm high, 4.8 cm i.d., 55 cm³ volume) were collected at the soil surface (0 – 10 cm) with volumetric rings.

The chosen wetting process was the capillary rise, which is used during soil water retention determinations. The procedure of wetting consisted initially in maintaining a level of water 0.3 cm from the bottom of the cylinder during 2 hours and after this the water level was elevated to just below the top of the cylinder. Forty eight hours were necessary to obtain complete saturation of soil samples by capillary rise in order to avoid entrapped air bubbles, which can cause slaking of soil aggregates, changing soil structure.

The procedure used to dry samples was the application of 4.0 MPa of pressure (P) on the saturated soil sample, driving away soil water retained at pressures below P (Klute, 1986), inside a Richards apparatus. Soil samples were submitted to none (T0WD) and nine (T9WD) W-D cycles. GCT images were obtained at fixed water contents, to avoid differences in soil images due to differences in the residual water content after each treatment.

The procedure used to obtain fixed water contents, after W-D cycles, was to maintain samples in contact with air until a residual value of θ. When samples, after T0WD and T9WD, reached this residual water content they were involved in plastic film, to minimize water loss, and submitted to CT scanning.

Mass attenuation coefficients were obtained using the method described in Ferraz and Mansell (1979) and the following results were obtained: 0.328±0.003 (soil) and 0.199± 0.001 cm² g⁻¹ (water). The calibration of GCT presented a high positive correlation coefficient (r=0.99). Qualitative analyses of changes in soil structure were obtained by soil image analysis (Figure 12).

From the GCT images (Figure 12) it was possible to visualize modifications in soil structure. In the T0WD sample (Figures 12a and 12b), the existence of compacted regions can be seen at the upper and at the lower layers (Layers A and F) of the sample. Higher ρ_s at layer A was a characteristic of the investigated sample while that at the bottom probably was due to sampling preparation that, in this case consisted in making the sample bottom flat with a sharp blade. However, after the application of nine W-D cycles (Figures 12c and 12d) to the same sample it is possible to observe that ρ_s values in the investigated layers decreased, with more evidence in the more compacted layers.

These results indicate that significant modifications in soil water retention characteristics can occur due to W-D cycles. The changes of the soil pore systems will affect water retention properties due to changes in ϕ. This result can represent a repair of soil structure, having as an impact increases in the water storing capacity, important for plant and root development.

A better analysis of changes in soil structure with the W-D cycles along depth can be obtained through quantitative analysis of ϕ variation (Figure 13). To investigate the effects of W-D cycles on ϕ, each investigated sample was divided in six regions, named from A to F as schematically presented in figure 12. In this particular experimental setting up, each subsequent layer was around 4.5mm apart one from the other.

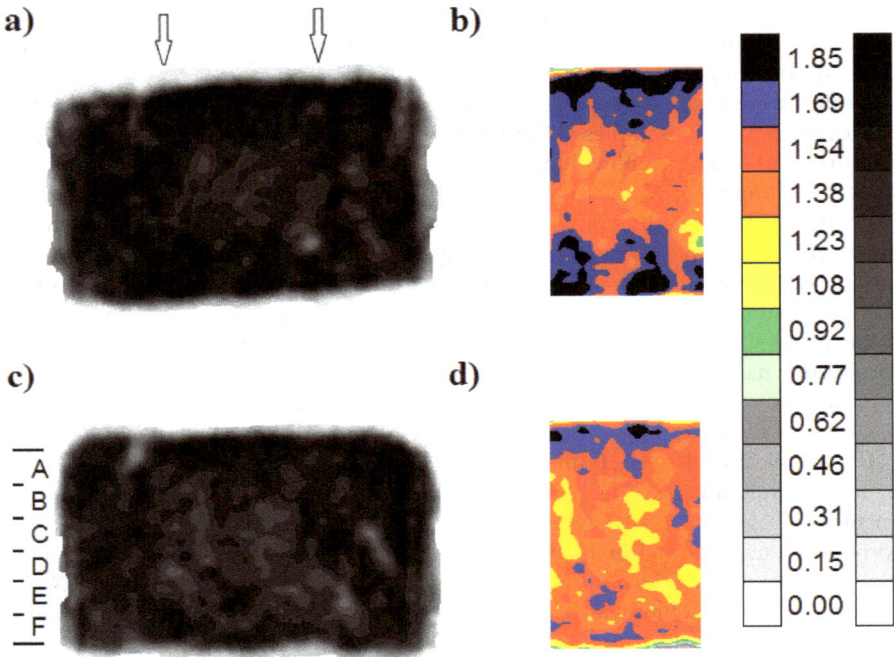

Fig. 12. (a) 2-D tomographic images of core samples used to evaluate soil bulk density (ρ_s) and porosity by image (ϕ) variations of samples not submitted to wetting and drying (W-D) cycles, (b) Tomographic unit (TU) distribution (matrix of 80x20) map of an area selected inside the sample presented in (a), (c) Soil image of the sample submitted to 9 W-D cycles by the capillary rise method, (d) TU distribution map of an area selected inside the sample presented in (c). The gray and color scales represent the distribution of ρ_s. For the gray scale white refers to the lowest ρ_s value and black to the largest. Arrows indicate the region (matrix of 1600 (80x20) TU values) of soil structure change analysis (b-d). Letters A to F represent soil layers defined for quantitative analysis.

As it can be seen, the application of W-D cycles caused increases in ϕ mainly for the layers (L-A and L-F) near to the border of samples (Figures 13a and 13f). This result is characterized by the increase in the frequency of higher ϕ values. The application of W-D cycles expands the ϕ distribution. This result means that the W-D cycles can induce the appearance of large macropores in the soil samples and a more heterogeneous distribution of ϕ. This result is particularly interesting to soil science because it represents an improvement of soil structure.

The analyses of results along depth show that the changes in ϕ for intermediate depths (L-C and L-D) are smoother (Figures 13c and 13d) than those for layers next to the sample border. This result can be explained by the soil sampling procedure and by the fact that the most significant changes in ϕ occur in the most compacted regions in figure 12 (layers A, E and F). It is expected that the most significant changes occur in the outer layers, because the soil in these regions can also freely expand with the W-D cycles.

Layer A (L-A)

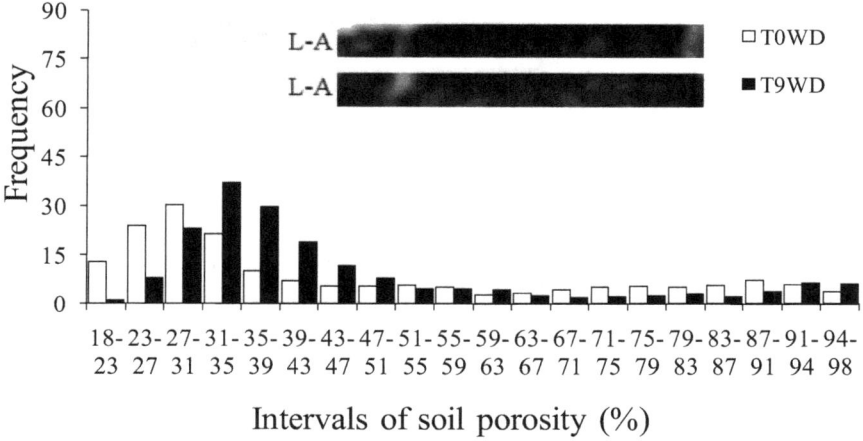

(a)

Layer B (L-B)

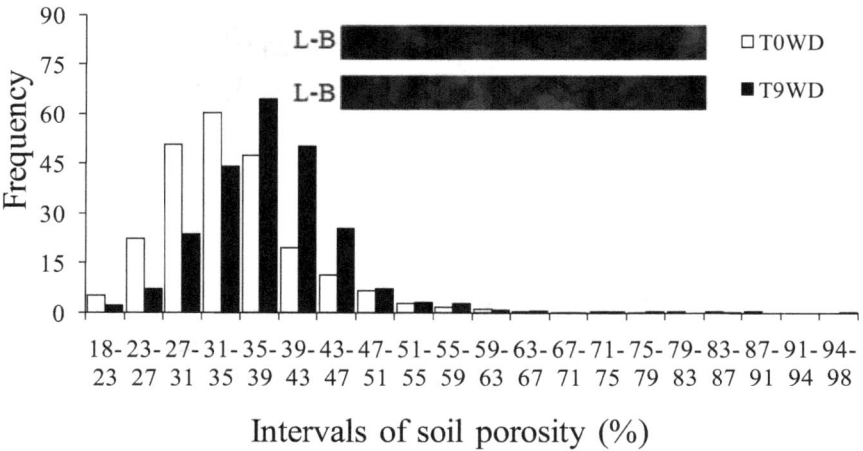

(b)

Layer C (L-C)

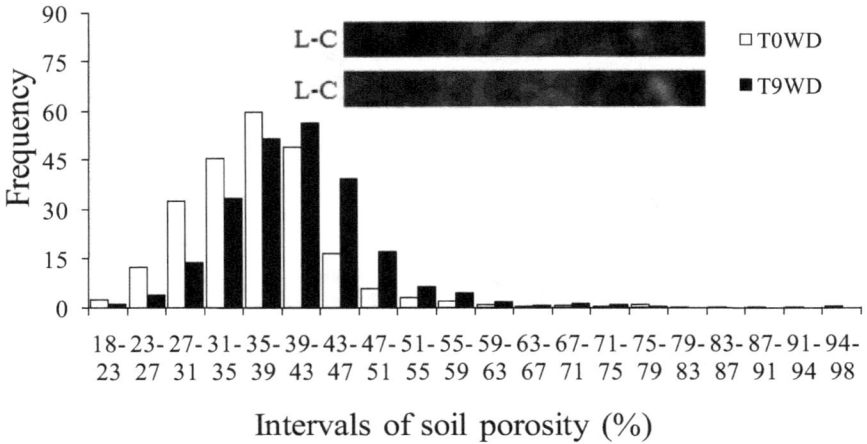

(c)

Layer D (L-D)

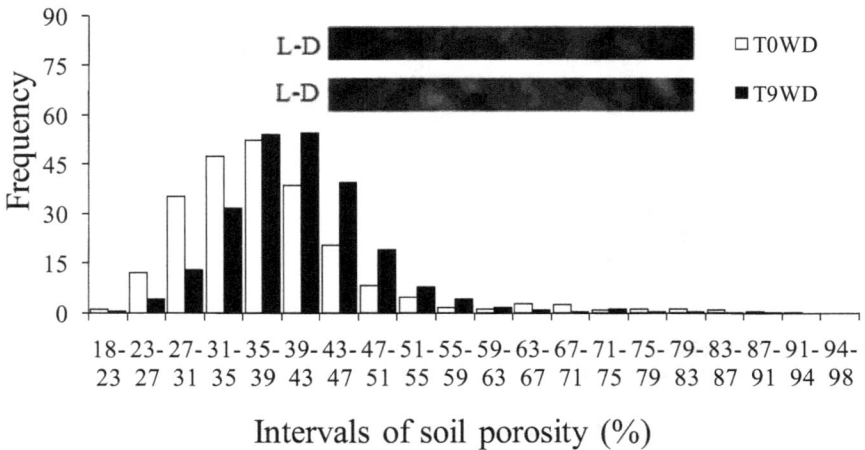

(d)

Layer E (L-E)

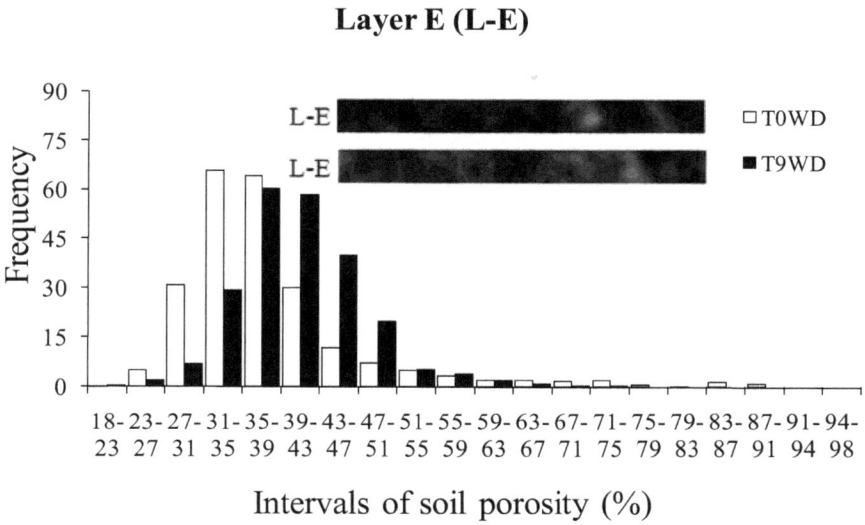

(e)

Layer F (L-F)

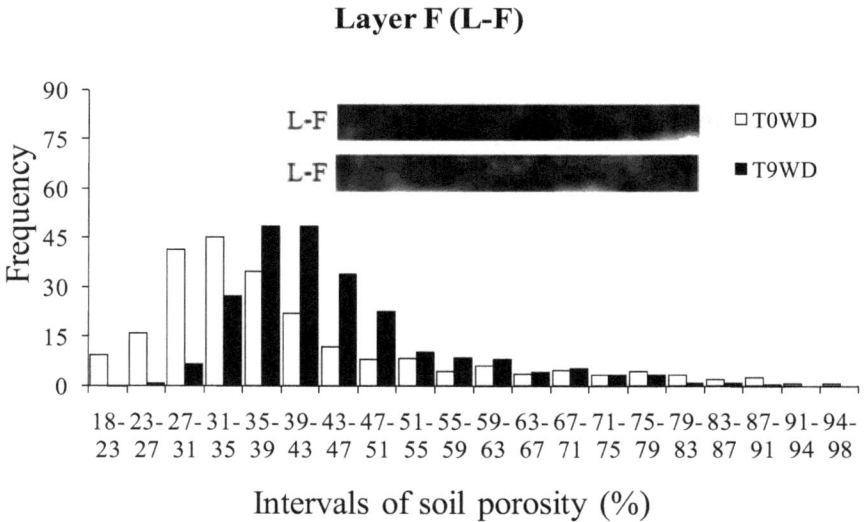

(f)

Fig. 13. (a-f) Changes in soil porosity (φ) along soil sample depth. T0WD and T9WD represents soil samples not submitted to wetting and drying (W-D) cycles and submitted to 9 W-D, respectively. Values of φ represent average of six replicates. The layer pictures (L slices) presented on the graphs is only illustrative for the specific sample presented in figures 12a and 12c.

5. Future expectations on the use of CT in soil physics

From the discussion on the GCT technique it can clearly be seen that it has been applied with success in the analysis of physical properties of soils. With the investments that have been made in equipment exclusively projected for this purpose it is expected that CT will gradually be able to yield more representative results of these properties.

New tomographic models based on the use of radiation from synchrotron light, positrons and neutrons may become interesting alternatives for the study of soil physical characteristics, opening the possibility of obtaining images of better resolution and also presenting greater sensitivity to monitor soil water content changes. The development of new microtomographs of 3rd and 4th generation for specific use in soil science can also be an interesting alternative for dynamic soil water studies.

Studies of the dynamics of root growth can also be carried out in a non invasive way using microtomographs. Systems that make use of X-ray or synchrotron light beams can be used with success in this type of investigation since they allow the analysis of samples of very large size such as 20 cm or more. Third generation scanners of X-rays and with micrometric resolution allow quick analyses of soil structure in 3D, which may be useful for dynamic processes that occur inside the soil.

The broadening of the use of the 3rd generation X-ray microtomography that work in soil science would certainly lead to new applications of CT that would bring new developments related to soil structure, like more realistic studies on tortuosity, connectivity, shape, size, and pore distribution. Such information, until now not well explored will help in a significant way the construction of models for flow processes involving hydraulic conductivity, solute infiltration, root development, and would produce more representative images for the numeric simulation of these important physical processes that take place in soils.

6. Acknowledgment

The authors would like to thank the Brazilian agency 'Conselho Nacional de Desenvolvimento Científico e Tecnológico' (CNPq) for the research fellowships to Klaus Reichardt, Luiz F. Pires and Osny O.S. Bacchi.

7. References

Appoloni, C.R., Macedo, A., Fernandes, C.P. & Philippi, P.C. (2002). Characterization of porous microstructure by X-ray microtomography. *X-Ray Spectrometry*, 31, 124-127

Balogun, F.A. & Cruvinel, P.E. (2003). Compton scattering tomography in soil compaction study. *Nuclear Instruments and Methods in Physics Research A*, 505, 502-507

Baumgartl, Th. (1998). Physical soil properties in specific fields of application especially in anthropogenic soils. *Soil and Tillage Research*, 47, 51-59

Baver, L.D., Gardner, W.J. & Gardner, W.R. (1973). *Física de suelos,* Union Tipográfica Editorial Hispano Americana, Mexico

Baveye, P., Rogasik, H., Wendroth, O., Onasch, I. & Crawford, J.W. (2002). Effect of sampling volume on the measurement of soil physical properties: simulation with X-ray tomography data. *Measurement Science Technology,* 13, 775-784

Biassusi, M., Pauletto, E.A. & Crestana, S. (1999). Estudo da deformação de um vertissolo por meio da tomografia computadorizada de dupla energia simultânea. *Revista Brasileira de Ciência do Solo,* 23, 1-7

Brandsma, R.T., Fullen, M.A., Hocking, T.J. & Allen, J.R. (1999). An X-ray scanning technique to determine soil macroporosity by chemical mapping. *Soil and Tillage Research*, 50, 95-98

Braz, D., Barroso, R.C., Lopes, R.T., Anjos, M.J. & Jesus, E.F.O. (2001). Evaluation of scatter-to-primary ratio in soil CT-imaging. *Radiation Physics and Chemistry*, 61, 747-751

Bresson, L.M. & Moran, C.J. (2003). Role of compaction versus aggregate disruption on slumping and shrinking of repacked hardsetting seedbeds. *Soil Science*, 168, 585-594

Brooks, R.A., Mitchell, L.G., O'Conner, C.M. & Di Chiro, G. (1981). On the relationship between computed tomography numbers and specific gravity. *Physics in Medicine and Biology*, 26, 141-147

Camponez do Brasil, R.P. (2000). Influência das técnicas de coleta de amostras na determinação das propriedades físicas do solo. Master Thesis, Universidade de São Paulo, Piracicaba, Brazil, 110p

Cesareo, R. & Giannini, M. (1980). Elemental analysis by means of X-ray attenuation measurements. *Nuclear Instruments and Methods*, 169, 551-555

Cesareo, R., Assis, J.T. & Crestana, S. (1994). Attenuation coefficients and tomographic measurements for soil in the energy range 10-300 keV. *Applied Radiation and Isotopes*, 45, 613-620

Chase, G.D. & Rabinowitz, J.L. (1968). *Principles of radioisotope methodology*, Burgess Publishing Co., Minneapolis, USA

Coles, M.E., Hazlett, R.D., Muegge, E.L., Jones, K.W., Andrews, B., Dowd, B., Siddons, P., Peskin, A., Spanne, P. & Soll, W. (1998). Developments in synchrotron X-ray microtomography with applications to flow in porous media. *SPE Reservoir Evaluation and Engineering*, 1, 288-296

Colgate, S.A. (1952). Gamma-ray absorption measurements. *Physics Review*, 87, 592-600.

Cormack, A.M. (1963). Representation of a foundation by its line with some radiological application. *Journal of Applied Physics*, 34, 2722-2727

Costa, J.C. (2011). Tamanho do colimador e espessura da amostra em medidas do coeficiente de atenuação de raios gama do solo. Master Thesis, Universidade Estadual de Ponta Grossa, Ponta Grossa, Brazil, 105p

Crestana, S., Mascarenhas, S. & Pozzi-Mucelli, R.S. (1985). Static and dynamic 3D studies of water in soil using computed tomographic scanning. *Soil Science*, 140, 326-332

Crestana, S., Cesareo, R. & Mascarenhas, S. (1986). Using a computed tomography miniscanner in soil science. *Soil Science*, 142, 56-61

Crestana, S., Cruvinel, P.E., Vaz, C.M.P., Cesareo, R., Mascarenhas, S. & Reichardt, K. (1992). Calibração e uso de um tomógrafo computadorizado em ciência do solo. *Revista Brasileira de Ciência do Solo*, 16, 161-167

Cruvinel, P.E., Cesareo, R., Crestana, S. & Mascarenhas, S. (1990). X- and gamma-rays computerized minitomograph scanner for soil science. *IEEE Transactions on Instrumentation and Measurement*, 39, 745-750

Dexter, A.R. (1988). Advances in characterization of soil structure. *Soil and Tillage Research*, 11, 199-238

Elliot, T.R. & Heck, R.J. (2007). A comparison of optical and X-ray CT technique for void analysis in soil thin section. *Geoderma*, 141, 60-70

Elzeftawy, A., Mansell, R.S. & Selim, H.M. (1976). Distribution of water and herbicide in Lakeland sand during initial stages of infiltration. *Soil Science*, 122, 297-307

Fante Júnior, L., Oliveira J.C.M., Bassoi, L.H., Vaz, C.M.P., Macedo, A., Bacchi, O.O.S., Reichardt, K., Cavalcanti, A.C. & Silva, F.H.B.B. (2002). Tomografia

Computadorizada na avaliação da densidade de um solo do semi-árido brasileiro. *Revista Brasileira de Ciência do Solo*, 26, 835-842

FAO. (1998). *World reference base for soil resources*, FAO, ISRIC and ISSS, Rome, Italy

Ferraz, E.S.B. (1974). Determinação simultânea de densidade e umidade de solos por atenuação de raios gama do [137]Cs e [241]Am. Free Teaching Thesis, Universidade de São Paulo, Piracicaba, Brazil,120p

Ferraz, E.S.B. & Mansell, R.S. (1979). Determining water content and bulk density of soil by gamma-ray attenuation methods. *Technical Bulletin*, 807, IFAS, Flórida, USA 51p

Flint, A.L. & Flint, L.E. (2002). The solid phase: Particle density. In: Dane, J.H. & Topp, G.C. (Eds.), *Methods of soil analysis. Part 4. Physical Methods*. ASA, SSSA, Madison, USA p.229-240

Gantzer, C.J. & Anderson, S.H. (2002). Computed tomographic measurement of macroporosity in chisel-disk and no-tillage seedbeds. *Soil and Tillage Research*, 64, 101-111

Hainsworth, J.M. & Aylmore, L.A.G. (1983). The use of computer-assisted tomography to determine spatial distribution of soil water content. *Australian Journal of Soil Research*, 21, 435-443

Herman, G.T. (1980). *Image reconstruction from projections*, Academic Press, London, UK

Horgan, G.W. (1998). Mathematical morphology for analyzing soil structure from images. *European Journal of Soil Science*, 49, 161-173

Hounsfield, G.N. (1973). Computerized transverse axial scanning (tomography). 1. Description of system. *British Journal of Radiology*, 46, 1016-1022

Hussein, J. & Adey, M.A. (1998). Changes in microstructure, voids and b-fabric of surface samples of a Vertisol caused by wet/dry cycles. *Geoderma*, 85, 63-82

Jégou, D., Brunotte, J., Rogasik, H., Capowiez, Y., Diestel, H., Schrader, S. & Cluzeau, D. (2002). Impact of soil compaction on earthworm burrow systems using X-ray computed tomography: preliminary study. *Soil Biology*, 38, 329-336

Jenkins, R., Gould, R.W. & Gedcke, D. (1981). *Qualitative X-ray spectrometry*, Marcel Dekker, New York, USA

Kak, A.C. & Slaney, M. (1988). *Principles of computerized tomographic imaging*, IEEE Press, New York, USA

Kaplan, I. (1963). *Nuclear Physics*, Addison-Wesley Publishing Co., Reading, USA

Klute, A. (1986). Water retention: laboratory methods. In: Black, C.A. (Ed.), *Methods of soil analysis. I. Physical and mineralogical methods*. ASA, SSSA, Madison, USA, p.635-662

Kutílek, M. & Nielsen, D.R. (1994). *Soil hydrology*, Catena Verlag, Berlin, Germany

Langmaak, M., Schrader, S., Rapp-Bernhardt, U. & Kotze, K. (2002). Soil structure rehabilitation of arable soil degraded by compaction. *Geoderma*, 105, 141-152

Li, D., Velde, B. & Zhang, T. (2004). Observations of pores and aggregates during aggregation in some clay-rich agricultural soils as seen in 2D image analysis. *Geoderma*, 118, 191-207

Lopes, R.T., Bessa, A.P., Braz, D. & Jesus E.F.O. (1999). Neutron computerized tomography in compacted soil. *Applied Radiation and Isotopes*, 50, 451- 458

Martz, H.E., Azevedo, S.G., Brase, J.M., Waltjen, K.E. & Schneberk, D.J. (1990). Computed tomography systems and their industrial applications. *Applied Radiation and Isotopes*, 41, 943-961

MICROVIS. (2000). *Programa de reconstrução e visualização de imagens tomográficas*, Embrapa Instrumentação Agropecuária, São Carlos, Brazil

Modolo, A.J., Fernandes, H.C., Naime, J.M., Schaefer, C.E.G.R., Santos, N.T. & Silveira, J.C.M. (2008). Avaliação do ambiente solo-semente por meio da tomografia computadorizada. *Revista Brasileira de Ciência do Solo*, 32, 525-532

Naime, J. de M. (1994). Projeto e construção de um minitomógrafo portátil para estudo de ciência do solo e plantas em campo. Master Thesis, Universidade de São Paulo, São Carlos, Brazil, 87p

Naime, J. de M. (2001). Um novo método para estudos dinâmicos, in situ, da infiltração da água na região não-saturada do solo. Ph.D. Thesis, Universidade de São Paulo, São Carlos, Brazil, 145p

Newman, A.C.D. & Thomasson, A.J. (1979). Rothamsted studies of soil structure: III. Pore size distributions and shrinkage processes. *Journal of Soil Science*, 30, 415-439

Oliveira, J.C.M., Appoloni, C.R., Coimbra, M.M., Reichardt, K., Bacchi, O.O.S., Ferraz, E., Silva, S.C. & Galvão Filho, W. (1998). Soil structure evaluated by gamma-ray attenuation. *Soil and Tillage Research*, 48, 127-133

Pagliai, M., La Marca, M. & Lucamante, G. (1987). Changes in soil porosity in remolded soils treated with poultry manure. *Soil Science*, 144, 128-140

Pagliai, M. & Vignozzi, N. (1998). Use of manure for soil improvement. In: Wallace, A. & Terry, R.E. (Eds.), *Handbook of soil conditions: Substances that enhance the physical properties of soil*. Marcel Dekker, New York, USA

Paulus, M.J., Sari-Sarraf, H., Gleason, S.S., Bobrek, M., Hicks, J.S., Johnson, D.K., Behel, J.K., Thompson, L.H. & Allen, W.C. (1999). A new X-ray computed tomography system for laboratory mouse imaging. *IEEE Transactions on Nuclear Science*, 46, 558-564

Pedrotti, A., Pauletto E.A., Crestana S., Cruvinel P.E., Vaz, C.M.P., Naime, J.M. & Silva, A.M. (2003). Planosol soil sample size for computerized tomography measurement of physical parameters. *Scientia Agricola*, 60, 735-740

Perret, J., Prasher, S.O., Kantzas, A. & Langford, C. (1999). Three-dimensional quantification of macropore networks in undisturbed soil cores. *Soil Science Society of America Journal*, 63, 1530-1543

Petrovic, A.M., Siebert, J.E. & Rieke, P.E. (1982). Soil bulk density analysis in three dimensions by computed tomographic scanning. *Soil Science Society of America Journal*, 46, 445- 450

Phogat, V.K., Aylmore, L.A.G. & Schuller, R.D. (1991). Simultaneous measurement of the spatial-distribution of soil-water content and bulk-density. *Soil Science Society of America Journal*, 55, 908-915

Pires, L.F., Bacchi, O.O.S. & Reichardt, K. (2004). Damage to soil physical properties caused by soil sampler devices assessed by gamma ray computed tomography. *Australian Journal of Soil Research*, 42, 857-863

Pires, L.F., Bacchi, O.O.S. & Reichardt, K. (2005). Gamma ray computed tomography to evaluate wetting/drying soil structure changes. *Nuclear Instruments and Methods in Physics Research B*, 229, 443-456

Pires, L.F., Arthur, R.C.J., Bacchi, O.O.S. & Reichardt, K. (2007). Application of gamma-ray computed tomography to evaluate the radius of influence of soil solution extractors and tensiometers. *Nuclear Instruments and Methods in Physics Research B*, 259, 969-974

Pires, L.F., Cooper, M., Cássaro, F.A.M., Bacchi, O.O.S., Reichardt, K. & Dias, N.M.P. (2008). Micromorphological analysis to characterize structure modifications of soil samples submitted to wetting and drying cycles. *Catena*, 72, 297-304

Pires, L.F., Borges, J.A.R., Bacchi, O.O.S. & Reichardt, K. (2010). Twenty-five years of computed tomography in soil physics: A literature review of the Brazilian contribution. *Soil and Tillage Research*, 110, 197-210

Pires, L.F., Cássaro, F.A.M., Bacchi, O.O.S. & Reichardt, K. (2011a). Non-destructive image analysis of soil surface porosity and bulk density dynamics. *Radiation Physics and Chemistry*, 80, 561-566

Pires, L.F., Arthur, R.C.J., Bacchi, O.O.S. & Reichardt, K. (2011b). Representative gamma-ray computed tomography calibration for applications in soil physics. *Brazilian Journal of Physics*, 41, 21-28

Pires, L.F., Cássaro, F.A.M., Saab, S.C. & Brinatti, A.M. (2011c). Characterization of changes in soil porous system by gamma-ray tomography. *Nuclear Instruments and Methods in Physics Research A*, 644, 68-71

Pla, I. (1985). A routine laboratory index to predict the effects of soil sealin on soil and water conservation. In. *International Symposium on the assessment of soil surface sealing and crusting*. Ghent, Belgium. ISSS. AISS. IBG, pp.154-162

Rajaram, G. & Erbach, D.C. (1999). Effect of wetting and drying on soil physical properties. *Journal of Terramechanics*, 36, 39-49

Rasiah, V. & Aylmore, L.A.G. (1998). Computed tomography data on soil structural and hydraulic parameters assessed for spatial continuity by semivariance geostatistics. *Australian Journal of Soil Research*, 36, 485-493

Rogasik, H., Crawford, J.W., Wendroth, O., Young, I.M., Joshko, M. & Ritz, K. (1999). Discrimination of soil phases by dual energy X-ray tomography. *Soil Science Society of America Journal*, 63, 741-751

Sartori, G., Ferrari, G.A. & Pagliai, M. (1985). Changes in soil porosity and surface shrinkage in a remolded, saline clay soil treated with compost. *Soil Science*, 139, 523-530

Stenstrom, M., Olander, B., Carlsson, C.A., Alm Carlsson, G., Lehto-Axtelius, D. & Hakanson, R. (1998). The use of computed microtomography to monitor morphological changes in small animals. *Applied Radiation and Isotopes*, 49, 565-570

Taina, I.A., Heck, R.J. & Elliot, T.R. (2008). Application of X-ray computed tomography to soil science: A literature review. *Canadian Journal of Soil Science*, 88, 1-20

Telfair, D., Gardner, M.R. & Miars, D. (1957). The restoration of a structurally degenerated soil. *Soil Science Society of America Journal*, 21, 131-134

Vandenbygaart, A.J. & Protz, R. (1999). The representative elementary area (REA) in studies of quantitative soil micromorphology. *Geoderma*, 89, 333-346

Viana, J.H.M., Fernandes Filho, E.I. & Schaefer, C.EG.R. (2004). Efeitos de ciclos de umedecimento e secagem na reorganização da estrutura microgranular de latossolos. *Revista Brasileira de Ciência do Solo*, 28, 11-19

Vontobel, P., Lehmann, E.H., Hassanein, R. & Frei, G. (2006). Neutron tomography: Method and applications. *Physica B*, 385/386, 475-480

Voronov, R.S., VanGordon, S.B., Sikavitsas, V.I. & Papavassiliou, D.V. (2010). Distribution of flow-induced stresses in highly porous media. *Applied Physics Letters*, 97, 24101-24103

Vaz, C.M.P., Crestana, S., Mascarenhas, S., Cruvinel, P.E., Reichardt, K. & Stolf, R. (1989). Using a computed tomography miniscanner for studying tillage induced soil compaction. *Soil Technology*, 2, 313–321

Wang, C.H., Willis, D.L. & Loveland, W.D. (1975). Characteristics of ionizing radiation, In: Wang, C.H., Willis, D.L. & Loveland, W.D. (Eds.), *Radiotracer methodology in the biological, environmental, and physics sciences*. Prentice-Hall, Englewood Cliffs, p.39-74

Wildenschild, D., Hopmans, J.W., Vaz, C.M.P., Rivers, M.L., Rikard, D. & Christensen, B.S.B. (2002). Using X-ray computed tomography in hydrology: systems, resolutions, and limitations. *Journal of Hydrology*, 267, 285-297

Wingler, B., Kahle, A. & Hennion, B. (2006). Neutron radiography of rocks and melts. *Physica B*, 385/386, 933-934

15

Scaling Index Method (SIM): A Novel Technique for Assessment of Local Topological Properties of Porous and Irregular Structures

Irina Sidorenko[1], Roberto Monetti[1], Jan Bauer[2],
Dirk Müller[2] and Christoph Räth[1]
[1]Max-Planck-Institut fuer extraterrestrische Physik
[2]Department of Radiology, Technische Universitaet Muenchen
Germany

1. Introduction

The development of high-resolution visualisation techniques, such as magnetic resonance (MR) and computer tomography (CT) opens the possibility for non-destructive studies of the inner structure of the objects of different nature and origin. The deterioration of the structure with time, deformations and loss of strength under the load and other processes lead to morphological and topological changes inside materials, which require both qualitative analysis and quantitative evaluation. Assessment and proper description of the topological and morphological characteristics of materials with porous and irregular architecture is of great importance for many scientific and engineering studies.

The Scaling Index Method (SIM) is a novel numerical tool for characterising the local topology of an arbitrary structure. By evaluating the local dimensionality of each point, the SIM indicates topologically different substructures: unstructured background, one-dimensional (rod-like) and two-dimensional (plate-like) elements. By changing the parameters of the SIM one can distinguish the outer surface from inner points of the structure, describe structures at different scales, and include anisotropic features of the tissue. This method can be applied to both binary and greyscale multidimensional images. To demonstrate the scientific performance of the method we apply numerical techniques based on the SIM to tree-dimensional µCT images of the bone tissue engineering scaffolds (as an example of designed porous structure) and to trabecular bone specimens taken from the human vertebrae in vitro (as an example of biological tissue with very irregular and complicated structure). A proper description of the global and local structural characteristics of the trabecular bone network, which carries and redistributes mechanical load inside the bone, helps to evaluate the deterioration of bone tissue caused by osteoporosis and to predict the most frequent complications of this disease, namely spine and hip fractures. Because of the porous and very irregular architecture of the trabecular bone tissue, a detailed assessment of such a structure requires the use of many texture measures derived from different morphological, biomechanical, topological, and statistical concepts. We show that the Scaling Index Method provides complementary information to the existing well-established techniques.

One of the most frequently used morphological parameter in classical three-dimensional morphometric analysis is the Structure Model Index (*SMI*). It quantifies the type of the structure by the estimation of the plate-to-rode ratio, which is calculated by means of three-dimensional differential analysis of the triangulated bone surface. Scaling Index Method proposes a new approach for the calculation of rode-plate ratio, leading to the novel approach of calculation *SMI*. Combination of the SIM, which describes the topology of the structure on a local level, with Finite Element Method (FEM), which models the biomechanical behaviour of the bone, gives a possibility to analyse redistribution of the stresses and deformations within topologically different structure elements. Minkowski Functionals (MF) supply global morphological information about any structure. According to integral geometry the topology of an arbitrary 3D body can be described by four quantities, known as the Minkowski Functionals, which represent the volume (MF_1), the surface (MF_2), the integral mean curvature (MF_3), and connectivity number (MF_4). The first and second Minkowski Functionals (MF_1 and MF_2) correspond to the bone volume fraction *BV/TV* and normalized bone surface area *BS/TV*, respectively. To extract global morphological characteristics of the trabecular structure, Minkowski Functionals are calculated from the binarized high-resolution image. In conventional approach binarization is made according to the grey level value. In our study we threshold 3D µCT images according to the local structure characteristic calculated by SIM. Such a nonlinear combination of the SIM and MF opens a possibility to calculate *global* topological properties for substructures selected according to their *local* topology.

We provide a detailed theoretical description of the Scaling Index Method with examples of its application in the second section. In the third section we demonstrate possible combinations of SIM with existing numerical techniques and compare the diagnostic performance of the numerical methods and their combinations with SIM by Pearson's correlation analysis with respect to the maximum compressive strength (MCS) measured in biomechanical tests. In the fourth section we summarize main conclusions and underline advantages and perspectives of the proposed Scaling Index Method.

2. Scaling Index Method (SIM)

The Scaling Index Method (SIM) characterises patterns of multi-dimensional point distributions by assessing local topological properties of the underlying structure. The method originated from the study of fractal measures of turbulent and chaotic systems (Benzi et al., 1984), onset of chaos (Jensen et al., 1985), scaling laws for chaotic attractors (Paladin & Vulpiani, 1987) and other multifractal objects (Grassberger et al., 1988). With the development of high-resolution image processing Scaling Index Method became an effective tool for analysis of different systems and structures in which nonlinear correlation plays an important role. It was successfully applied to texture detection and discrimination (Räth & Morfil, 1997), cosmological large-scale structures analysis (Räth et al., 2002), fluctuations in the cosmic microwave background (Rossmanith et al., 2009) and trabecular bone network assessment in the context of osteoporosis (Monetti et al., 2003, 2007; Mueller et al., 2006).

2.1 Theoretical background

In SIM a 3D binary image is described as a set of points $\vec{p}_i$ with spatial coordinates x, y, z:

$$I(x,y,z) = \{\vec{p}_i\}, i = 1,...,N_{voxels}.$$ (1)

Scaling Index Method (SIM): A Novel Technique for Assessment of Local Topological
Properties of Porous and Irregular Structures

303

In a 3D greyscale CT or MR image a discrete grey value $g_i(x_i, y_i, z_i)$ of each voxel plays the role of a fourth dimension. Thus, both space and intensity information are combined in a 4D space vector and the image can be regarded as a set of points $\vec{p}_i(x_i, y_i, z_i, g_i)$ in a virtual 4D space. For each point $\vec{p}_i$ we estimate the number of points of the structure in the vicinity with radius r, which determines the length scale on which the structure is analysed. We assume a power law behaviour for the cumulative point distribution function ρ

$$\rho(\vec{p}_i, r) \propto r^{\alpha_i(r)} \tag{2}$$

with exponent $\alpha(r)$, which is called scaling index and has the meaning of a dimensionality of the object. For ordinary shapes like one-dimensional lines and two-dimensional surfaces scaling index α coincides with the usual topological dimension. By varying the scaling radius r one can characterise the same object with different scaling indices α.

In the analysis of nonuniform structures and tissues scaling exponent varies from point to point and it is meaningful to consider pointwise scaling measure, which can be defined as the logarithmic derivative of ρ

$$\alpha_i(r) = \frac{\partial \log \rho(\vec{p}_i, r)}{\partial \log r} = \frac{r}{\rho} \frac{\partial \rho(\vec{p}_i, r)}{\partial r} . \tag{3}$$

In order to calculate scaling indices α one needs to define the number of points within a multidimensional ball with radius r and centre $\vec{p}_i$, i.e. to determine the cumulative point distribution ρ. In principle, any differentiable function and any distance measure between two points can be used for calculation of scaling indices α. In our applications we assume a Gaussian shaping function to weight the cumulative point distribution

$$\rho(\vec{p}_i, r) = \sum_{j=1}^{N} e^{-(d_{ij}/r)2} , \tag{4}$$

where d_{ij} indicates a distance measure between two points in the multidimensional space (3D in case of binary image, or 4D in case of greyscale image). Because of the exponential form of the function ρ the impact of each point is weighted according to its distance d_{ij} from the central point $\vec{p}_i$. This causes SIM to be a local method: the value of the scaling index depends on the number of neighbours in a small vicinity of radius r of the point for which α is calculated, while contributions of points with $d_{ij} > r$ are negligible. For the case of isotropic scaling indices we use the Euclidean distance between two points

$$d_{ij} = \left\| \vec{p}_i - \vec{p}_j \right\|_2 = \sqrt{(x_i - x_j)^2 + (y_i - y_j)^2 + (z_i - z_j)^2} . \tag{5}$$

Anisotropic features of the tissue can be taken into account by using a generalized quadratic distance measure of the form

$$d_{ij} = \sqrt{\lambda_x \left(x_i - x_j\right)^2 + \lambda_y \left(y_i - y_j\right)^2 + \lambda_z (z_i - z_j)^2} , \tag{6}$$

where λ_x, λ_y, λ_z are the weighting factors of the tree orthogonal spatial directions, respectively. In the case of human vertebrae with natural vertical loading along z-axis we set

$\lambda_x = \lambda_y = 5$ $\lambda_z = 1$. The Scaling Index Method is well suited for quantifying topological aspects on a local level, especially to discriminate substructures with different dimensionality: values of $\alpha \approx 1$ correspond to rod-like components, $1.5 < \alpha < 2.5$ correspond to sheet-like substructure and $\alpha \approx 3$ describe tree-dimensional elements. By means of the SIM a topological characteristic is assigned to each point of the structure, which describes dimensionality of the local neighbourhood. In order to evaluate global topological features based on the local representation of the structure the values of scaling indices can be compiled into the probability density function (pdf)

$$P(\alpha) = prob\big(\alpha \in [\alpha, \alpha + \Delta\alpha]\big).$$ (7)

Combining all points of the structure with the same value of scaling index α one obtains structural decomposition of the object according to the local dimensionality of each point.

2.2 Bone tissue engineering scaffolds

One of the most essential features of the Scaling Index Method is its possibility to vary the length scale of the topological decomposition. We demonstrate the scaling flexibility of the SIM by applying to bone engineering scaffolds (Kerckhofs, 2008, 2010), which are examples of designed porous structures. Evaluation of the morphology, mechanical behaviour, material erosion and structural deterioration of such objects is of great importance for many applications in biology, medicine, pharmacy, engineering and other sciences. Regular architecture of the scaffolds gives us exact knowledge of the strut thickness, which we use as a base length for the choice of scaling radius r. For numerical calculations we use µCT images of scaffolds with a resolution of 14 µm. The scaffolds have a strut thickness of 178 µm on average, what corresponds to 12 - 13 pixels length (Fig. 1).

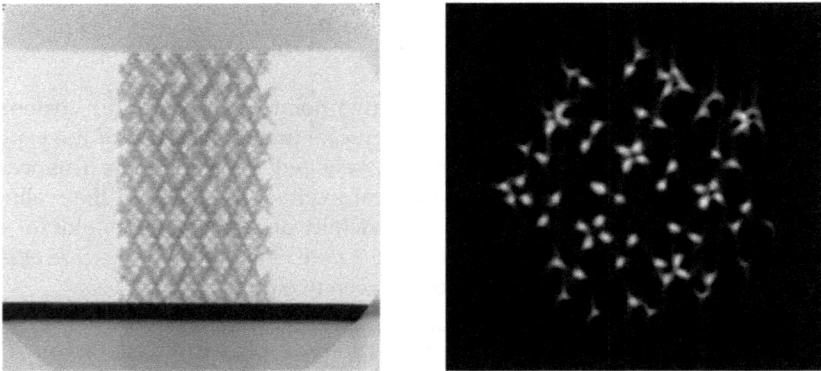

Fig. 1. Original µCT images of the bone engineering scaffolds. Left: side view; right: top view.

In Table 1 we show results of two calculations: with scaling radius $r = 12$ pixels and $r = 2$ pixels. When the scaling radius is comparable with the strut thickness ($r = 12$ pixels, second column of Table 1), all pixels except nodes have $\alpha \in [1,2]$ (blue and green colours), i.e. cylindrical struts are recognised as "thick" one-dimensional elements and the probability distribution function $P(\alpha)$ reaches its maximum at $\alpha \approx 1.7$. When the scaling radius is much

Scaling Index Method (SIM): A Novel Technique for Assessment of Local Topological
Properties of Porous and Irregular Structures

305

Cross section $y=y_{max}/2$		
Cross section $z=z_{max}/2$		
Probability distribution function $P(\alpha)$		
Parameters of computations	*Scaling radius: r=12 pixels;* *CPU time: 14 hours;* *P(α) mean=1.88;*	*Scaling radius: r=2 pixels;* *CPU time: 12min;* *P(α) mean=2.80;*

Table 1. Scaling index representation of the bone tissue engineering scaffolds. Colour coding: blue $1 < \alpha < 1.5$, green $1.5 < \alpha < 2$,yellow $2 < \alpha < 2.5$, red $2.5 < \alpha < 3$.

smaller than the average strut thickness ($r = 2$ pixels, third column of Table 1), SIM provides a very good decomposition of structure elements on the surface and inner body voxels: all inner strut voxels have $\alpha \approx 3$ (red colour on images and the largest peak on the $P(\alpha)$ curve) and surface voxels have $\alpha \approx 2.6$ (yellow colour on images and second large peak on the $P(\alpha)$ curve). Such a α-decomposition can be used in studies of surface erosion, structure deformation under mechanical loading and other applications.

2.3 Trabecular bone

Different biological tissues with irregular structure are the most challenging objects for topological description. In our present paper we use specimens of cancellous bone as a typical example of such a tissue. We base our numerical analysis on 151 μCT images of trabecular network taken from the human vertebrae as previously described in Räth et al., 2008. The scans were acquired for the central 6 mm in length of the specimen using a μCT scanner (Scanco Medical, Bassersdorf, Switzerland). The resulting μCT grey-value images with isotropic spatial resolution of 26 μm were segmented using a fixed global threshold equal to 22% of the maximal grey value to extract the mineralised bone phase. After scanning the 12 mm bone samples were tested by uniaxial compressive experiment and maximum compressive strength (MCS) was determined as the first local maximum of the force-displacement curve. The value of the MCS was used in correlation analysis to assess the diagnostic performance of different numerical methods and their combinations.

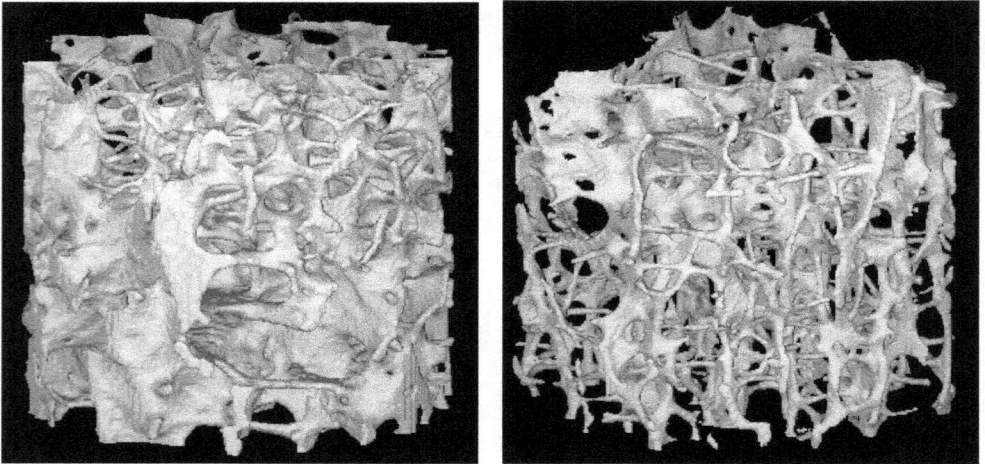

Fig. 2. Original μCT images of the trabecular bone specimens taken from the human vertebrae. Left: strong bone with $BV/TV=0.17$ and $MCS=157.00\ N$; right: weak bone with $BV/TV=0.07$ and $MCS=17.87\ N$.

The topological structure of the trabecular network is different for every specimen and reflects its biomechanical features. Typical characteristics of the strong bone (left image on Fig. 2) are following: large amount of plate-like structures, high values of bone mineral content (described by BV/TV) and large fracture load in biomechanical test (described by

MCS). Weak bone (right image on the Fig. 2) has rarefied trabecular network with a lot of rod-like trabecular elements and very small amount of plates, which consequently reflects in low bone mass and fracture load. We apply the Scaling Index Method both with isotropic and anisotropic distance measures d_{ij}, using scale radius r comparable to the average trabecular thickness. For anisotropic SIM we choose the natural direction of vertical loading of human vertebrae (in our notations z-coordinate) as a preferential direction. Analysing the $P(\alpha)$ spectrum of the trabecular structure (Fig. 3) one can distinguish between strong (green curve) and weak (red curve) bones. For specimens with strong trabecular structure the position of the maximum of the $P(\alpha)$ distribution is typically shifted to higher values of α. This systematic shift reflects the fact that strong bones have more plate-like structures and weak bones consist mainly of rod-like elements. This shift in $P(\alpha)$ spectrum is observed both for isotropic and anisotropic SIM and can be used as a structure texture measure for differentiation between strong and weak bones. The additional advantage of the anisotropic approach is the possibility to describe structures in different directions. From the anisotropic $P(\alpha_z)$ spectrum (right plot on Fig. 3) one can conclude that strong bone (green curve) has much more plates along z direction (the largest peak around $\alpha \approx 2.8$) than on the horizontal plane (second maximum around $2 < \alpha < 2.2$). The weaker bone (red curve) has a large amount of horizontal plates, but less vertically elongated plates.

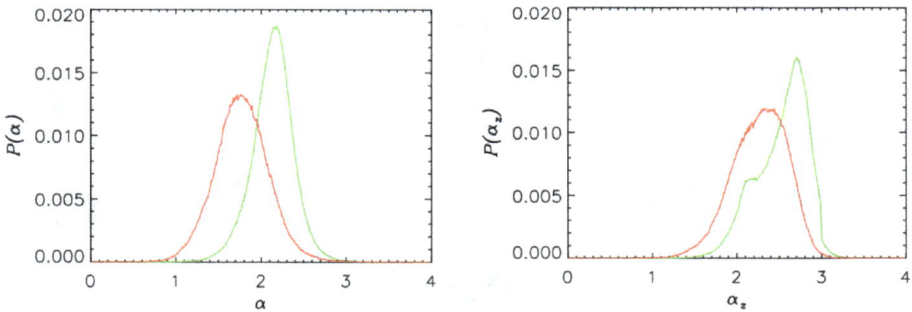

Fig. 3. Probability distribution function of isotropic (left) and anisotropic (right) scaling indices for strong (green curves) and weak (red curves) bones.

The Scaling Index Method provides very clear topological decomposition of the irregular porous structure. Combining all voxels with $\alpha_z < \alpha_{th}$ (Fig. 4) or $\alpha_z > \alpha_{th}$ (Fig. 5) we choose substructures with special topological characteristics and compare trabecular bone elements with different dimensionality. Starting with the small threshold value $\alpha_{th} = 1.7$ we select thin rod-like trabecular elements (first row of Fig. 4). Most of them are horizontally oriented and work for stability of the structure. Increasing threshold value up to $\alpha_{th} = 2$ we can observe all rod-like trabecular elements with any thickness (second row of Fig. 4). By slight increase of threshold value over 2 ($\alpha_{th} > 2.2$, third row in Fig. 4) we add thin horizontal plates into consideration.

$\alpha_z < 1.7$

$\alpha_z < 2$

$\alpha_z < 2.2$

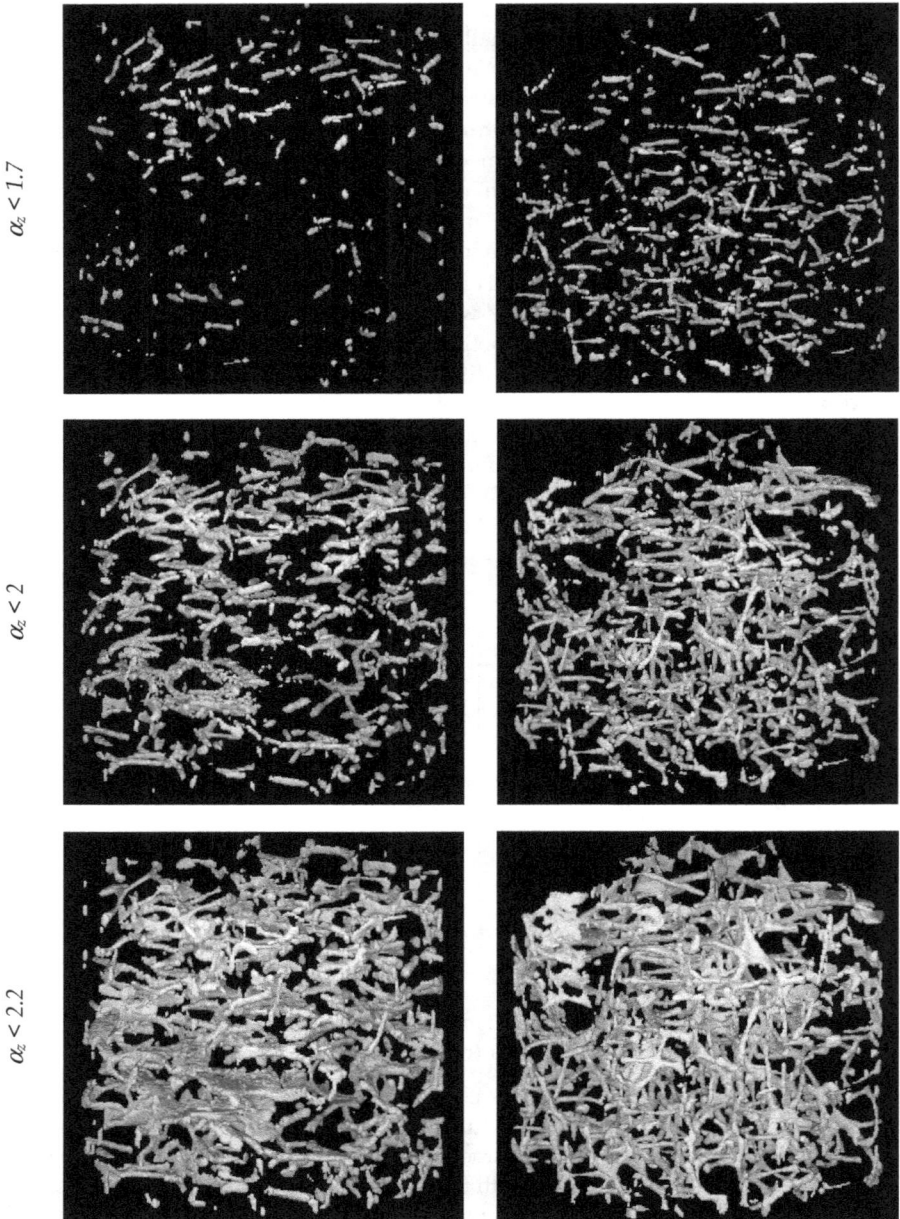

Fig. 4. Topological decomposition of the trabecular bone structure based on the anisotropic scaling index α_z. Substructures are described by voxels with $\alpha_z < \alpha_{th}$. Left: strong bone with *BV/TV=0.17* and *MCS=157.00 N*; right: weak bone with *BV/TV=0.07* and *MCS=17.87 N*.

Scaling Index Method (SIM): A Novel Technique for Assessment of Local Topological
Properties of Porous and Irregular Structures

309

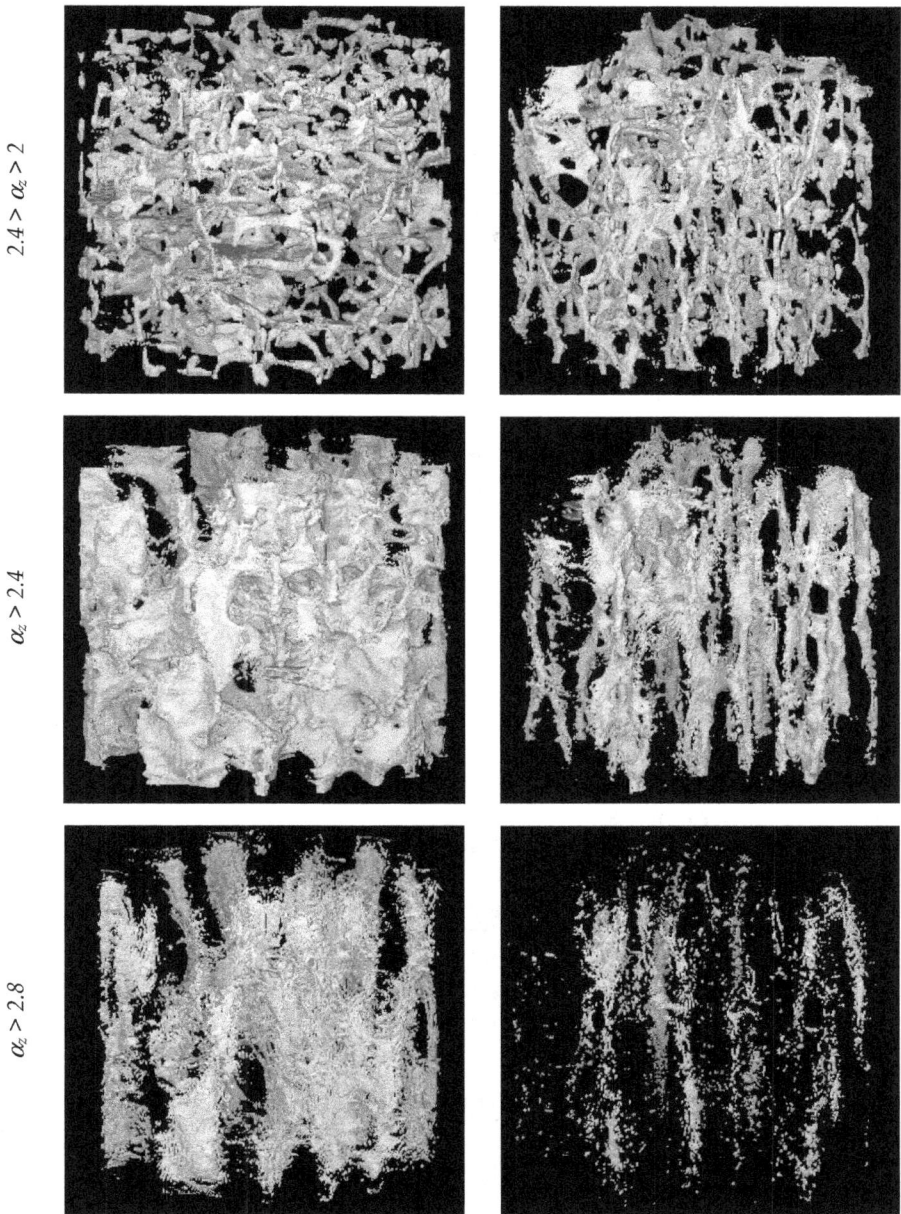

Fig. 5. Topological decomposition of the trabecular bone structure based on the anisotropic
scaling index α_z. Substructures are described by voxels with $\alpha_z > \alpha_{th}$. Left: strong bone with
BV/TV=0.17 and *MCS=157.00 N*; right: weak bone with *BV/TV=0.07* and *MCS=17.87 N*.

Assessment of the plate-like structure can be done by choosing all voxels with $\alpha_z > \alpha_{th}$ (Fig. 5). By taking $2 < \alpha_z < 2.4$ we extract thin plate elements (first row in Fig. 5) and by increasing threshold we get more massive, almost three dimensional plates (second and third rows in Fig. 5). Comparison of the vertebrae specimens based on the topological decomposition of the trabecular structure demonstrates several differences in microarchitecture of the strong and weak bones. The microstructure of strong bones has less strut elements and more plates. Both strength and stability are provided by plate-like elements. Thick plates in direction of natural loading (left image of third row in Fig. 5) are main load bearing elements of the structure, while thin horizontal plates (left image of first row in Fig. 5) are responsible for stability of the bone. The trabecular network of weak bones consists of a large amount of rod-like elements oriented in all directions (right column in Fig. 4) and thin plate-like trabecular elements (right column in Fig. 5). Strength of the weak rarefied bones is ensured by both rod- and plate-like elements oriented along natural loading of the structure, while stability of the structure is provided by horizontal thin struts.

3. Combination of the SIM with different numerical methods

Structure analysis of the tissues with porous and irregular architecture is a very complicated task, which requires the application of a large variety of mathematical concepts. In the present section we show that the Scaling Index Method provides complementary information to the existing morphological and biomechanical methods. As an example, we demonstrate that including local topological characteristics into the analysis of the microarchitecture of the cancellous bone, improves qualitative understanding and quantitative evaluation of the trabecular network strength. We assess the diagnostic performance of the numerical techniques by means of Pearson's correlation analysis with respect to the maximum compressive strength (MCS) obtained in biomechanical experiments.

3.1 Morphometric parameters

Morphometric parameters are an efficient numerical tools, which are widely implemented in the standard software delivered by the µCT scanner manufacture. They are determined from the 3D binary images by direct evaluation of typical mean space distances without assumptions of the particular structure model type (Hildebrand & Rüegsegger, 1997a; Hildebrand et al., 1999). Mean Trabecular Thickness (Tb.Th.) and mean Trabecular Separation (Tb.Sp.) are calculated by filling maximal spheres into the bone mineral tissue or bone marrow, respectively. Trabecular Number (Tb.N.) is defined as the number of plates per unit length and can be obtained as the inverse of mean distance between the mid-axes of the structure. Another important morphometric parameter is the Structure Model Index (SMI) (Hilderbrand & Rüegsegger, 1997b; Hildebrand et al., 1999; Ding & Hvid, 2000):

$$SMI = 12 \cdot \frac{\varepsilon + \varepsilon^2}{1 + 4(\varepsilon + \varepsilon^2)}. \tag{8}$$

The SMI characterises the observed structure by estimating the plate-to-rode ratio ε, which is calculated by means of differential analysis of the triangulated bone surface.

In this work we implement a new approach for the estimation of the relative amount of plates to rods. We use the topological decomposition of the trabecular network based on the

Scaling Index Method (SIM): A Novel Technique for Assessment of Local Topological
Properties of Porous and Irregular Structures

311

scaling indices described in section 2.3. For the threshold value of the scaling indices α_{th} we define rods and plates as voxels with $\alpha < \alpha_{th}$ and $\alpha > \alpha_{th}$, respectively. Plate-to-rod ratio is then defined as:

$$\varepsilon = \frac{\sum_{i=1}^{N_{voxels}} H(\alpha_i - \alpha_{th})}{\sum_{i=1}^{N_{voxels}} H(\alpha_{th} - \alpha_i)}.$$ (9)

Here N_{voxels} is number of voxels composing the observed structure and $H(x)$ is the Heaviside step function:

$$H(x) = \begin{cases} 0, & x < 0 \\ 1, & x \geq 0 \end{cases}.$$ (10)

Calculating plate-to-rod ratio ε for different threshold value α_{th} we obtain novel parameters $SMI\alpha$ and $SMI\alpha_z$ as function of α_{th}.

Pearson's correlation analysis with respect to the experimental MCS demonstrates (Table 2) that among classical morphometric parameters the best correlation coefficient $|r_p| = 0.43$ is shown by $Tr.N.$ and SMI. By the novel nonlinear combination of SMI and scaling indices α or α_z we can significantly improve prediction of bone strength and achieve a much higher value of the correlation coefficient: $r_p = -0.74$. The observed improvement in diagnostic performance can be explained by the fact that we combine local topological and global morphometric characteristics in one parameter ($SMI\alpha$ or $SMI\alpha_z$ in Table 2).

Tb.Th.	Tb.Sp.	Tr.N.	SMI	SMIα	SMIα_z
0.3	-0.41	0.43	-0.43	-0.73	-0.74

Table 2. Pearson's correlation coefficient r_p for classical morphometric parameters and novel combination of SMI with isotropic ($SMI\alpha$) and anisotropic ($SMI\alpha_z$) Scaling Index Method.

Analysing $r_p(\alpha_{th})$ curves for the novel parameters $SMI\alpha$ and $SMI\alpha_z$ (Fig. 6) one can see, that the diagnostic performance of both parameters depends only slightly on the amount of thin horizontal rod-like trabecular elements (up to the threshold $\alpha_{th} \approx 1.8$ for $SMI\alpha$ and up to the threshold $\alpha_{zth} \approx 2$ for $SMI\alpha_z$ value of the r_p stays constantly high), but the underestimation of amount of plates (i.e. taken $\alpha_{th} > 2$) in the structure drastically decrease correlation coefficient. An additional important observation is the increase of the correlation coefficient within the range $2 < \alpha_{zth} < 2.2$ for anisotropic $SMI\alpha_z$ (right plot in Fig. 6). This region corresponds to the thin horizontal plates (last row in Fig. 4), which are important for stability of the bone, but do not work as load bearing elements. This means that the best diagnostic performance of the novel morphological parameter $SMI\alpha_z$ is obtained when we separate structure not only according to the morphological form of trabecular elements (plates or rods), but rather according to their mechanical functionality within the structure (bearing of load or support of stability).

3.2 Minkowski Functionals (MF)

Minkowski Functionals (MF) provide a global morphological and topological description of structural properties of multidimensional data (Mecke et al., 1994). According to integral geometry n-dimensional body can be completely characterized by $n+1$ functionals, which

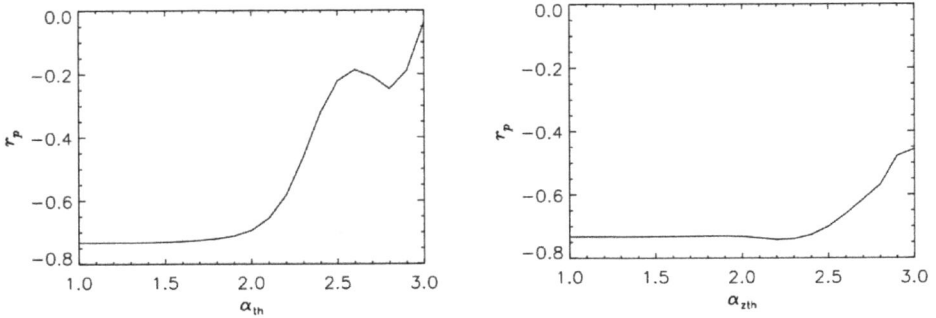

Fig. 6. Pearson's correlation coefficient r_p as a function of threshold value α_{th} for novel combination of SMI with isotropic (left) and anisotropic (right) scaling indices.

evaluate both size and shape of the object. In a three-dimensional space they represent the volume (MF_1), surface area (MF_2), integral mean curvature (MF_3) and integral Gaussian curvature (MF_4). Minkowski Functionals are derived from the theory of convex sets and expressed as volume integral for MF_1 and surface integrals over boundary S with principal radii of curvature R_1 and R_2 for other functionals.

$$MF_1(v_{th}) = \int_{I(v_{th})} dV , \qquad MF_3(v_{th}) = 1/2 \int_{\partial I(v_{th})} (\frac{1}{R_1} + \frac{1}{R_2}) dS$$

$$MF_2(v_{th}) = \int_{\partial I(v_{th})} dS , \qquad MF_4(v_{th}) = \int_{\partial I(v_{th})} \frac{1}{R_1 R_2} dS \qquad (11)$$

The first two functionals MF_1 and MF_2 describe morphology of the structure and coincide with morphometrical parameters bone volume BV/TV and surface BS/TV fractions. The fourth integral is also known as Euler characteristic χ, which characterises topological connectivity of the structure and can be expressed in terms of Betti numbers β_0 (number of connected components), β_1 (number of tunnels), β_2 (number of cavities):

$$\chi = \beta_0 - \beta_1 + \beta_2 . \qquad (12)$$

In the case of binary images we have exactly four global characteristics, which can be used as texture measures for diagnostic of bone strength. For greyscale CT or MR images the bone mineral network must be segmented according to the intensity threshold value v_{th}. Thus, Minkowski Functionals become a function of an excursion set $I(v_{th})$, which is determined by all voxels with $v > v_{th}$ or $v < v_{th}$. The calculation of the MF for the binary or images thresholded at a certain threshold v_{th} can be reduced to the calculation of open vertices (n_v), edges (n_e), faces (n_f) and number of the voxels (n_p), that belong to the excursion set $I(v_{th})$ (Michielsen & Raedt, 2001).

$$MF_1(v_{th}) = n_p , \qquad MF_3(v_{th}) = 3n_p - 2n_f + n_e$$

$$MF_2(v_{th}) = -6n_p + 2n_f , \qquad MF_4(v_{th}) = -n_p + n_f - n_e + n_v \qquad (13)$$

Scaling Index Method (SIM): A Novel Technique for Assessment of Local Topological
Properties of Porous and Irregular Structures

313

In the common approach an excursion set $I(\nu_{th})$ is defined as the union of image voxels, which have a grey level g below or above a threshold $\nu_{th} = g_{th}$. Different values of threshold g_{th} describe different tissues of the bone. Scaling Index Method offers a new possibility for binarizing images before calculation of MF (Monetti et al., 2009). Taking a scaling index α_{th} as a threshold variable ν_{th} for excursion set I, we compose excursion set $I(\alpha_{th})$ with the structure elements which are selected according to their local topological properties (i.e. rod-like and plate-like substructures). Thus we combine both local and global characteristics and for each Minkowski Functional $MF_{1,2,3,4}$ obtain a new texture measures $MF\alpha_{1,2,3,4}$ and $MF\alpha_{z1,2,3,4}$. In Table 3 we demonstrate diagnostic performance of MF and their combination with isotropic and anisotropic SIM. We compare standard linear multiregression analysis and novel nonlinear combination of global (MF) and local (SIM) topological approaches. One can observe significant improvement of correlation coefficient for the third and the forth Minkowski Functionals (up to the value $r_p = 0.74$), when they are calculated in combination with anisotropic SIM ($MF\alpha_{z3}$ and $MF\alpha_{z4}$). In general nonlinear combination global and local topological characteristics improves correlation with experimental MCS more significantly, than standard linear multiregression analysis. The best correlation with experimental MCS is obtained by choosing substructure with $\alpha_z > 2.8$, what corresponds to thick vertical plate-like trabecular elements (last row in Fig. 5).

Conventional ($MF_{1,2,3,4}$)			0.73	0.6	0.06	0.38
Linear combination of MF with SIM	isotropic		0.73	0.65	0.59	0.60
	anisotropic		0.73	0.67	0.62	0.63
Nonlinear combination of MF with SIM	isotropic ($MF\alpha_{1,2,3,4}$)		0.71	0.70	0.69	0.47
	anisotropic ($MF\alpha_{z1,2,3,4}$)		0.72	0.73	0.73	0.74

Table 3. Correlation coefficient for conventional Minkowski Functionals (first row), linear combination of MF with isotropic and anisotropic SIM (second row) and novel nonlinear combination of MF with isotropic ($MF\alpha$) and anisotropic ($MF\alpha_z$) SIM (third row).

3.3 Finite Element Method (FEM)

Finite Element Method is the most powerful method in the description of biomechanical behaviour of structures under the external load (Rietbergen et al., 1995). The obvious advantage of the method is that by converting voxels of μCT images into finite element mesh it takes into account exact microarchitecture of the object and thus allows to study both apparent and tissue level biomechanical stresses in structures. In present section we show that the combination of tissue level biomechanical characteristics obtained by FEM with local topological measures calculated by SIM provides complementary understanding of load redistribution between topologically different structure elements. We apply the linear elastic approach described by generalized Hook's law with the fundamental assumption that deformations are under the yield level. Bone mineral tissue is described as isotropic and elastic material with Young's modulus $Y = 10$ GPa and Poisson's ratio $\nu = 0.3$. According to the biomechanical experiments we apply Dirichlet boundary conditions to simulate a high friction compressive test in the uniaxial direction (we call it z direction) with constant strain $\varepsilon_z = 1\%$ prescribed on the top surface. As a main mechanical characteristic on tissue level we use the effective strain (Pistoia et al., 2002)

$$\varepsilon_{eff} = \sqrt{2U/Y} \, , \qquad (14)$$

which is calculated from the strain energy density

$$U = 1/2\left(\sigma_{xx}\varepsilon_{xx} + \sigma_{yy}\varepsilon_{yy} + \sigma_{zz}\varepsilon_{zz}\right) + \sigma_{xy}\varepsilon_{xy} + \sigma_{xz}\varepsilon_{xz} + \sigma_{yz}\varepsilon_{yz} \qquad (15)$$

normalised to Young's modulus Y of the bone mineral material. The energy density U (15) describes the stored energy associated with elastic deformation caused by the external loading. Also linear elastic model is valid only below the yield limit and does not describe development of fractures, the numerically estimated failure load

$$L_{cv} = F_r \cdot k_{cv} \qquad (16)$$

is often used as a predictive parameter in correlation analysis with respect to the experimentally measured MCS (Pistoia et al., 2002). We calculate failure load L_{cv} from the apparent total reaction force F_r at the top face A^t

$$F_r = \int \sigma_{zz}^t dA^t \qquad (17)$$

by multiplying with a linear scaling factor k_{cv}, which depends on the distribution of the effective strain ε_{eff} in the trabecular bone network

$$k_{cv} = 1/\sum_{i=1}^{N_{voxels}} H(\varepsilon_{eff} - \varepsilon_{cv}) \, . \qquad (18)$$

Here N_{voxels} is number of voxels composing the observed structure and $H(x)$ is Heaviside step function (10). Absolute value of the failure load L_{cv} depends on the critical value of the effective strain ε_{cv}. The best Pearson's correlation coefficient $r_p = 0.76$ with respect to the MCS is obtained for critical value $\varepsilon_{cv} = 0.002$, which takes into account both large and small deformations in the trabecular bone under the vertical load.

We generate a finite element model by converting bone voxels into equally sized and oriented hexahedral elements and calculate effective strain (14) for each voxel of the trabecular structure. Thus SIM and FEM propose alternative representation of the structure on tissue level. Each voxel can be characterised by two new properties: effective strain ε_{eff} obtained by FEM and scaling index α (or α_z) obtained by SIM. Combination of SIM and FEM allows to analyse the redistribution of the deformation energy stored during compressive loading between the trabecular elements with different topological dimensionality. We calculate the average effective strain $<\varepsilon_{eff}>$ for voxels having the same values of scaling indices (Fig. 7). Both in strong and weak bones maximum average effective strain $<\varepsilon_{eff}>$ is accumulated in substructures with $\alpha > 2$ (isotropic SIM) or $\alpha_z \approx 2.5$ (anisotropic SIM), which corresponds to plate-like trabecular elements, but according to the $P(\alpha)$ spectrum (Fig. 3) the amount of plates in weak bones is smaller than in strong ones. This means that plates along the direction of natural loading are the main load bearing substructure of the trabecular network and the relative amount of vertical plates plays the most important role for bone strength on a global level, while thin horizontal rod and plate structure elements play stabilizing role under different shear loading.

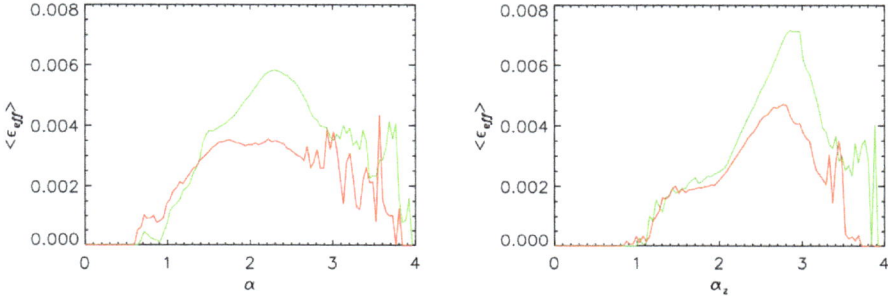

Fig. 7. Effective strain ε_{eff} calculated with FEM averaged over the voxels with the same value of scaling indices calculated with SIM (left: isotropic, right: anisotropic). Red lines: weak bone, green lines: strong bone.

		MF_2	MF_3	MF_4	SMI
	Conventional methods	0.60	0.06	0.38	-0.43
Combination with SIM	isotropic (α)	0.70	0.69	0.47	-0.73
	anisotropic (α_z)	0.73	0.73	0.74	-0.74

Table 4. Increase of the Pearson's correlation coefficient r_p due to the nonlinear combination with the isotropic (α) and anisotropic (α_z) Scaling Index Method.

	FEM	MF1	$MF\alpha_{z1}$	$MF\alpha_{z2}$	$MF\alpha_{z3}$	$MF\alpha_{z4}$	$SMI\alpha_z$
MCS	0.76	0.73	0.72	0.73	0.73	0.74	-0.74
FEM	1	0.94	0.95	0.94	0.94	0.94	-0.94

Table 5. Pearson's correlation coefficient for the seven strongest numerical methods with respect to the experimental MCS and numerical failure load estimated by FEM.

3.4 Prediction of bone strength with different numerical methods

We assess the diagnostic performance of the numerical methods described in the previous sections by means of correlation analysis with respect to the maximum compressive strength (MCS) experimentally measured in uniaxial compressive test. High values of the Pearson's correlation coefficient r_p are demonstrated only by two texture measures: failure load L_{cv}

estimated by FEM ($r_p = 0.76$) and first Minkowski Functional MF_1, which represents mineral bone volume fraction BV/TV ($r_p = 0.73$). Second Minkowski Functional MF_2, which coincides with bone surface fraction BS/TV and texture measures based on the isotropic and anisotropic Scaling Index Method (Räth et al., 2008) demonstrate only moderate correlation with MCS (0.6, 0.55 and 0.52 respectively). Morphological parameters, provided by standard software delivered by the μCT scanner manufacture, *Tb.Th., Tb.Sp., Tb.N.* and *SMI*, as well as MF_3 and MF_4 correlate very weak ($r_p < 0.5$) with experiment, but in combination with local topological information provided by isotropic and anisotropic SIM, correlation coefficient significantly increases (Table 4). Thus, we have a group of seven methods (Table 5), which have good diagnostic performance in differentiating between strong and weak trabecular bone structure. They have high Pearson's correlation coefficient with respect to the experimental MCS ($r_p > 0.7$) and correlate very well with the best numerical texture measure, which is failure load estimated by FEM ($r > 0.94$). General feature of these methods is that all of them provide texture measures based both on structure quality and size.

4. Conclusions

Our study clearly shows that in order to give comprehensive description of materials and tissues with porous and irregular structures it is not sufficient to use only global methods. Local topological measures provide complementary information to the global characteristics and their proper evaluation is of a great importance for many scientific purposes. To the best of our knowledge, Scaling Index Method is a unique technique for assessing local topological properties of arbitrary structures. It is well suited for quantifying topological aspects on a local level, especially to discriminate substructures with different dimensionality or separate the inner body and the surface of the object. It can be applied both to greyscale and binary images. By varying the scaling parameter of the method one can characterise the same structure on different levels of dimensionality. SIM provides complementary information to biomechanical (FEM), morphological (SMI) and global topological (MF) methods. Nonlinear combination of SIM with existing numerical techniques improves both qualitative understanding and diagnostic performance of the methods. Calculation of SMI and MF based on the scaling index decomposition of the μCT images of human trabecular bone, which represent a typical example of the biological tissue with irregular structure, significantly improves the correlation with the experimentally measured MCS (Table 4). Comparison on the tissue level of the effective strain calculated by the FEM and scaling indices provided by SIM, shows that the plate-like elements in direction of natural loading are the main load bearing substructure of trabecular network both in strong and weak bones, but the amount of plates in weak bones is reduced in comparison with strong ones, which leads to the global decrease of the bone strength and stability on the global level.

5. Acknowledgments

This study was supported by the Deutsche Forschungsgemainschaft (DFG) under the grant MU 2288/2-2. The authors are very thankful to E. Rummeny (Klinikum Rechts der Isar, Technical University Munich, Germany), F. Eckstein (Institute of Anatomy and Musculoskeletal Research, Paracelsus Medical Private University Salzburg, Austria), M. Matsuura (Institute of Anatomy, Ludwig Maximillians University Munich, Germany), E.-M.

Scaling Index Method (SIM): A Novel Technique for Assessment of Local Topological
Properties of Porous and Irregular Structures

317

Lochmueller (Department of Gynecology I, Ludwig Maximillians University Munich, Germany) and P. Zysset (Institute for Lightweight Design and Structural Biomechanics, Vienna University of Technology, Austria) for μCT images of human trabecular bones and data of biomechanical experiments. The authors are grateful to P. Salmon (Skyscan NV, Kontich, Belgium) and G. Kerckhofs (Katholieke Universiteit Leuven, Belgium) for the μCT images of bone tissue engineering scaffolds. The authors thank Andrew Burghardt (University of California, San Francisco, USA) for collaboration in benchmarking of the FEM numerical code with commercial software "Scanco FE Software v1.12" developed by Dr. B. van Rietbergen and provided by Scanco Medical AG, Bruettisellen, Switzerland.

6. References

Benzi, R.; Paladin, G.; Parisi, G. & Vulpiani, A. (1984). On the multifractal nature of fully developed turbulence and chaotic systems. *J. Phys. A: Math.Gen.*, Vol. 17, pp. 3521-3531

Ding, M. & Hvid, I. (2000). Quantification of age-related changes in the structure mdoel type and trabecular thickness of human tibial cancellous bone. *Bone*, Vol.26, No. 3, pp. 291-295

Grassberger, P.; Badii, R. & Politi, A. (1988). Scaling laws for invariant measures on hyperbolic and nonhyberbolic atractors. *Journal of Statistical Physics*, Vol. 51, No. 1/2, pp. 135-178

Hildebrand, T. & Rüegsegger, P. (1997a). A new method for the model-independent assessment of thickness in three-dimensional images. *J Microsc*, Vol. 185, Pt 1, pp. 67-75

Hildebrand, T. & Rüegsegger, P. (1997b). Quantification of bone microarchitecture with the Structure Model Index. *CMBBE*, Vol.1, pp.15-23

Hildebrand, T.;Laib, A.; Müller, R.; Dequeker, J. & Rüegsegger, P. (1999). Direct three-dimensional morphometric analysis of human cancellous bone: microstructural data from spine, femur iliac crest, and calcaneus. *J Bone Miner Res*, Vol. 14, No. 7, pp.1167-1174

Jensen, M.; Kadanoff, L.P. & Libchaber, A. (1985). Global universality at the onset of chaos: results of a forced Rayleigh-Benard experiment. *Phys. Rev. Lett.* Vol. 55, No. 25, pp. 2798-2801

Kerckhofs, G.; Schrooten, J.; Elicegui, L.; Van Bael, S.; Moesen, M.; Lomov, S. & Wevers, M. (2008). Mechanical characterization of porous structures by the combined use of micro-CT and in-situ loading. *Proceedings of World Conference on Non-Destructive Testing (WCNDT)*, Shanghai, China, 25-28 October 2008

Kerckhofs, G.; Pyka, G.; Loeckx, D.; Van Bael, S.; Schrooten, J. & Wevers, M. (2010). The combined use of micro-CT imaging, in-situ loading and non-rigid image registration for 3D experimental local strain mapping on porous bone tissue engineering scaffolds under compressive loading. *Proceedings of European Conference for non-Destructive Testing (ECNDT)*, Moscow, Russia, 7-11 June 2010

Mecke, K.R.; Buchert, T. & Wagner, H. (1994). Robust morphological measures for large-scale structure in the Universe. *Astron. Astrophys.*, Vol. 288, pp. 697-704

Michielsen, K. & Raedt, H. (2001), Integral-geometry morphological image analysis. *Physics Reports*, Vol.347, pp.461-538

Monetti, R.A.; Boehm, H.; Mueller, D.; Newitt, D.; Majumdar, S.; Rummeny, E.; Link, T.M. & Raeth, C. (2003). Scaling Index Method: a novel nonlinear technique for the analysis of high-resolution MRI of human bones. *Proceedings of Medical Imaging Conference of SPIE*, Vol. 5032, pp. 1777-1786

Monetti, R.A.; Bauer, J.; Mueller, D.; Rummeny, E.; Matsuura, M.; Eckstein, F.; Link, T. & Raeth, C. (2007). Application of the Scaling Index Method to μ-CT images of human trabecular bone for the characterization of biomechanical strength. *Proceedings of Medical Imaging Conference of SPIE*, Vol. 6512, pp. 65124H

Monetti, R.A.; Bauer, J.; Sidorenko, I.; Mueller, D.; Rummeny, E.; Matsuura, M.; Eckstein, F.; Lochmueller, E.M.; Zysset, P. & Raeth, C. (2009). Assessment of the human trabecular bone structure using Minkowski Functionals. *Proceedings of Medical Imaging Conference of SPIE*, Vol. 7262, pp. 7262ON1-7262ON9

Mueller, D.; Link, T.M.; Monetti, R.; Baur, J.; Boehm, H.; Seifert-Klauss, V.; Rummeny, E.J.; Morfill, G.E. & Raeth, C. (2006). The 3D-based scaling index algorithm: a new structure measure to analyze trabecular bone architecture in hifh-resolution MR images in vivo. *Osteoporos. Int.*, Vol. 17, pp. 1783-1493

Paladini, G. & Vulpiani, A. (1987). Anomalous scaling laws in multiftactal objects. *Phys Reports*, Vol. 156, No. 4, pp. 147-225

Pistoia, W.; van Rietbergen, B.; Lochnueller, E.-M.; Lill, C. A.; Eckstein, F. & Ruegsegger, P. (2002). Estimation of distal radius failure load with micro-finite element analysis models based on three-dimensional peripheral quantitative computed tomography images. *Bone*, Vol. 30, No. 6, pp. 842-848

Räth, C. & Morfill, G. (1997). Texture detection and texture duscrimination with anisotropic scaling indices. *J. Opt. Soc. Am. A*, Vol. 14, No. 12, pp. 3208-3215

Räth, C.; Bunk, W.; Huber, M.B.; Morfill, G.E.; Retzlaff, J. & Schuecker, P. (2002). Analysing large-scale structure –I. Weighted scaling indices and constrained randomization. *Mon. Not. R. Astron. Soc.*, Vol. 337, pp. 413-421

Räth, C.; Monetti, R.; Bauer, J.; Sidorenko, I.; Mueller, D.; Matsuura, M.; Lochmueller, E.-M.; Zysset, P. & Eckstein, F. (2008). Strength through structure: visualization and local assessment of the trabecular bone structure. *New Journal of Physics*, Vol. 10, pp. 125010-125027

Rietbergen, B.; Weinans, H.; Huiskes, R. & Odgaard, A. (1995). A new method to determine trabecular bone elastic properties and loading using micromechanical finite-element models. *J. Bioemchanics*, Vol. 28, No. 1, pp. 69-81

Rossmanith, G.; Räth, C.; Banday, A. J. & Morfill, G. (2009). Non-Gaussian signatures in the five-year *WMAP* data as identified with isotropic scaling indices. *MNRAS*, Vol. 399, No. 4, pp.1921–1933

Permissions

The contributors of this book come from diverse backgrounds, making this book a truly international effort. This book will bring forth new frontiers with its revolutionizing research information and detailed analysis of the nascent developments around the world.

We would like to thank Luca Saba MD, for lending his expertise to make the book truly unique. He has played a crucial role in the development of this book. Without his invaluable contribution this book wouldn't have been possible. He has made vital efforts to compile up to date information on the varied aspects of this subject to make this book a valuable addition to the collection of many professionals and students.

This book was conceptualized with the vision of imparting up-to-date information and advanced data in this field. To ensure the same, a matchless editorial board was set up. Every individual on the board went through rigorous rounds of assessment to prove their worth. After which they invested a large part of their time researching and compiling the most relevant data for our readers. Conferences and sessions were held from time to time between the editorial board and the contributing authors to present the data in the most comprehensible form. The editorial team has worked tirelessly to provide valuable and valid information to help people across the globe.

Every chapter published in this book has been scrutinized by our experts. Their significance has been extensively debated. The topics covered herein carry significant findings which will fuel the growth of the discipline. They may even be implemented as practical applications or may be referred to as a beginning point for another development. Chapters in this book were first published by InTech; hereby published with permission under the Creative Commons Attribution License or equivalent.

The editorial board has been involved in producing this book since its inception. They have spent rigorous hours researching and exploring the diverse topics which have resulted in the successful publishing of this book. They have passed on their knowledge of decades through this book. To expedite this challenging task, the publisher supported the team at every step. A small team of assistant editors was also appointed to further simplify the editing procedure and attain best results for the readers.

Our editorial team has been hand-picked from every corner of the world. Their multi-ethnicity adds dynamic inputs to the discussions which result in innovative outcomes. These outcomes are then further discussed with the researchers and contributors who give their valuable feedback and opinion regarding the same. The feedback is then collaborated with the researches and they are edited in a comprehensive manner to aid the understanding of the subject.

Apart from the editorial board, the designing team has also invested a significant amount of their time in understanding the subject and creating the most relevant covers. They scrutinized every image to scout for the most suitable representation of the subject and create an appropriate cover for the book.

The publishing team has been involved in this book since its early stages. They were actively engaged in every process, be it collecting the data, connecting with the contributors or procuring relevant information. The team has been an ardent support to the editorial, designing and production team. Their endless efforts to recruit the best for this project, has resulted in the accomplishment of this book. They are a veteran in the field of academics and their pool of knowledge is as vast as their experience in printing. Their expertise and guidance has proved useful at every step. Their uncompromising quality standards have made this book an exceptional effort. Their encouragement from time to time has been an inspiration for everyone.

The publisher and the editorial board hope that this book will prove to be a valuable piece of knowledge for researchers, students, practitioners and scholars across the globe.

List of Contributors

Tatsurou Tanaka
Department of Oral Diagnostic Science, Kyushu Dental College, Kitakyushu, Japan

Yasuhiro Morimoto, Tatsurou Tanaka, Shinji Kito,Shinobu Matsumoto-Takeda, Masafumi Oda, Nao Wakasugi-Sato and Kozue Otsuka
Department of Oral Diagnostic Science, Kyushu Dental College, Kitakyushu, Japan

Ayataka Ishikawa, Kou Matsuo and Yuji Seta
Department of Oral Bioscience, Kyushu Dental College, Kokurakita-ku, Kitakyushu, Japan

Shinya Kokuryo, Noriaki Yamamoto, Manabu Habu, Ikuya Miyamoto, Masaaki Kodama, Yoshihiro Yamashita, Tetsu Takahashi and Kazuhiro Tominaga
Department of Oral and Maxillofacial Surgery, Kyushu Dental College, Kitakyushu, Japan

Shunji Shiiba
Department of Control of Physical Functions, Kyushu Dental College, Kokurakita-ku, Kitakyushu, Japan

Izumi Yoshioka
Department of Sensory and Motor Organs, Faculty of Medicine, Miyazaki University, Miyazaki, Japan

Yasuhiro Morimoto
Center for Oral Biological Research, Kyushu Dental College, Kitakyushu, Japan
Department of Oral Diagnostic Science, Kyushu Dental College, Kitakyushu, Japan

Vincent Degos, Thomas Lescot and Louis Puybasset
Neuro-ICU Unit, Department of Anesthesiology and Critical Care, Groupe Hospitalier Pitié-Salpêtrière, APHP, Université Pierre et Marie Curie, Paris, France

Stephen Hughes
Department of Physics, Queensland University of Technology, Brisbane, Queensland, Australia

Ahmet Mesrur Halefoglu
Sisli Etfal Training and Research Hospital Radiology Department, Sisli, Istanbul, Turkey

Cem Onal and Ezgi Oymak
Baskent University Faculty of Medicine/ Department of Radiation Oncology, Turkey

Roberto Monetti
Max-Planck-Institut für extraterrestrische Physik, Garching, Germany

Irina Sidorenko and Christoph Räth
Max-Plack-Institut für extraterrestrische Physik, Garching, Germany

Jan Bauer, Thomas Baum and Dirk Müller
Institut für Röntgendiagnostik, Technische Universität München, München, Germany

Felix Eckstein
Institute of Anatomy and Musculoskeletal Research, Paracelsus Private Medical University, Salzburg, Austria

Thomas Link
Magnetic Resonance Science Center, Department of Radiology, UCSF, San Francisco, CA, USA

Quoc P. Nguyen
The University of Texas at Austin, USA

F. de Carlos and J. Cobo
Departamentos de Cirugía y Especialidades Médico-Quirúrgicas (Section of Odontology) Instituto Asturiano de Odontología, Oviedo, Spain

Alvarez-Suárez
Construcción e Ingeniería de la Fabricación (Section of Mechanic Engineering), Spain
Instituto Asturiano de Odontología, Oviedo, Spain

S. Costilla
Medicina (Section of Radiology), Spain

I. Noval
Servicio de Radiología, Hospital Universitario Central de Asturias, Oviedo, Spain

J. A. Vega
Morfología y Biología Celular (Section of Anatomy and Human Embryology), Universidad de Oviedo, Spain

Gabriela R. Pereira
Non-destructive Testing, Corrosion and Welding Laboratory, Department of Metallurgical and Materials Engineering COPPE/UFRJ Federal University of Rio de Janeiro, Rio de Janeiro/RJ, Brazil

Ricardo T. Lopes
Nuclear Instrumentation Laboratory, Department of Nuclear Engineering COPPE/UFRJ, Federal University of Rio de Janeiro, Rio de Janeiro/RJ, Brazil

Tetsuya Suekane and Hiroki Ushita
The University of Tokushima, Japan

Peter Johnston
University of Auckland, New Zealand

Volkan Arısan
Department of Oral Implantology, Faculty of Dentistry, Istanbul University, Turkey

Luiz Fernando Pires and Fábio Augusto Meira Cássaro
State University of Ponta Grossa, Department of Physics, Brazil

Osny Oliveira Santos Bacchi and Klaus Reichardt
Center for Nuclear Energy in Agriculture, Laboratory of Soil Physics, Brazil

Irina Sidorenko, Roberto Monetti and Christoph Räth
Max-Planck-Institut fuer extraterrestrische Physik, Germany

Jan Bauer and Dirk Müller
Department of Radiology, Technische Universitaet Muenchen, Germany